SM99000191
10/99
£19.95

Undertaking Midwifery Research

D0245094

✓

CARLISLE

WITHDRAWN

WITHDRAWN

CARLISLE LIBRARY
ST MARTINS SERVICES LTD.

0443052301

For Tom and Laura

For Churchill Livingstone:

Editorial Director: Mary Law
Project Development Editor: Dinah Thom
Project Manager: Valerie Burgess
Project Controller: Pat Miller/Derek Robertson
Design Direction: Judith Wright
Sales Promotion Executive: Hilary Brown

Undertaking Midwifery Research

A Basic Guide to Design and Analysis

Carolyn M. Hicks BA MA PhD PGCE C Psychol

Senior Lecturer in Psychology, School of Continuing Studies, The University of Birmingham, UK

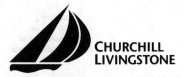

CHURCHILL
LIVINGSTONE

NEW YORK, EDINBURGH, LONDON, MADRID, MELBOURNE, SAN FRANCISCO AND TOKYO 1996

CHURCHILL LIVINGSTONE
An imprint of Harcourt Brace and Company Limited

© Pearson Professional Limited 1996
© Harcourt Brace and Company Limited 1998

✦ is a registered trademark of Harcourt Brace and
Company Limited

All rights reserved. No part of this publication may be
reproduced, stored in a retrieval system, or transmitted in
any form or by any means, electronic, mechanical,
photocopying, recording or otherwise, without either the
prior permission of the publishers (Harcourt Brace and Company
Limited, 24–28 Oval Road, London NW1 7DX, UK), or a licence
permitting restricted copying in the United Kingdom issued by
the Copyright Licensing Agency Ltd, 90 Tottenham Court Road,
London W1P 0LP.

First published 1996
   Reprinted 1998

ISBN 0 443 05230 1

British Library Cataloguing in Publication Data
A catalogue record for this book is available from the British
Library.

Library of Congress Cataloging in Publication Data
A catalog record for this book is available from the Library
of Congress.

Medical knowledge is constantly changing. As new information
becomes available, changes in treatment, procedures, equipment
and the use of drugs become necessary. The author and
publishers have, as far as it is possible, taken care to ensure that
the information given in this text is accurate and up-to-date.
However, readers are strongly advised to confirm that the
information, especially with regard to drug usage, complies with
latest legislation and standards of practice.

The
publisher's
policy is to use
**paper manufactured
from sustainable forests**

Produced by Addison Wesley Longman China Limited, Hong Kong
GCC/02

Contents

Preface

The last decade has witnessed radical changes to the UK National Health Service. Curbs in public sector spending together with an increasing need for open accountability within health care delivery have meant that treatments can no longer be based on ritual and tradition but instead have to be justified by scientifically derived evidence. As a result, there have been numerous initiatives to create a research culture within the NHS. This, of course, is not intended to mean that all health care practitioners should become instant data collectors and active researchers, but rather that they become more *research minded*. Inherent in this aim is the assumption that a significant number of health care professionals will start to question the validity of their practice either by conducting their own research or by critically evaluating published research findings and in this way will facilitate cost-effective, systematic and appropriate health care.

Unassailable though this argument is, there has been well-documented concern in recent years that the quality and quantity of published research within nursing and midwifery have not been sufficiently high to enhance the scientific knowledge base of these professions. Furthermore, even where sound research exists it appears to be only partially effective in influencing service delivery. Numerous reasons have been put forward to account for the shortfall in well-conducted research. Professional ideologies which promote the midwife as caring, nurturing, reactive and intuitive are not only deeply entrenched but are diametrically opposed to the stereotypic

perceptions of the detached, objective, hard-nosed researcher. Consequently, for midwives to accept research as a routine part of their role means that they have to abandon, at least in part, their traditional professional persona. Enmeshed within this is a common understanding within the hospital hierarchy that research has historically been the rightful territory of doctors, and for midwives and allied personnel to engage in this activity has been construed by many as professional trespassing. Anecdotal evidence abounds which testifies to the tensions which are caused by those midwives who propose research studies or modifications to existing care interventions based on scientific evidence collected by health care professionals other than doctors.

Moreover, many midwives qualified before research skills were included in the core curriculum of the basic training and therefore do not have the necessary competencies to undertake research at any level. This inevitably means that their capacity both to conduct research or to evaluate published research findings is limited. While numerous research methodology courses exist, their provision is often haphazard and not tailored to meet local needs, with the end result that many midwives are falling through this particular continuing professional education net.

Other, more personal, obstacles to research have also been identified. A lack of confidence to carry out or assess research has frequently been noted, as has a disregard for any research studies which have been conducted by peer professionals. This latter point corroborates the earlier argument that research has not been universally or traditionally acknowledged to be an integral part of the midwife's role, and therefore that research which *is* conducted is perceived by some to be an amateurish first attempt by novices.

The foregoing evidence paints a negative picture of the current status of midwifery research, but to concentrate on this whilst ignoring the very significant research activities in midwifery would be misleading. Indeed, one glance through MIDIRS, the midwifery research data base, or MIRIAD, the compendium of ongoing midwifery research, should be enough to convince even the most sceptical that many midwives are engaging in valuable research. However, there remain numerous midwives who, because they lack the opportunity and knowledge, feel unable to address research at any level. It is for them that this text is primarily intended.

In parallel with the national changes in health care delivery has been the publication of many books on research methodologies. However, such is the resistance to research within some members of the core professions that a *general* text on research may not suffice. What is needed instead is a text which translates the sometimes unfamiliar concepts which are fundamental to research into contexts and examples which are directly relevant to the reader. In this way, the present book differs from the majority currently on the market, in that the essential terms, ideas and principles are tailored specifically for midwives. Corroboration of the value of this customised approach comes from my many years of teaching research skills to a variety of professional groups, who can more readily make sense of new and alien ideas when these are related to examples deriving from their own work experience. However, I should emphasize that I am not a midwife and that, apart from two episodes of first-hand experience of the profession, my only point of contact has been through many years of teaching on pre- and post-registration midwifery courses. This lack of professional experience, of course, may have resulted in the use of some odd examples throughout the book. If

this is the case, I would request the reader's forbearance.

Because I am not a statistician either, I share the terror experienced by many intending researchers when faced with an unfamiliar mathematical formula or a dense table of numbers. I hope that this has enabled me to simplify and make clear some of the issues which are central to research and statistical analysis. I have also attempted to avoid jargon as far as possible. Some is inevitable, but that which seems unnecessary, I have omitted in favour of more familiar phrases and words. Criticism could be levelled against me for this. Every discipline has its own terminology, often functioning to preserve the professional boundaries and thereby maintaining restricted access to the knowledge base. However, I do not subscribe to the view that research is the exclusive domain of academics but rather should be accessible to any professional who is interested in advancing the scientific basis of their practice.

In a continued search for lucidity, I have also deliberately left out as much statistical theory as possible. Whilst I acknowledge the value of a sound understanding of the theoretical background to a subject discipline, my experience when teaching research methodology has shown that including anything other than the most essential bits of the theory has served only to quell any interest and enthusiasm the student might have had in the topic and has therefore been completely counter-productive. I now believe that it is not crucial for a researcher to know the derivation of a statistical formula. What is critical, however, is that the midwife knows how to design, run, analyse and interpret a useful research study; it is possible to achieve this without an excess of theoretical input. This text, then, is a *practical* guide to conducting and evaluating research.

Lastly, the main emphasis of this book is *experimental* research methodology. The reasons for this are two-fold. Firstly, there is a demand for midwifery research which involves comparison – of treatment procedures, of effectiveness of interventions, of responses of different women. The experimental method is central to this comparative approach to research. Secondly, there are several texts already on the market which address survey methods, interviews, question-naires and other qualitative techniques in health care research, while relatively few deal with experimental designs. This book hopefully will fill the gap. However, this is not to suggest that I consider experimental methods superior to other research approaches. What I do believe is that some research questions are better answered using this technique. However, the various research methodologies can, and should, be complementary and mutually informative, and so the experimental methods included in this text should be viewed in conjunction with the others. To facilitate this, I have included sections on some of the other principal approaches which are useful to the midwife researcher and which should broaden the spectrum of available research tools.

The book has been divided into two sections. The first includes an introduction to some of the most useful methods in midwifery research, followed by a more detailed explanation of the principles involved in designing experimental studies. At the end of the first section are chapters intended to aid the publication of research as well as the evaluation of published research articles — both of which are critical stages in increasing the research-base of midwifery. The second part of the book comprises a number of statistical techniques for analysing data. In addition there is a glossary of terms and a refresher section of some basic mathematical principles. Exercises and activities are scattered throughout the book as a means of testing and consolidating understanding.

Finally, I would like to thank the many people who helped in the production of this book. My gratitude goes to my secretary, Anne Hollows, who made her way through my maze-like manuscripts with dedication and skill. I am also indebted to Mary Nolan who read the final draft of the book for errors, nonsense and clarity with typical thoroughness and goodwill. Her attention to detail and advice were invaluable, and without her help many grammatical errors and odd examples would pepper the book. Lastly, I would like to express my thanks to my husband, Professor Peter Spurgeon, whose own research skills have been a constant source of information and inspiration and to my children, Tom and Laura, whose arrival was responsible for sparking my interest in midwifery.

Birmingham 1996   C.M.H.

Acknowledgements

I am indebted to the following sources for granting permission to reproduce the statistical tables in Appendix 2 of this book:

Tables A2.1, A2.5 and *A2.6* from Lindley D V, Scott, W F 1995 New Cambridge Statistical tables, 2nd edn. Cambridge University Press, Cambridge.

Table A2.2 from Wilcoxon F, Wilcox R A 1949 Some rapid approximate statistical procedures. American Cyanamid Company. Reproduced with the permission of the American Cyanamid Company.

Table A2.3 from Friedman M 1937 The use of ranks to avoid the assumptions of normality implicit in the analysis of variance. Reprinted with the permission of the Journal of the American Statistical Association. Copyright (1937) by the American Statistical Association. All rights reserved.

Table A2.4 from Page E E 1963. Reprinted with the permission of the Journal of the American Statistical Association. Copyright (1963) by the American Statistical Association. All rights reserved.

Table A2.7 from Runyon R P, Haber A 1976 Fundamentals of behavioural statistics, 3rd edn. Addison Wesley, Reading, Mass.

Table A2.8 from Kruskal W H, Wallis W A 1952 The use of ranks in one-criterion variance analysis. Reprinted with the permission of the Journal of the American Statistical Association. Copyright (1952) by the American Statistical Association. All rights reserved.

Table A2.9 from Jonckheere A R 1954 A distribution-free k-sample test against ordered alternatives. Biometrika 14 (Biometrika Trustees)

Table A2.10 from Olds E G 1949 The 5% significance levels for sums of squares of rank differences and a correction. Annals of Mathematical Statistics 20 (The Institute of Mathematical Statistics)

Table A2.11 from Table VII (p. 63) of Fisher R A, Yates F 1974 Statistical tables for biological, agricultural and medical research. Longman Group Ltd, London (previously published by Oliver and Boyd Ltd, Edinburgh). I am grateful to the Literary Executor of the late Sir Ronald Fisher, FRS, to Dr Frank Yates and to Longman Group Ltd, London for permission to reprint Table VII from their book Statistical tables for biological, agriculture and medical research, 6th edn, 1974.

Table A2.12 adapted from Friedman M 1940 A comparison of alternative tests of significance for the problem of m rankings. Annals of Mathematical Statistics.

SECTION 1

An introduction to some basic principles in research

1

Introduction

THE NEED FOR RESEARCH IN MIDWIFERY

The current state of midwifery knowledge is the result of a steady accumulation of experience and information which has been gathered over centuries. Pre-, peri- and post-natal mortality are steadily declining, midwifery is now seen as a discrete profession and not a sub-section of nursing — is there any need to promote research and statistics in an area clearly already working effectively and to capacity?

Objections to the increasing profile of research within midwifery are regularly voiced both by members of the profession themselves as well as by those allied to it. The basis of their opposition stems from the fact that midwifery is fundamentally based on care, individual treatment, intuition and support, in which research, with its detached, objective, scientific, quantifying procedures, has no place. To introduce control and rigour of the sort necessary for good research risks dehumanizing the very procedures and values on which midwifery is founded.

It is impossible not to have some sympathy with this point of view. However, the changing nature of health care delivery world-wide and in the United Kingdom in particular, means that the limited resources currently available for health services must be used as judiciously as possible, whilst at the same time ensuring that the quality of patient care is enhanced. This means that ritualistic treatment or unchallenged procedures selected on the basis of prejudice

3

or assumption can no longer be justified. What is needed instead is a corpus of scientifically derived knowledge which can inform practitioners as to the best types of intervention for any woman. This is the role of research within midwifery and it is one which is clearly not incompatible with the delivery of high quality care.

Research is about asking questions and finding answers to those questions in a systematic way. Midwives should routinely challenge the effectiveness of their own practice in order both to improve the quality of care and to support their choice of treatment. Knowing how to question practice in a scientific way is the first stage in the research process.

However, despite wide-scale acceptance of the importance of evidence-based care, a considerable number of procedures are routinely used which have been shown by research to have no value. Oft quoted examples include the use of salt water baths to relieve perineal pain, shaving the pubic area prior to delivery and the excessive and inconsistent use of blood pressure monitoring, all of which have been demonstrated either to have no value or to be counter-productive. Such research results have the potential to streamline service delivery, but to do that they have to be read, evaluated and implemented in practice. Critical evaluation skills are therefore essential to the midwife. However, these skills are founded on a sound working knowledge of research methodologies and data analysis.

These two points — the generation and execution of sound research projects which question practice and the use of published research findings to modify existing policy and service delivery — are central to enhancing and systematizing midwifery and for these reasons alone the value of research must be self-evident. However, there is a further argument in support of research. Midwifery has experienced radical changes over recent years which have moved it from being a side-shoot of nursing to being a profession in its own right. This, together with the fact that basic training now incorporates some form of academic accreditation, requires that midwifery must have its own body of professional knowledge, developed by midwives, for midwives, to be used by midwives. Therefore, it is imperative that a prevailing research culture is fostered within the profession.

I hope that you can see from these arguments that research is essential if midwifery is to be systematized and optimized. In the current era of increasing pressure on resources, hit and miss policies of treatment based on opinion and preference rather than hard evidence are too wasteful of time and money to be justified. Therefore it is crucial for midwives to evaluate their procedures systematically to make the profession even more efficient, cost-effective and successful. To do this, a knowledge of research methods and data analysis is essential.

USING STATISTICS

Statistics are a crucial part of research. Whenever someone carries out an experiment it is essential that the results are analysed and presented in a way that can be understood by other interested parties. Statistics are one means by which this is achieved. For example, if an experiment had been carried out to compare two forms of assisted labour on a range of neonatal outcomes, it is insufficient just to present a table of figures showing a number of measures for each baby following delivery and expecting the reader to make sense of it. The data have to be analysed and interpreted using statistical methods, so that an objective conclusion can be reached in terms of which of the two modes of delivery is better.

However, many people are put off research because of the statistical procedures that are required. They see a page of formulae and figures, panic and slam the book shut. This suggests the first and most important rule of statistics — *do not panic!* Inability to understand statistics is rarely an intellectual problem, but an *emotional* one, and anyone who feels diffident in the face of figures should remember this. As long as you approach the statistical analysis systematically and in a step-by-step manner, there should be few problems.

Another point should be raised here. Do not imagine that the object of statistical analysis is to test your long multiplication and division — it is not. Statistics are no more than a tool for analysing data. So, always use a calculator — it is quicker and usually more reliable than even the quickest mind.

And lastly, remember that you do not need to memorize formulae — as long as you know where to look them up and how to use them there is no need to commit them to memory. Further, at the risk of being hammered by the purists, I would also add that there is no need to understand how the formula was derived from statistical theory. While many statisticians would vehemently disagree with that rather bald statement, I would liken statistical analysis to any other tool or piece of apparatus — you do not need to understand the workings of a car or television in order to use it. If that were the case, only garage mechanics would be allowed to drive cars. Many would argue, of course, that if you do understand the mechanism, then you are able to put it right if the apparatus goes wrong. However, if you know *when*, *why* and *how* to use a statistical method, and if you follow the procedure step-by-step, then the statistical tool will not break down. It is the when, why and how of statistics that this book aims to explain.

STRUCTURE OF THE BOOK

The book has been divided into two sections, the first of which is devoted to designing experiments and other research studies and the second section to statistical procedures. I would recommend that anyone who feels unsure of themselves mathematically should read Appendix 1 at the end of the book. Others may wish just to refresh their memories on some basic rules of mathematics. These are presented briefly in the next section. Once you have read as far as Chapter 9 you should have a sound idea of how to design experiments and which analysis to use on any data resulting from them. In Section 2 the chapters are devoted to outlining the procedures involved in particular statistical tests. You should read the relevant chapter as and when required. For this reason, these chapters are independent of each other and so may contain common material. I make no apologies for this repetition, since I find nothing more irritating than to open a sta-

tistics book at the relevant chapter only to discover that certain essential elements have been covered earlier, necessitating the reading of additional chapters in which I have little immediate interest. For this reason, the chapters on statistical tests are virtually self-contained.

Throughout the book, too, there are exercises to test your understanding of a particular principle. If you decide to do these, you will find the answers at the back of the book. Also, within each chapter, at appropriate intervals, there are 'Key Concept' boxes, which summarize the most important points. These can be used to refresh your memory without having to plough through pages of typescript to find what you want.

Finally, there are not a lot of laughs in statistics. Many students find the topic dry, so I have tried to make the style as chatty as possible. Nonetheless, jokes are hard to come by, but do persevere — statistics are an essential part of research life.

So, I hope you will find that this book equips you with the basic elements you need for your research.

P.S. All the experiments and data in the book are entirely fictitious!

P.P.S. Please note that all the calculations in the examples and activities have been worked to three decimal places throughout.

And a final word from a student: 'If I only had one day to live I would spend it in my statistics class. It would seem so much longer'.

SOME BASIC MATHS

Most of us have forgotten many of the basic mathematical concepts we learnt for 'O' or GCSE level, simply because we do not use them very often. Even though you are advised to use a calculator to compute the statistical tests in this book, it is still essential that you are familiar with the basic mathematical principles, for two main reasons. Firstly, even though a calculator will do all the most complex multiplying, dividing and square-rooting for you, you will need to know the *order* in which these processes are carried out, because, as you will no doubt remember, some types of computation must be done before others. This will be clarified later. Secondly, even though you will be using a calculator, it is still quite possible to come up with some odd results, either because some information has been entered wrongly, or simply because on occasions, calculators have been known to go haywire. So you need to be able to 'eyeball' the results of your calculations to see if they *look* right. If you have any doubts or reservations about any of this, read on.

This section is just a brief reminder of some of the basic principles you will need. These principles are discussed in greater detail in Appendix 1, so if you are unsure of any of them, turn to page 208.

Some basic rules

1. If the formula contains brackets, you must carry out all the calculations inside them first.
2. If the formula contains brackets within brackets, you must do the calculations in the innermost brackets first.
3. If the formula contains no brackets, do the multiplications and divisions first.
4. If the formula contains only additions and subtractions, work from left to right.
5. Adding two negative numbers results in a negative answer.
6. Adding a plus number to a minus number is the same as taking the minus number from the plus number.
7. Multiplying two positive numbers gives a positive answer.
8. Multiplying a positive number and a negative number gives a negative answer.
9. Multiplying two negative numbers gives a positive answer.
10. Dividing a positive number by a negative number (or vice versa) gives a negative answer.
11. Dividing two negative numbers gives a positive answer.
12. The square of a number is that number multiplied by itself. It is expressed as ^{2}.
13. The square root of a given number is a number which when multiplied by itself

gives the number you already have. It is expressed as $\sqrt{}$.

14. To round up decimal points, start at the extreme right hand number. If it is 5 or more, increase the number to its left by 1. If it is less than 5, the number to its left remains the same.

You might like to do the following exercises just to satisfy yourself that you are happy with these rules.

Activity 1.1 (Answers on page 233)

Calculate the following:

1. $14 + 8 + 27 - 3$
2. $14 + 8 - (27 - 3)$
3. $17 + (30 - 4)$
4. $11(19 + 4)$
5. $19 \times 3 + 8$
6. $12 + (14 \times 3) - 5$
7. $6[(4 + 8) - 3]$
8. $15 - 4 \times 4 + 12$
9. $(49 - 1) + 7 \times 8$
10. $36 - (12 - 6) + 17$
11. $-18 + 22 - 10$
12. $24 + 16$
13. $12 \times +4$
14. $-18 - 26$
15. 14×-3
16. $-51 + 3$
17. $51 - (+3 \times +2)$
18. $+17 - 4 - 26$
19. $-19 + 11 + 15$
20. $-5 (4 \times 12)$

SYMBOLS IN STATISTICS

You will find the following symbols appearing in formulae throughout the book. Although they will be explained when they appear, this page can serve as a quick reference point.

Σ = sum or total of all the calculations to the right of the symbol e.g. $3^2 + 6^2 + 4^2 = 61$

x = an individual score

$\bar{x}$ = the average score

$\sqrt{}$ = the square root of a figure or calculations,

e.g. $\sqrt{89} = 9.434$

$$\sqrt{17 + 15 + 86} = 10.863$$

$$\sqrt{15 \times 3} + 4 = 12.369 + 4$$

$$= 16.369$$

N = the total number of scores in an experiment

^{2} = the number times itself,
e.g. $8^2 = 8 \times 8$
$= 64$

$<$ = less than,
e.g. $5 < 7$ (5 is less than 7)

$>$ = more than,
e.g. $10 > 2$ (10 is more than 2)

C = the number of conditions in the experiment

n = the number of scores in a sub-group or condition.

2

Approaches to research design and statistics: some basic concepts

Whenever you engage in research, you will end up measuring something — Apgar scores, blood pressure, hours in labour, pain, etc. These measurements are called *data*. In order for the research to have some value, the meaning of these data has to be presented in ways that other research workers can understand. For example, there is no point in carrying out a well-designed experiment to compare the effectiveness of two pain relief techniques in labour, if the data on this is just left a jumbled mass of figures. In other words, the researcher has to make sense of the results.

There are various ways of making sense of the results, but for the midwife two methods are of major importance. The first approach is called *descriptive statistics*, whereby the researcher collects a set of data, usually from a form of survey and then describes it in terms of its most important features, e.g. average scores, range of scores etc.; the second approach is called *inferential statistics* in which the data, which has usually been collected from an experiment, is subjected to statistical analysis using tests which allow the researcher to make inferences beyond the actual data in front of him/her. The differences between these approaches will be discussed briefly now, and then in more detail in later chapters.

DESCRIPTIVE STATISTICS

As has already been mentioned, descriptive statistics are often used in conjunction with *survey* methods. A survey is a research approach which involves collecting information from a large number of people using interviews or question-naires, in order that an overall picture of that group can be described in terms of any character-istics which are of interest to the researcher. Examples are take-up of ante-natal services, use of parentcraft classes, health states, vaccination rates etc. The information that is collected can be analysed using techniques of *descriptive statistics* in order to highlight some of the most interesting findings. The way in which a survey is carried out will be described in more detail in the next chapter. However, some general introductory points about survey methods and descriptive statistics will be described here in order that the reader can get an overview of how descriptive and inferential statistics differ.

Let us take an example. Supposing you are interested in the general topic of community midwifery. You could easily gather a vast quan-tity of data on this topic, e.g.

1. The number of community midwives currently employed in a particular district.
2. The number of calls made on average per week within the district over the last year.
3. The types of clients seen (their ages, ethnic origin, social class, etc.) over the last year.
4. The average amount of time spent treating a particular category of client.
5. Any changes in the execution of community midwifery over the previous 10-year period could be noted, e.g. any increase in provision to a particular client group.

From all this survey data, you could gain the following sorts of information:

● what is going on in a particular area (type and extent of community midwifery provision)
● identification of areas of existing or potential problems (e.g. lesser provision in some geographical areas or for some categories of client)
● measurement of the extent of these problems
● the generation of possible explanations for them.

In addition to all this, the survey could identify past trends and so could be used to predict future patterns (e.g. with the growing trend towards

home-deliveries, the need for greater provision of community midwifery services together with any special skills or equipment needs might be highlighted).

The outcome of such surveys can radically influence major, as well as minor, policy deci-sions. And if such policy changes are imple-mented, survey techniques may be used to evaluate the impact these changes have. (For further information on survey methods see Cartwright (1983).) It will be useful at this point to look at some of the ways in which descriptive statistics might be useful to the midwife, by means of a more specific illustration.

Suppose that you are the head of a college of midwifery. Obviously, in this role you will be concerned about the standards of student performance, both clinical and theoretical, in your college. In particular, you may want to find out (a) whether these standards are dropping or rising from year to year and (b) how they com-pare with other colleges throughout the country. To do this you need to employ some common mathematical techniques in order to highlight certain features of the data, in other words, des-criptive statistics. Let us take the first example. To find out whether the standards are changing from year to year, you could take the average mark in both final theory and clinical exams over, say, the last 10 years. From this you can draw a

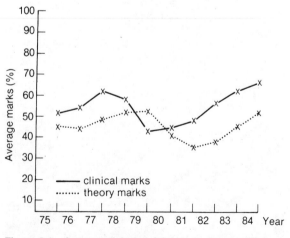

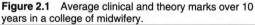

Figure 2.1 Average clinical and theory marks over 10 years in a college of midwifery.

graph to get the general picture of the standards of performance. You might end up with something like Figure 2.1.

From such a graph of average marks, you can get the general picture of the trend of performance and also the comparative performance on clinical and theory exams.

To solve your second problem of how your college compares with others, you can collect the average marks from all the other colleges for 1995, and compare yours with these. You might obtain the data shown in Table 2.1.

Your own averages (66% for theory, 52% for clinical — see Fig. 2.1) can be compared with the other colleges to find out how well your college does. It can be seen, then, from this information that your college comes 3rd in the theory exams, but only 7th in the clinical exams. From the above information, too, you can see that although college E has the best marks on theory, they have the biggest discrepancy between theory and practice, while college H appears to be the most consistent. In other words, you can glean a considerable amount of information from such data.

It should be pointed out that there are many ways of describing your data besides the methods illustrated above. However, the three most commonly used forms of descriptive statistics are *graphs*; *measures of central tendency*, which present data in terms of the most typical scores and results, and *measures of dispersion*, which present data in terms of the variation in the scores. Each of these will be discussed in Chapter 5, 'Techniques of descriptive statistics.'

Descriptive statistics, then, are used when the researcher has collected a large quantity of data, usually from a survey of some sort, and wishes to extract certain information from it in order to provide a description of the data. It is important to recognize that descriptive statistics allow you to make statements about features of your data that are of interest but they do not allow you to *infer* anything beyond the results you have in front of you. In other words, if you were measuring post-natal stress incontinence in a group of 20 elderly primips, you could use descriptive statistics to make statements about the incontinence data of that particular group of women in terms of frequency of incontinence, amount of urine voided, stressors etc. What you could not do would be to infer anything about the incontinence of elderly primips as a whole, simply on the basis of the data from your particular group. To be able to do that you have to use techniques called inferential statistics.

INFERENTIAL STATISTICS

Prior to every election, we are bombarded with the results of opinion polls which tell us how well one political party is likely to do compared with the others. In order to obtain this sort of information, a *sample* of the general public is questioned, since it would be impossible to ask the opinions of every member of the electorate. From the responses given by this sample, the attitudes of the rest of the voters are predicted, or *inferred*. However, we all know that these opinion polls may be quite incorrect. For example, if the opinion pollsters only went to a polo match in Surrey and asked the views of the spectators, they would be likely to get a very different picture of the prevailing political opinion than if they *only* went to a rugby match in South Wales. In other words, if the opinion poll is to have any value in predicting the outcome of an election, the sample of potential voters selected for the poll must be representative of the population as a whole and not representative of just one section of it.

The usual method of selecting a sample which is representative of the population from which it is drawn is a technique called *random sampling*.

Table 2.1 Average exam marks from all the colleges of midwifery in 1995

College	Average theory mark (%)	Average clinical mark (%)
A	63	58
B	45	55
C	48	59
D	57	45
E	70	50
F	52	60
G	54	61
H	67	66

For a sample to be random, it must have been selected in such a way that every member of the relevant population had an equal chance of being chosen. For example, if six playing cards are to be randomly selected from a pack, the pack is first shuffled and any six cards are chosen. Assuming the dealer did not hide any or keep his thumb on some, then these six cards will be a random sample because every one of the 52 cards had an equal chance of selection. Now, there are two important points here. Firstly, if these cards are not replaced and a second random sample is drawn from the same population, it will not be the same; so, if another set of six cards is selected from the pack, they will be different from the first set because there is only one ace of clubs, seven of hearts etc. in a pack. Similarly, any two groups of recurrent miscarriage patients, if randomly drawn from a population of recurrent miscarriage patients, will not be identical in their characteristics (age, height, fitness etc.) Secondly, the larger the random sample drawn, the more likely it is that it will be fairly representative of the population from which it comes. So, a random sample of three recurrent miscarriage patients out of a total population of 60 will stand less chance of being representative than a random sample of 35. More information about the ways in which the researcher can select a random sample in practice are given in Chapter 3. Returning to the opinion poll, even if the sample is representative of the whole population, there will still be an element of error in the predictions about the election (because some voters subsequently change their views, fail to vote or misunderstand the questions etc.).

Nonetheless, if the voters selected for the poll have been chosen randomly, according to certain statistical principles, then this degree of error can be calculated using a branch of statistics known as inferential statistics. Essentially what this approach enables the researcher to do is to select a small sample of people for study, and from the results of that study to make inferences about the larger group from which that sample was drawn. In other words, techniques of inferential statistics allow the researcher to move from what they *know* to be the case, as indicated by the data they have collected, to what they *predict* will be the case in other similar situations. In case this sounds a rather complex procedure, it should be stated that these inferential techniques are used by everyone on a daily basis. For example, your children, for as long as you can remember, have had cereal for breakfast. This is your data, the facts that you know are true. On this basis, then, you anticipate that this morning they will again want cereal so you put the packets out for them on the assumption that this is what they will want. This is your *inference*, based on the information collected from previous mornings and generalized to another similar situation. There are doubtless numerous examples that you can think of, where your knowledge about one situation leads you to make assumptions about other comparable situations. The actual techniques of inferential statistics are rather more complex than this, but the basic idea is the same.

The proper scientific procedure for making these inferences involves formulating a hypothesis, setting up an experiment to test the hypothesis and using inferential statistics to analyse the results of your experiment to see if your hypothesis has been supported. Thus, inferential statistics are used in testing hypotheses. It should be pointed out at this stage, that there are two main types of research design which are used to test hypotheses: experimental designs and correlational designs. They will be described in detail in Chapter 6.

One classic way in which the midwife might use the experimental approach is in the comparison of different treatment techniques with clients. Let us suppose you were interested in trying to alter the position of breech presentation foetuses in the third trimester of pregnancy. You have two exercise techniques, A and B, and you want to find out which is more effective. For a host of practical reasons, you cannot test *every* breech presentation foetus, and so you select a random sample of, say, 20 women with known breech presentations and assign them to Treatment A and a further random sample of 20 breech presentations and assign them to Treatment B. Both groups are managed in exactly the same way except for the nature of their treatment, and at the end of a given period, you compare the groups in terms of the presentation of the foetus. Suppose you find that the incidence of breech presentation is less (i.e. improved) for Treatment A group than for Treatment B. Now you would expect that there would be some differences between the groups anyway, simply because of chance factors, like the general exercise level of the women, chances of spontaneous change in presentation, current state of health, fatigue etc, but the question is whether the difference between the two groups in terms of the foetal presentation can be accounted for by these chance factors, or whether the difference is due to the relative effectiveness of the treatments. If the experiment has been carried out properly and in accordance with certain prerequisite conditions (see Chapters 7 and 8 for details on this), then statistical tests can be used to analyse the data and to conclude whether the difference between the groups is, in fact, attributable to the type of treatment or not. If it is found to be due to the treatment procedure, then you would conclude that Treatment A is more effective with this group. If you have selected your sample of patients randomly from women with breech presentation foetuses as a whole, then you could reasonably infer that Treatment A is likely to be more effective than Treatment B with other similar women, and hence you would recommend it to other midwives. In other words, you have selected a small sample for study and from the results of this study, you can make inferences about the whole population from which the sample was drawn. This is the basis of inferential statistics.

KEY CONCEPTS

Data from research must be presented in a way that can be understood by the reader. There are two main ways of doing this:

- Descriptive statistics, which summarize the main features of the results from a survey by describing the average scores etc.
- Inferential statistics, which are used in testing hypotheses. This involves selecting a small sample of people for study and from the results of this, allowing the researcher to make inferences about the population from which the sample was drawn.

In other words, descriptive statistics allow the researcher to make statements *only* about the results obtained, but do not permit any assumptions to be made beyond the data collected, whereas inferential statistics allow the researcher to make assumptions *beyond* the set of data in front of her/him.

3

Questionnaires, surveys and sampling

It was noted in the last chapter that surveys often use questionnaires as a means of collecting information about a group of people. However, while questionnaires are commonly used in this way, they can also be used in other designs, and as such are an invaluable method of data collection. This chapter will look at the basic principles of questionnaire design, as well as providing more details on carrying out surveys.

QUESTIONNAIRE DESIGN

Designing a good questionnaire is a skilled business and does not involve simply jotting a few questions down on paper.

The design of a good questionnaire should follow six steps:

1. Identifying the general topics to be covered by the questionnaire, which will reflect the objectives the researcher has in mind.

2. Initial draft of the questions covering all these topics.

3. Piloting the questionnaire i.e. giving out the questionnaire to a number of people (who do not necessarily come from the population at whom the questionnaire is targeted) in order to collect feedback on unclear or insensitive questions, ambiguous instructions etc.

4. Modification of the questionnaire using the information collected from the pilot trial.

5. A second pilot trial to establish whether or not the earlier problems have been ironed out.

6. Final administration of the questionnaire in

the actual study or survey. The completed questionnaire can then be analysed in a variety of different ways.

ASKING THE QUESTIONS

Questions come in two main forms — open and closed. Open-ended questions are those questions which allow respondents free range when supplying their answers. They are questions which do not provide boundaries or constraints on the answers. Closed questions, on the other hand, do just that — they allow the respondent only a limited choice of how to answer the question. To illustrate the difference between the two, let us take a simple enquiry that any midwife might make about a pregnant woman's health. She might ask the client

'How do you feel today?'

or alternatively

'Are you feeling any better today?'

The first is an open-ended question since the woman is being given the opportunity to make statements about her pain levels, appetite, anxiety level or whatever. The second example is a closed question, since the patient can really only answer 'yes' or 'no'. This example is a simplistic one, but it does illustrate the different ways in which questions can be used to elicit information. As with every other aspect of research, both types of question have their pros and cons. Open ended questions allow the respondent more flexibility and consequently much more information can be derived, often of a type the researcher had not thought of. On the debit side, though, such answers are difficult to analyse objectively which means that it can be difficult to compare one person's answer with another's. In consequence, the analysis may be much wider, less informative and more unsophisticated. Also, open-ended questions are more time consuming to complete and without answer guidelines many respondents may miss the point completely and provide responses which are neither relevant nor useful.

Closed questions overcome a lot of these diffi-

culties, since the structured response format means that answers can be completed quickly, analysed easily and direct comparisons between people can be made. The level of analysis can also be more sophisticated and useful. [This point will be discussed in more detail later in this chapter as well as in Chapter 4]. However, the value of such questions is largely governed by the skill of the question setter, who needs both to ask sound questions, devoid of ambiguities and bias and to provide a comprehensive and appropriate answer structure. Too often respondents get irritated by answer formats which do not meet their needs and consequently they refuse to fill in their replies.

These points raise two particularly important issues in questionnaire design — how to word the questions and how to structure a response format for closed questions.

Wording the questions

Asking the right questions is a skilled science and is not a topic which can be covered adequately in part of a chapter. I would therefore refer the reader to Oppenheim's (1966) seminal text 'Questionnaire Design and Attitude Measurement' which remains a leader in the field.

However, some guidelines can be given here as a starter-pack. Good question design is dictated by a list of do's and don'ts, each of which will be illustrated in turn:

1. *Don't* use complex sentence structures.
   Do keep your sentences clear and simple.

   For example,

   Don't ask 'Do you think that infertility, which is a distressing, frustrating and debilitating condition and one which causes untold anxiety, misery and pain to couples and families alike, should be given top priority in terms of government funding for health care?'

   Do ask 'Do you think that infertility is a sufficiently distressing condition to merit top priority for government funding for health care?'

2. *Don't* use medical or professional jargon.

Do use words and phrases that the respondents will understand.

For example,

Don't ask 'How adequate did you find the inhalation analgesia?'
Do ask 'How adequate did you find the gas and air?'

3. *Don't* confuse the respondent by asking about more than one thing at a time.
   Do keep to one idea per sentence.

For example,

Don't ask 'Do you experience any pain while going to the toilet or walking?'
Do ask 'Do you experience any pain while going to the toilet?'
and 'Do you experience any pain while walking?'

4. *Don't* assume everyone will know what you mean.
   Do keep your questions unambiguous.

For example,

Don't ask 'Do you do your exercises regularly?'
Do ask 'Do you do your pelvic floor exercises at least 20 times a day?'

5. *Don't* use double negatives.
   Do ask questions positively.

For example,

Don't ask 'Have you ever not wanted to take your iron tablets as a result of not wanting to get constipated?'
Do ask 'Do you avoid taking your iron tablets because of fear of constipation?'

6. *Don't* ask leading questions.
   Do ask questions in an unbiased unemotional way.

For example,

Don't ask 'Do you agree that women who have the filthy habit of smoking should be given bottom priority for care?'

Do ask 'Do you think that women who smoke should be given lower priority for care?'

Instructions on how to complete the questionnaire should also be clear and unambiguous. In addition, it may be necessary to enclose a definition of what the essential terms are to avoid misunderstanding; for example:

> 'Doing your exercises' should be taken to mean: 'Doing all the pelvic floor exercises you have been shown in the way they were demonstrated and for the time suggested'.

Remember that if the questionnaire is piloted in the way suggested earlier, then many of these potential problems can be ironed out.

Response formats for closed-ended questions

The way in which the response options are structured is important in questionnaire design, since it can dictate how honestly the respondent answers as well as the value and amount of information that can be derived from the questionnaires. These response formats can be thought of as ways of measuring a person's reply to your question and these measurements range from simple through to sophisticated scales. The whole area of *scales or levels of measurement* is an essential one in all sorts of research and is dealt with in Chapter 4 in much more detail. However, a brief introduction will be given here.

Let us imagine you have been treating a group of post-partum women for stress incontinence, and you wish to send them a follow-up questionnaire 6 months after the delivery to find out how they are progressing. One question you want to ask is:

Do you still suffer any incontinence?

You can structure the possible answers to this in a number of ways, for example:

(a) Do you still suffer any incontinence?
   Yes ☐   No ☐

(b) Do you still suffer any incontinence?

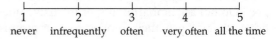

| 1 | 2 | 3 | 4 | 5 |
| never | infrequently | often | very often | all the time |

(c) Do you still suffer any incontinence?

Never	☐
Once a day	☐
Twice a day	☐
Three times a day	☐
Four times a day	☐
Five times a day	☐
More than five times a day	☐

(Please state)

The first response format is a simple one and gives us only basic information. For instance, a respondent who ticks the 'Yes' box might suffer stress incontinence once a month or once an hour, but this sort of answer format does not provide that level of detail.

The second answer format is somewhat more sophisticated, since it allows us to collect a range information on the overall frequency of incontinence. However, the descriptions 'infrequently', 'often' etc are open to subjective interpretation and while they provide more information about the woman's level of incontinence than the previous format, they are still lacking in objectivity and precision.

The last response format is the most sophisticated of the three, since it gives us detailed and accurate information about how often the patient is incontinent, in absolute terms.

These different types of response need different techniques to analyse them and this point is referred to in some detail later. As a rule of thumb, it is better, where possible, to use the most sophisticated and objective response formats as they supply a lot more information about your respondents.

It is also important to note, that respondents are not always honest in their answers, not necessarily because they deliberately wish to deceive the researcher, but simply because they want to present themselves in the best possible light. This tendency is known as a social-desirability response set and topics which are sensitive or emotive are particularly vulnerable to this type of bias.

Finally, do treat your respondents with respect. Do not ask embarrassing or intrusive questions, do not use their replies to compromise them, do not mislead them in any way and if you tell them their responses are anonymous or confidential, mean it.

ADVANTAGES AND DISADVANTAGES OF THE QUESTIONNAIRE

The main advantage of the questionnaire is that it can be designed and customized for any purpose or group of people. In addition, because a questionnaire does not have to be administered by the researcher in person, it means that a large sample of people can participate in the study by posting the questionnaire to them. This has added advantages. Firstly, posting a questionnaire is considerably cheaper than the time and travel expenses which would be incurred either by transporting the individual participants into the project centre, or by the researcher travelling to meet the participants. Secondly, if questionnaires are to be posted, the possibility of the researcher influencing the respondent's answers either unwittingly or deliberately is reduced considerably.

However, questionnaires have their disadvantages too. If the questionnaires are sent by post there is a very high chance that a lot of recipients will not return them. While this non-return rate can be reduced somewhat by the inclusion of stamped addressed envelopes, it does, nonetheless, mean that the researcher usually has to send out considerably more questionnaires than are actually needed in order to compensate for the non-returners, and this, of course, adds to the cost. Additionally, it has been found that sending out reminders to respondents can increase the response rate (e.g. Cartwright, 1983) but also increases the cost. Furthermore, whether a questionnaire is administered in person or by post there is still a high probability that some questions will be ignored, or incorrectly completed, instructions may be misinterpreted and some answers will be inadequately detailed. Also, while it seems obvious, it is still a point which is commonly overlooked by a lot of researchers — the respondent should be able to read the questions. This means that issues of visual impairment, non-English speakers and illiteracy must be considered. This having been said, questionnaires are still a very popular and very useful technique of data collection within the health care area.

KEY CONCEPTS

1. Questionnaires are a very useful way of collecting data in the health care area.
2. Asking the appropriate questions is a very skilled task and requires consideration of a number of issues.
3. Questions can be open-ended or closed-ended, both of which have advantages and disadvantages.
4. Closed-ended questions require structured answers, and the way in which the questioner sets out the answer structures is an important consideration.

SURVEYS

In the last chapter a survey was described as a research technique which involves collecting data from a large number of people, so that a general overview of the group can be obtained. Surveys usually use questionnaires or interviews as a means by which information is gathered, but since a key characteristic of the survey is the large number of people who take part, it is often quicker and much cheaper to use questionnaires rather than interviews. Indeed, so costly is it to interview hundreds of people that it is often outside the scope of most researchers. Consequently, this section will not cover issues concerning interviews. If you would like to find more about interview techniques, Polgar and Thomas (1991) and Cartwright (1983) both provide useful overviews.

GENERAL PRINCIPLES OF A SURVEY

The first stage in designing a survey is to establish its aims. In other words — what questions do you want answered? So, for example, you may want to describe the services of a satellite antenatal clinic, and consequently might want to ask:

1. How many women use it in the course of a year?
2. Where do they come from?
3. How many primigravidas use the clinic?
4. How many multigravidas use the clinic?
5. What are the ethnic origins of the users?
6. What are the ages of the users?
7. What are the occupations of the users?
8. What is the length of time women have to wait at the clinic?
9. How do the users rate the quality of care they receive at the clinic?
   etc.

You then have to decide the best ways of finding answers to these questions; in other words you have to design your survey.

THE DESIGN OF THE SURVEY

Two commonly used survey designs are *prospective designs* and *retrospective designs*. Prospective designs involve identifying the group of people you want to study and then collecting the information you require when they use the particular service. So, for example, you might want to focus on elderly primigravidas using the clinic. As soon as such women enter the clinic the researcher would collect the *relevant information* from them. However, by far the most common survey approach is the *retrospective design* which focuses particularly on past events. For example, you might identify from the medical records department in the clinic, patients who have undergone chorionic villus sampling or amniocentesis. You would then contact these patients to collect the information you require, such as their subsequent problems, perceptions of care etc. The main problem with this approach is the fact that when people are asked to recall events their memory may be selective and consequently this might bias the data you collect. Once you have decided on the design, you then have to identify the people who will take part in your survey.

SELECTING THE PEOPLE TO TAKE PART IN THE SURVEY

Finding the appropriate number and type of people to take part in your study is called *sampling*. This is an essential part of good research design of any sort, whether it be surveys or experimental approaches. While some reference has already been made to sampling in the earlier section on Inferential Statistics (Chapter 2) it is sufficiently important to merit a section on its own.

Sampling

When you carry out a piece of research it is impossible to involve every person who might be of interest to you, both for practical and financial reasons. For example, you might want to conduct some research on women who had episiotomies, but as there must be many thousands of these women within the UK it would be completely impossible to study them all. Consequently, you would select just some of them to take part in your study. These women would be your *sample.*

However, if the data collected from the sample is to be of any value, the sample must be representative of episiotomy patients as a whole. This entire group of *all* the episiotomy patients in the UK is called the *population*. The population can be defined as all those people (or even events) who possess the characteristic(s) in which the researcher is interested. Thus, the *sample* of episiotomy patients is a subset of the *population* of episiotomy patients as a whole. To take another example, you may wish to look at the Apgar scores of babies born to mothers who had Entonox during labour, within a Regional Health Authority. *All* the mothers who had Entonox in that authority would constitute the *population* and you might select a *sample* of 50 of them for your study.

However, if you are to collect any useful information from your sample, you have got to try to ensure that the sample is pretty well representative of the population from which it is drawn. If it is not, then the conclusions you reach from your study cannot readily generalize to the rest of the population and might lead you to make invalid assumptions about that population.

Let us illustrate this idea with an example. Supposing you wanted to conduct a survey looking at breast feeding practices, perhaps with a view to targeting health education information

more precisely. You devise your questionnaire and send it out to every woman within two postal districts who delivered at your hospital within the last 12 months. When you get the returns and analyse the data, you find to your amazement that 80% of the respondents breast fed for at least 6 months. You then assume that 80% of all mothers in your region breast feed for at least 6 months and you throw away your health education literature as it is not now the priority activity you had previously assumed. However, 2 years later you notice that there has not been the anticipated reduction in gastroenteritis, serious infections, obesity and eczema that would normally be associated with high breast feeding rates. Did something go wrong with your original survey data?

One possible reason might lie with the way in which you selected your survey sample. When you go back to check this, you realize that a very high proportion of professional women live in the two postal areas which you chose. You are aware of the extensive literature which shows that social class 2 women are more likely to breast feed. Moreover, you also learn that the La Leche League had just set up two new groups, one in each of the areas you sampled and were flourishing at the time of the survey. Small wonder, then, that your survey results suggested an incredibly high incidence of extended breast feeding. It also becomes clear why the associated benefits of breast feeding (such as the reduction in gastro-enteritis) were not noted across the region as a whole. In short, your assumptions about general breast feeding practices were based on a very biased sample of women.

Consequently, it is imperative that the sampling techniques employed in any study, be it survey or experimental, must be sound if you are to draw valid conclusions from your data. The most commonly used sampling methods in scientific and health research are *incidental sampling* and *random sampling*.

Incidental sampling

Incidental sampling involves selecting the most easily accessible people from your population and consequently it is relatively easy to do. Let us imagine that you are interested in doing a survey of client satisfaction with ante-natal care and you ask a community midwife to give the questionnaire you are using to all the women she sees in her area. This is undoubtedly an easy way of accessing a sample, but it may not give you a representative selection of mothers. For example, the community midwife may only see those women who have very straightforward pregnancies because those women with severe problems may be under the consultant obstetrician. In other words, this incidental sample may or may not be representative of the population and unless you had a lot more information about the population of pregnant women in that area, then you would not know whether the sample was biased or representative. In the above example, satisfaction with care may be intricately linked with the extent and nature of the care given. Consequently, those women with straightforward pregnancies might report a higher level of satisfaction than those women who had difficulties.

One way round this is to use a variation of incidental sampling called *quota sampling*. Suppose you know that 40% of all pregnant women in your selected area had non-proteinuric hypertension, 20% had breech presentations, 10% were multiple pregnancies, and 15% were Rhesus negative. You would have the information shown in Table 3.1.

Having this information you would then collect your sample of pregnant women by quota, ensuring that:

1. 40% of the women in your sample had non-proteinuric hypertension.

2. 20% of the women in your sample had breech presentations.

Table 3.1

Problem	Percentage of pregnant women suffering from the specified problem
Non-proteinuric hypertension	40
Breech presentation	20
Multiple pregnancy	10
Rhesus negative	15

3. 10% of the women in your sample had multiple pregnancies.

4. 15% of the women in your sample were Rhesus negative.

However, this approach means that you must know what particular characteristics are likely to be important in your study and secondly, you have to know what proportions of the pregnant woman population come into these categories. Both pieces of information may be difficult or even impossible to obtain, and this makes proper quota sampling problematic.

Random sampling

This is perhaps the most commonly used and best way of selecting a sample. The basic concepts were referred to under the heading 'Inferential statistics' in the previous chapter (pages 11–13) and consequently only a review will be presented here. The fundamental principle underpinning random sampling is that every member of the target population should have an equal chance of being selected for study. There are a number of ways in which this can be achieved. For instance, you can put the names of all members of the population into a hat and then draw out the number you need for your sample — just like a raffle. Alternatively you can use *random number tables*. This involves giving a number to every member of the population and then using a set of random number tables to select the sample size you need. (Random number tables can be found in a number of research texts e.g. Robson, 1974).

Essentially, the process works like this. Random number tables consist of the numbers 0–99 occurring with the same probability at any point in the table. If you wanted to select 25 twin pregnancies from a population of 100 such pregnancies then you would number the population from 0–99, shut your eyes and stick a pin into the random number table. From that number you work in any direction you like, making a note of the first 25 different numbers you encounter. You then tally these up with the corresponding numbers assigned to your clients and you have your random sample. Remember not to change direction once you have started; also, if you need to select another random sample then you should enter the table at a different point and move in another direction.

Random samples have an important advantage over other sampling techniques in that the sample, because it is more representative of the population, does not have to be a large one. (Sample size will be dealt with later in this chapter). However, there are major disadvantages. The researcher must know the names of all the population members before a random sample can be selected. If we think about the prospect of doing this with the topic of ultrasound screening, the task becomes impossible. Allied to this is the cost; it is much cheaper to find subjects for an incidental sample simply because it is by definition, easily accessible.

Two variations of random sampling are worth a brief mention: *stratified random sampling* and *systematic sampling*.

Stratified random sampling is akin to quota sampling in that it involves the researcher defining relevant sub-groups of the population. A random sample, using either of the above techniques would then be drawn from each sub-group. This approach ensures that all the important sub-sets of a population are represented in the sample but like random sampling it requires the names of every member of the population and is therefore costly, difficult and time consuming.

Systematic sampling involves choosing every third, seventh, thirteenth or whatever, member of the population. While this is not a truly random technique, it usually provides a sample which is adequately representative of the population.

When you have chosen an appropriate method for selecting your sample you then have to decide how many people you want to survey.

Sample size

Many would-be researchers are deterred from undertaking research because they believe they need hundreds of people to participate. This is not necessarily so and indeed in many situations it may be inadvisable to have crowds of people taking part, particularly if painful procedures or ethical issues are involved. There is no easy way of establishing the best size of sample since this decision depends very largely on the research which is being undertaken. However, as a general rule of thumb, a larger sample is more likely to be representative of the population than a smaller one and secondly, where techniques of inferential statistics are being used, small sample sizes are corrected by an increase in the stringency with which the analysis is conducted. In crude terms, then, if you have only a small sample, your results have to be 'better' before you can draw any conclusions from them. This will be discussed in more detail later in the text.

Once you have collected your results you then have to make sense of them. Some ways in which this can be done are described in the next chapter.

It may be worth pointing out that decisions concerning surveys or any other type of research approach can never be perfect; because of the practical difficulties and complexities of field and applied research, compromises in design always have to be made. However, it is important that the researcher knows what the pros, cons and implications of any decision are before implementing it and this text is an attempt to provide some of this basic information.

If you are interested to find out more about health surveys, Cartwright's (1983) book may be useful.

KEY CONCEPTS

1. Surveys are a research approach which involves collecting data from a large number of people, either by questionnaires or interviews, so that an overview of that group can be obtained.
2. Surveys can be *prospective* in design or *retrospective*. Retrospective surveys are more commonly used, but as they rely on people's recall of events may be flawed by selective or inadequate memory.
3. Deciding on who takes part in your study is called *sampling*. The general idea behind sampling is that you can generalize the results from your sample to the rest of the population from which it was drawn.
4. There are a number of different sampling methods, each of which has its own advantages and disadvantages.
5. The appropriate size for the sample is not easy to determine, since it depends very much on the topic being studied, as well as on the researcher's knowledge of the relevant population's characteristics.

4

The nature of the data

LEVELS OF MEASUREMENT

Whatever sort of research you are interested in, whether a survey or an experiment, you will be involved in measuring something, e.g. exam performance, degree of tear, reported pain levels, blood pressure and so on. These measurements form your *data* or results. If we look at the above examples a bit more carefully, we can see that each involves a different sort of measurement:

- exam performance may be measured as marks out of 20 or 100
- degree of tear may be classified as 1st, 2nd or 3rd degree
- reported pain levels may be measured on a subjective pain scale
- blood pressure is measured as systolic over diastolic pressure.

You can doubtless think of other sorts of measures that might be involved in midwifery research and it might be useful to make a list of these.

However, any measurement you use belongs to one of four main *categories of measurement*. It is important to be able to distinguish which category your data belongs to because it will affect the way in which you analyse your results, since different analyses can only be used with different categories of measurement.

The four categories of measurement are called levels of measurement and each category gives us a different amount of information:

1. **N**ominal level: the most basic level which gives us least information.
2. **O**rdinal level: the next level which provides all the information of the nominal scale plus some additional information.
3. **I**nterval level: a higher level of measurement which provides all the information of the nominal and ordinal scales but which offers additional information.
4. **R**atio level: the highest level of all which provides all the information of the nominal, ordinal and interval scales but which offers further information still.

For the purposes of statistical analysis, the interval and ratio scales are combined to form a single category, and this is how we will be dealing with them in this book.

Before we go on to look at what these levels actually mean, you may find it useful to remember the mnemonic *NOIR* (as it becomes most students' 'bête noir' trying to understand which category is which) to help you with the order of the different levels.

KEY CONCEPTS

When you carry out research you will be involved in measuring something. These measurements form your data or results and fall into one of four main categories of measurement. You need to be able to identify which category your own measurements come into, because this will affect the way in which you analyze your data, since some statistical tests can only be used with certain categories of measurement.

NOMINAL LEVEL

Let us take the nominal level first of all. As you may have guessed, this is simply a naming category, in that it only gives names or labels to your data without implying any order, quality or dimension. So, for example, you might want to ascertain how many of the applicants for places on a direct entry Diploma in Midwifery Course are mature students and how many are school leavers. You have two categories then, 'mature' and 'school leaver', and you simply count up how many applicants fall into each

category. This is a *nominal* level of measurement, because it has simply allowed you to allocate your data into one of two named categories.

Two important points are worth noting here. I have just said that this level of measurement has no implication for degree, order or quality of the data, which means that we could very easily alter the headings of the categories in any way, without affecting the results. So, for instance, 'mature' could just as easily have been called 'adult' 'chronologically challenged' or whatever, since it will not affect the number of applicants who fall into that category.

Secondly, the categories are mutually exclusive, in that an applicant can only be classified as 'mature' or 'school leaver' and cannot be both. Thus, once we have allocated a subject to one particular category, she cannot be allocated to any other category.

Let us take an example. If you were looking at the final exam success of two different courses of midwifery, you might take College A and College B and count up the number of fails and passes in each.

What you are measuring here is exam success, but all you have done is to use two labels — *pass* and *fail* — and you have counted up how many students in each school achieved more than 50% (pass category) and how many achieved less (fail category). You might end up with the data in Table 4.1.

A student who comes into the pass category cannot also come into the fail category and so this sort of level of measurement involves mutually exclusive categories.

This level of measurement gives us very little information about our data. You do not know *how* well the students have passed: all College A's pass students may have achieved over 90%, while all College B's passes may have been between 50–55%. You also do not know how

Table 4.1

	Pass	Fail
College A	29	11
College B	33	7

bad the fails are — 0% or 49% — all you know is that a certain number of students can be labelled 'pass' and a certain number 'fail'. Therefore, this is a nominal level of measurement, and as you can see, it does not tell us a great deal. For example, if you had to recommend one of these courses on the basis of nominal data, you would probably suggest College B because it achieved 33 passes to College A's 29. But if College A had average pass marks of over 90% as opposed to College B's 50–55%, you might want to change your recommendation. However, you would not know this from nominal data alone, since all this category allows you to do is to classify your data under the broad headings of pass and fail.

Political opinion polls which simply categorize people into Conservative, Labour, Liberal Democrats and Don't Knows are nominal scales. Voting on a particular issue in a meeting categorizes people into For, Against and Abstain and so is a nominal scale. We do not know *how* Conservative a respondent in a poll is, or how Against a voter in a meeting is — we just know that they can be allocated to a particular category.

The following are also examples of the nominal level of measurement:

• The number of mature vs. school leaver applicants for direct entry midwifery at School A may be 29 mature candidates and 43 school leavers. You do not know how old the mature applicants are, how good their 'A'-level results are, or how suitable they are, all you know is that you have 29 mature applicants and 43 school leavers.

• You send a questionnaire to all the women attending ante-natal clinics in a given district asking them to indicate:

Do you smoke?   Yes _____   No _____

You get a set of replies, which suggests that 42 people smoke, and 101 do not. But you do not know how *many* cigarettes the smokers smoke — it may be five a day or 65. All you know is that 42 pregnant women attending ante-natal clinics in a particular district smoke and 101 do not.

It is worth noting that the nominal level of measurement is referred to as 'categorical data' in some text books.

Activity 4.1   (Answers on page 233)

Look at the following measures you might use in a piece of research, and indicate how these might be converted into a nominal category of measurement:

1. improvement in stress incontinence following therapy
2. reduced incidence of breech presentations following breathing exercises
3. reduction in perineal pain following a warm water bath
4. keeping appointments at an ante-natal clinic
5. perceptions of the quality of midwifery care.

ORDINAL LEVEL

The next category of measurement is the *ordinal scale* which tells us a bit more about our data. The ordinal scale allows us to *rank order* our data according to the dimension we are interested in, for example:

most preferred — least preferred
most improved — least improved
most competent — least competent.

Suppose you asked a clinical mentor to rank order a set of students on their competence during a placement, because you wanted to see if clinical performance was related to entry grades. The mentor might come up with the list in Table 4.2.

What we have is a rank ordering of these students in terms of the dimension we are interested in — their competence. We still do not have a great deal of information about them, however, because we do not know *how* much better Catherine A. is than Jane C. or how much worse Susan D. is than the rest (or in fact, whether any of them is competent at all). All we know is that Catherine A. *is* better than Jane C. who in turn *is* better than Jackie S.; but we don't know how much better. In other words, we have a *relative* and not an *absolute* measure of competence. It

Table 4.2   Students arranged in order of competence

Competence position		Student
1	(Most competent)	Catherine A.
2		Jane C.
3		Jackie S.
4		Carol R.
5	(Least competent)	Susan D.

is also important to note that the differences between each pair of ordinal positions are not necessarily the same, i.e. the difference in competence between Catherine A. and Jane C. may not be the same as the difference between Jane C. and Jackie S.

Another example of an ordinal scale of measurement is the use of a point scale. For example, in the previous study, you might alternatively have asked the clinical mentor to indicate on the following scale how competent each student was:

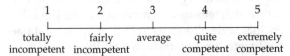

Here we have a dimension of most competent to least competent on a 5-point scale, (although we could use fewer or more than 5 points) and on which each student may be rated. Therefore, had we asked the clinical mentor to assess the students using this scale, we might have found the results shown in Table 4.3.

Again, the difference between each pair of scores must not be assumed to be the same; the difference in competence between:

5 (extremely competent)
and
4 (quite competent)

may not be the same as between:

1 (totally incompetent)
and
2 (fairly incompetent)

In our earlier example on the smoking questionnaire, you could modify your question from:

Do you smoke?   Yes _____ No _____

Table 4.3

Competence score	Student
5	Catherine A.
4	Jane C.
3	Jackie S.
2	Carol R.
1	Susan D.

to:

What sort of smoker would you classify yourself as:

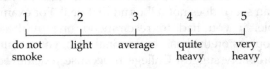

Again, we do not know whether the woman who selects 'very heavy' smokes 60 or 100 cigarettes a day, but we do know that she smokes more than the light smoker. Similarly, someone who scores 4 may not smoke *twice* the number of cigarettes as someone who scores 2. All we know is that someone with a score of 4 does smoke more than someone with a score of 2. We can see particularly clearly from this example how the ordinal scale gives us more information than the nominal scale. If we use this rank ordering technique, we can count up the number of *non-smokers* (anyone who scores 1) and the number of *smokers* (those who score 2, 3, 4 and 5) and this gives us the information provided by the nominal scale. However, the ordinal scale adds a *dimension* to the label of 'smoker', in that it allows us to measure people according to whether they are heavy, average or light smokers. In other words, it gives us a bit more information than the nominal level. It should be noted, though, that the ordinal scale is a rather imprecise measurement. It is commonly used to assess things like pain, attitudes, levels of agreement etc; consequently it relies on very subjective interpretations and so cannot be assumed to have any absolute meaning.

> **Activity 4.2** (Answers on pages 233–234)
>
> Look back at the examples given on page 25 and convert each of these to an ordinal level of measurement.

INTERVAL/RATIO LEVEL

The interval level or scale of measurement is like the ordinal scale, except that it does assume equal intervals in its measurement. Interval scales are measures such as percentage in an exam, range of movement etc. Interval and ratio measurements have two things in common. Firstly, they assume *equal* intervals, such that it is possible to say that the *difference* between scores of 30% and 60% (i.e. 30%) is half the difference of that between scores of 30% and 90% (i.e. 60%). Similarly, the *difference* between marks of 40% and 50% on an exam is exactly the same as the difference between 80% and 90% (i.e. 10%). If we look back to the ordinal scale of measurement, we cannot make these statements, because we simply do not know whether the difference between scores of 1 and 3 on a 5-point scale is the same as the difference between 3 and 5. In other words the gap between 'no smoker' and 'average smoker' is not necessarily identical to the gap between 'average smoker' and 'very heavy smoker' (see above).

The second point to note is that the interval scale does not have an absolute zero point although sometimes one is arbitrarily imposed. This means that a zero score on an interval scale does not necessarily mean an absence of the quality being measured. A good example of this is temperature where zero temperature does not mean an *absence* of temperature, but rather the temperature is at freezing point. The ratio level of measurement is like the interval level except that it does have an absolute zero. It includes measures such as distance, height, weight, time etc. Do not worry about this point, because for the purposes of statistical tests, interval and ratio scales are treated as the same. From now on, these two levels of measurement will be collapsed to form one category, which will be referred to as the interval/ratio level.

If, then, we look back at the example of students' competence on clinical placement, our clinical mentor could have given the students a test (marks out of 50, say), rather than rank ordering them. The results might have looked like Table 4.4.

Table 4.4 Test marks of students

Mark	Student
44	Catherine A.
39	Jane C.
30	Jackie S.
22	Carol R.
11	Susan D.

From these data, we can see that the difference between Catherine A. and Carol R. is twice the difference between Carol R. and Susan D. In addition, from these data we could rank order the scores to find each student's position in the group (ordinal level of measurement) and also we could classify the students into pass/fail (nominal level of measurement). Therefore, the interval/ratio level of measurement gives us more information than the ordinal scale, which in turn tells us more than the nominal scale. Again, if we look at our smoking example, we could modify our questionnaire again and simply ask 'How many cigarettes do you smoke per day?' We might get a range of answers from 0 to 60, and from this, we can say that someone who smokes 60 daily, smokes twice the amount of the person who smokes 30, three times the amount of the person who smokes 20, four times the amount of the person who smokes 15, and so on. We could also:

- rank order the replies from heaviest smoker to lightest (ordinal scale)
- classify the replies into smokers and non-smokers (nominal scale)

As a result, it can be seen that the interval/ratio level of measurement gives us all the information of the nominal and ordinal levels, plus a bit more. Other examples of interval/ratio data include temperature, blood pressure, time measures, length, weight, volume and heart rate.

It should be mentioned here that sometimes researchers treat point-scales as though they were interval rather than ordinal scales, because when constructing the point-scale they have *assumed* equal intervals between the points. Sometimes this is entirely legitimate, for example, when analysing questionnaire data. As a broad rule-of-thumb, if you construct a point-scale with at least 7 points on it, and are assuming that the distances between the points are comparable, then you may wish to classify this as an interval scale for the purposes of analysis.

This point is highlighted by the visual analogue method of measuring pain. This commonly used technique involves presenting patients with an unmarked line of exactly 10 cm, with 0 cm representing no pain and 10 cm representing excruciating pain:

| No pain | Excruciating pain |

The patient is then asked to mark on this line how much pain she is experiencing. The line up to the mark is then measured. In this way, one patient may report 54 mm of pain, and another 19 mm and so on. The problem then emerges of how to classify the data. Pain is subjective, so should this be called an ordinal scale? However, length measurement in cm, mm or whatever is an interval/ratio scale so how can the issue be resolved? There is no right answer here and it must be left to the researcher. However, as a general rule of data collection, it is usually advisable to use the most sophisticated level of measurement you can, since more detailed analyses can be performed. Therefore, it may be preferable to treat visual analogue data as interval/ratio.

Activity 4.3   (Answers on page 234)

1–5 Look back at the five examples given on page 25 and convert the measures to interval/ratio scores.

6   Look at the following data, and construct a:
    nominal
    ordinal
    interval/ratio
    level of measurement for each one, e.g. to look at the incidence of low back pain among primigravidas after 16 weeks' gestation, you would measure:

(i) How many had experienced low back pain and how many had not experienced low back pain after the 16 week gestation point (nominal).

(ii) Frequency of back pain using a 5-point scale by asking the question: How often have you experienced back pain since you reached 16 weeks' gestation? (ordinal):

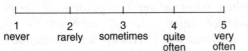

| 1 | 2 | 3 | 4 | 5 |
| never | rarely | sometimes | quite often | very often |

(iii) Frequency of back pain using absolute number of incidents (interval/ratio): How many times have you experienced back pain since the 16 weeks' gestation point?

Using the same format, construct nominal, ordinal and interval/ratio levels of measurement for the following:

(i)   efficiency of breast shells as a method of improving inverted nipples.
(ii) improvement in carpal tunnel syndrome 3 months after delivery.
(iii) experience of pain during stitching of an episiotomy.

7 Look at the following measurements and say whether they are nominal, ordinal or interval/ratio:

(i)   Number of attenders vs. non-attenders at an ante-natal clinic.
(ii) Mothers' ratings of the degree of confidence they have in their midwife, on a 7-point scale.
(iii) Number of work hours lost through stress in delivery suite midwives.
(iv) Percentage of face and neck covered by chloasma.
(v)   Recovery time in days following caesarean section.

Remember that you need to be able to distinguish between nominal, ordinal and interval/ratio levels of measurement, because the level of measurement will affect how you analyse your data. More information about this will be given throughout the text. And finally, it is generally advisable to use the highest levels of measurement you can (i.e. interval/ratio rather than ordinal, ordinal rather than nominal) because not only do the higher levels provide you with more information than the lower levels, but also the type of analysis that can be carried out with the higher levels is more detailed and sophisticated. Clearly, there will be occasions when you have no choice but to use nominal or ordinal levels of measurement. For instance, if you are collecting information about the number of medio-lateral J-shape and midline episiotomies performed, you would have to use the nominal categories of 'medio-lateral', 'J-shape' and 'midline' since nothing else would be appropriate. However, as a general rule-of-thumb, use the higher levels of measurement whenever you can.

KEY CONCEPTS

There are four levels of measurement, each of which gives us a different amount of information about our data.

- Nominal scales give us least information and simply allow our data to be labelled or categorized, e.g. pass/fail, male/female, over 40/under 40, improvement/no improvement.
- Ordinal scales give us a bit more information in that they allow us to put our data into a rank order, according to the dimension we are interested in, e.g. most competent to least, heaviest smoker to lightest, greatest pain to least etc.
- Interval/ratio scales give us more information, in that they deal with actual numerical scores, e.g., weight, height, time, percentage, pressure, capacity etc., which allow direct mathematical comparisons to be made.
- The interval and ratio levels are combined to form a single category for the purposes of data analysis.

5

Techniques of descriptive statistics

The information or *data* collected from your project has got to be interpreted, in order to make sense of it. It was noted in Chapter 2 that there are two main techniques you can use to interpret your data: *inferential statistics* which are used to check whether your results support your hypothesis, and *descriptive statistics* which are methods of describing your results in terms of their most interesting features. Techniques of descriptive statistics are commonly used to make sense of survey data, where large quantities of information are collected. Once this data have been organized and presented in a more accessible way, it is then possible for the researcher to formulate hypotheses from it. These can then be tested using the appropriate inferential statistics. In this way, descriptive statistics are sometimes thought of as the first stage in analysing results from surveys or whatever, and inferential statistics the second stage. This chapter is concerned with some frequently used techniques of descriptive statistics.

ORGANIZING DATA INTO A TABLE

It is very difficult to make any sense out of a large amount of information simply by looking at the raw data. However, if these data are organized into a table, then it is much easier to understand. Let us imagine you have been conducting a survey of the uptake of ante-natal services at a hospital clinic over a one month period and you have a mass of information concerning the women, their age, parity, occupation, address, medical

Table 5.1 Frequency of attenders at an ante-natal clinic by catchment area

Catchment area	Frequency
Harcourt	52
Mossway	21
Kings Chapel	11
Edgeheath	14
Norton	19
Quinbourne	9
Total	126

problems etc. This information can be tabulated to make the key points clearer. Let us focus, for an example, on geographical location of the women who attend. The first set of information you have is the number of women coming from the various catchment areas i.e. *nominal data*. This information can be represented as in Table 5.1.

From this table, you can see at a glance where most of the attenders came from. In order to construct this sort of table, then, you must group the data into the important nominal categories, which here were the catchment areas. The number of women coming from each category is counted up and information is then represented in a table.

You then decide to look at the attenders' reported satisfaction with ante-natal care. In order to collect this data you have asked every woman to rate how satisfied she is, using a 5-point ordinal scale:

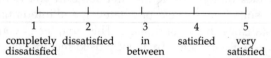

You tabulate these data and find the following: (Table 5.2)

Table 5.2 Frequency of reported satisfaction levels among attenders at an ante-natal clinic

Satisfaction level	Frequency
Completely dissatisfied (score of 1)	0
Dissatisfied (score of 2)	5
In between (score of 3)	29
Satisfied (score of 4)	76
Completely satisfied (score of 5)	16
Total	126

Therefore, to construct this table, you need to count up all the patients in each ordinal satisfaction category and these figures are then presented in table form.

The next set of data you need to interpret is the number of weeks' gestation of women attending the clinic. The raw data ranges from 4 weeks to 41 weeks. You may recall from the previous chapter that time measurements are of an interval/ratio type. This is organized as in Table 5.3.

Again, to arrive at this table, you would need to count up the total number of women falling into each gestational state; these stages should be arranged *in order* from lowest to highest and then set out accordingly. However, if there are a lot of intervals, as there are above, then the table can be large and unwieldy and rather difficult to interpret. Consequently, it may be better in such cases to *group* the intervals (Table 5.4).

While this is a neater table, it should be noted that a lot of detailed information is lost by collapsing the intervals in this way. If you decide to combine your data intervals like this, you should ensure that the grouped intervals are of an equal size.

It can be seen by looking at the above tables that they provide at-a-glance information about the women in your care and consequently they are a valuable technique of describing your

Table 5.3 Frequency of gestational stage of women attending an ante-natal clinic

Gestational stage (in weeks)	Frequency
4	1
6	3
8	5
12	8
14	13
16	16
18	16
20	12
24	15
28	11
30	15
34	5
36	3
38	1
41	2
Total	126

Table 5.4 Frequency of gestational stages of women attending an ante-natal clinic

Gestational stage (in weeks)	Frequency
0–12 weeks	17
13–24 weeks	72
25–36 weeks	34
37+	3
Total	126

Table 5.5 Incidence of various types of abortion

Type of abortion	No of women
Threatened	15
Complete	32
Incomplete	26
Missed	10
Recurrent	6

results. Remember, though, that all tables should be clearly labelled and self-explanatory.

GRAPHS

Sometimes it is easier to make sense of a set of data if it is presented as a graph rather than as a table of results. While a graph tells you no more than a table of figures, it often shows trends and other features of the data more clearly. Since we have all drawn graphs in school and elsewhere, the principles pertaining to graph drawing will be outlined only briefly here. For the purpose of midwifery research the frequency distribution graph is probably the most important. A frequency distribution refers to how often a particular event occurs; for instance, how many women in the second trimester have heart rates of the order of:

60–65 beats per minute,
66–70 beats per minute, or
71–75 beats per minute.

The most common forms of frequency distribution graph are the *histogram* (and related *bar graphs*) *pie charts* and the *frequency polygon*. The features of each will be outlined shortly, and some general rules for drawing graphs will be presented at the end of this section.

Histograms and bar graphs

These two graphical techniques are very similar, though many people feel the bar graph is clearer. Bar graphs are typically used to present *nominal and ordinal* data, and histograms for interval/ratio data. Each technique presents the data in a series of vertical rectangles, with each rectangle

representing the number of scores in a particular category. However with the histogram, the vertical bars are directly adjacent to one another, whereas with the bar graph there are spaces between them. These techniques can best be demonstrated by illustrations. Suppose you want to find out what the incidence of various types of abortion is within your particular hospital; you might come up with the figures in Table 5.5.

The frequencies for these nominal categories can be represented as a bar graph as in Figure 5.1.

Note that the categories of event go along the horizontal or *X axis* and the frequency with which they occur along the vertical or *Y axis*.

If the categories along the horizontal axis have no natural order, then they may be arranged in order of size, with the greatest frequency distri-

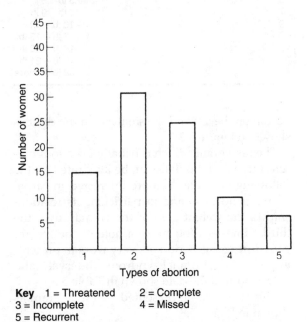

Key 1 = Threatened   2 = Complete
3 = Incomplete   4 = Missed
5 = Recurrent

Figure 5.1 Bar graph showing distribution of types of abortion in a given hospital.

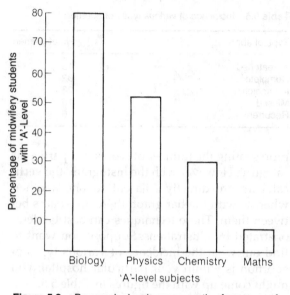

Figure 5.2 Bar graph showing comparative frequency of 'A' level subjects among midwifery degree students.

Table 5.6 Body weight of women with carpal tunnel syndrome

Number of women	Body weight
0	less than 3 lb
3	3 lb – 5 lb
7	6 lb – 9 lb
9	10 lb – 12 lb
15	13 lb – 15 lb
23	16 lb – 18 lb
38	19 lb – 21 lb
47	22 lb or more

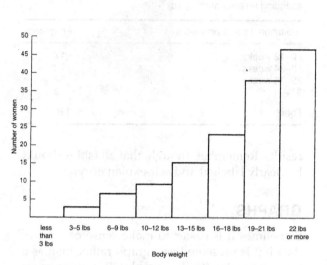

Figure 5.3 Histogram showing the weights of women presenting with carpal tunnel syndrome.

Table 5.7 Percentage of type of abortion

Type of abortion	Number	Percentage
Threatened	15	16.85
Complete	32	35.96
Incomplete	26	29.21
Missed	10	11.24
Recurrent	6	6.74
Total	89	100.00

bution on the left and the smallest on the right as shown in Figure 5.2.

The histogram, which is usually used to represent interval/ratio data, can be illustrated by the following example. You are interested in carpal tunnel syndrome, and in particular its relationship to the weight gain of the woman over the third trimester. You make a note of the weight gain during this period of every woman presenting with carpal tunnel syndrome (interval/ratio data) and find the data shown in Table 5.6.

This table can be presented as a histogram as shown in Figure 5.3.

It should be noted that the individual weight gains of women have been allocated to categories

for the purpose of simplifying the data and drawing the histogram. Clearly the category size should be appropriate for the range of data available; a small number of categories will lose much of the detailed information of the data, while too many will complicate the table or graph. No more than nine categories are used as a rule.

Pie charts

Nominal data can also be represented graphically using *pie-charts*. A pie-chart is a circle which is divided into sections, each section representing proportionately the number in each category or event. In order to do this, the figures in each category must be converted to percentages of

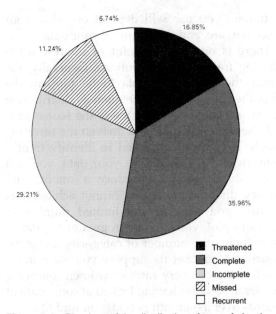

Figure 5.4 Pie-chart of the distribution of type of abortion in a given hospital.

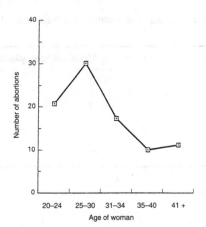

Figure 5.5 Frequency polygon showing age of women presenting with abortion within a given hospital.

Frequency polygons

Data of an interval/ratio type can also be plotted as a *frequency polygon*, in which the frequency of occurrence of each unit or event on the horizontal axis is plotted at the midpoint of the unit, and these points are then joined by a continuous straight line. Imagine that your survey of abortions has also included the age of the women presenting at the hospital with abortions (interval/ratio data) as in Table 5.8.

These can be represented by a frequency polygon, as in Figure 5.5.

In the above example the graph does not touch the horizontal axis. Some people are of the opinion that this gives a rather odd appearance to the graph, and so, in cases where it is appropriate, you can add a class to either end of the units with scores on the horizontal axis. Thus, to give an example, you might wish to plot the frequency of average final examination marks across a number of colleges of midwifery for 1994. The results you obtain are shown in Table 5.9.

Your graph might look like Figure 5.6.

There are no colleges which achieve an average mark of 31–40% or of 91–100%. Therefore, to give this graph a more complete appearance, the line can be extended to the values for the categories 31–40% and 91–100% (dotted line in Fig. 5.6).

Obviously, more than one set of data can be plotted on a frequency polygon, so that direct comparisons can be made. In the above example,

the *total* number first. So let us imagine you wish to represent Table 5.7 as a pie-chart rather than as a bar graph, you would need to convert the figures for each type of abortion into a percentage of the total number of abortion patients in the hospital.

The pie-chart would look like Figure 5.4.

To construct this pie-chart, the percentages for each type of abortion must be converted to degrees. Each 1% equals 3.6° since 100% is the equivalent of 360°. The value of a pie-chart lies in its immediate visual appeal and the ease with which proportions can be compared. However, if there are a lot of categories pie-charts can be confusing and difficult to construct and interpret accurately.

Table 5.8 Age of women presenting with various types of abortion at a given hospital

Age of woman	number of abortions
20–24	21
25–30	30
31–34	17
35–40	10
41+	11
Total	89

Table 5.9 Average final exam marks in colleges of midwifery

Average final exam mark	No of colleges attaining mark
31–40	0
41–50	1
51–60	3
61–70	4
71–80	1
81–90	1
91–100	0

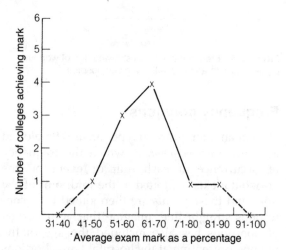

Figure 5.6 Frequency polygon showing distribution of average final examination marks across a number of colleges of midwifery for 1994.

you might want to plot the average marks for the year 1993 as well, so that you can compare performance.

Whether you decide to use a histogram, bar graph, pie chart or a frequency polygon depends on the nature of the data you wish to present. Nominal data, for instance, should not be plotted as a frequency polygon, but rather as a bar chart. Generally, the frequency polygon is more suitable if two or more sets of frequencies are to be compared, since a number of lines can be represented in different colours or styles on the same graph. A similar comparison using bar graphs or histograms is very confusing, since it will involve overlapping rectangles. However, that being said, lay people often find histograms and bar graphs easier to interpret, when they are not familiar with the subject area. In short, which

technique you use will depend on what your objectives are, and the nature of your data.

There is one further point of interest when plotting frequency distributions. Generally, the larger the amount of data to be plotted, the smoother the resulting frequency distribution curve and conversely, the fewer the scores plotted, the more irregular and uneven the resulting graph. If you are concerned to identify trends, patterns and regularities in your data, you will obviously be keen to produce a smooth frequency distribution. If you cannot achieve this because you have only a limited number of scores to plot, you can obtain greater regularity by reducing the number of categories along the horizontal axis. Let us suppose you were interested in the recovery rates of women following caesarean sections; having looked at some patient records over a 6-month period, you find that:

4 women were discharged after 4 days
6 women were discharged after 5 days
10 women were discharged after 6 days
13 women were discharged after 7 days
10 women were discharged after 8 days
9 women were discharged after 9 days
15 women were discharged after 10 days
3 women were discharged after 11 days
5 women were discharged after 12 days
2 women were discharged after 13 days

If these data are plotted as it is presented, we get the graph shown in Figure 5.7.

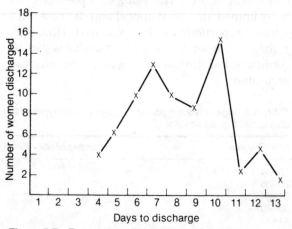

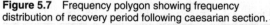

Figure 5.7 Frequency polygon showing frequency distribution of recovery period following caesarian section.

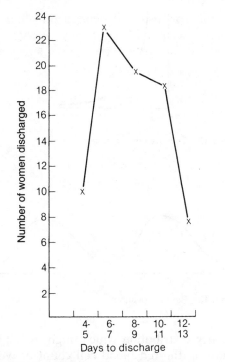

Figure 5.8 Frequency polygon showing frequency distribution of recovery period following caesarian section.

However, if we collapse the categories along the horizontal axis as shown in Figure 5.8, we achieve a rather smoother graph.

You can see from the above illustration that reducing the categories along the horizontal axis makes the graph appear more regular, and in so doing allows you to get a clearer idea of the trends in the data. (A word of caution, though! Reducing the categories in this way may also distort your data, and obscure important features).

Ten rules for drawing graphs of frequency distributions

1. The horizontal axis, also known as the X-axis, must be used to represent the categories or events.

2. The vertical axis, also known as the Y-axis, must be used to represent the frequencies with which each event occurs.

3. The intervals along the axes must be of a suitable size, so that the graph may be drawn and interpreted accurately.

4. The intersection point of the axes conventionally should be zero. If this does not suit your purposes ensure you make a note of this so that it is clear to the reader.

5. All graphs should be clearly labelled and self explanatory. Both axes should also be labelled.

6. Nominal and ordinal data are usually described in bar graphs or pie charts.

7. Interval/ratio data are usually described in histograms and frequency polygons.

8. Interval/ratio data can be combined so that the graph can be inspected for *trends*.

9. If the categories are to be combined to form larger sub-groups you should not use too many groups, otherwise the graph may be difficult to interpret. Similarly, you should not use too few sub-groups, otherwise a lot of information will be lost.

10. If you sub-group your data, the sub-groups should be of equal size, otherwise you will distort the information.

KEY CONCEPTS

- Data can be represented by drawing graphs.
- Histograms and bar charts can describe frequency distributions by columns or vertical bars to represent the numbers obtained in each category or event.
- Pie-charts can represent data pictorially by using a circle, which is divided into segments, the size of which represents the numbers in each category or event.
- Frequency polygons are graphs which use a single line to connect the numbers in each event.
- Nominal and ordinal data are best described using bar charts and pie charts.
- Interval ratio data are best described using histograms and frequency polygons.

Shapes of frequency distribution curves

If you plot a large number of graphs over a period of time, you will notice that some shapes of frequency distribution tend to occur time and again. It may be useful to outline some of these briefly.

Normal distribution (Fig. 5.9) is probably the most important frequency distribution shape of

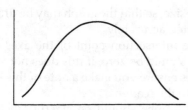

Figure 5.9 Normal distribution.

all and has numerous implications for statistics. So important is it that the next section will be devoted entirely to a more detailed description of it. Suffice it to say for the time being that it is typically a symmetrical bell-shaped curve, and were we to plot heights or heart-rates of a population in this way, we would find that both are normally distributed.

Skewed distribution (1): positive skew (Fig. 5.10) is skewed to the left and is the sort of graph that might result from an overly difficult exam, i.e. too many students achieved marks near the bottom end of the score range.

Skewed distribution (2): negative skew (Figure 5.11) is skewed in the opposite direction and might have been derived from a set of results from an exam that was too easy.

J-shaped distribution (Fig. 5.12) is the sort of

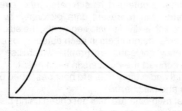

Figure 5.10 Skewed distribution (1) – also known as positive skew.

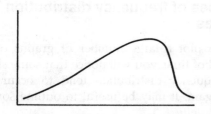

Figure 5.11 Skewed distribution (2) – also known as negative skew.

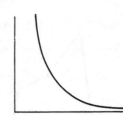

Figure 5.12 J-shaped distribution.

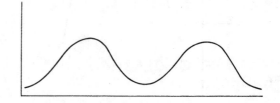

Figure 5.13 Bimodal distribution.

frequency distribution which might result from monitoring the red blood cell count of women with multiple pregnancies throughout their gestation. At the start of the pregnancies, the red blood cell count would be high and this might show a steep drop as pregnancy progresses, such that towards term the red blood cell count is very low.

Bimodal distribution (Fig. 5.13) is characterized by two distinct peaks and might have been obtained by plotting the neonatal birth weights of a mixed group of mothers with diabetes and those with placental insufficiency. The neonatal birth weights of women with placental insufficiency would be represented by the left-hand peak, while those of mothers with diabetes, and larger babies would be represented by the right-hand peak.

Activity 5.1   (Answers on pages 234–235)

In order to look at the consistency of measurements of fundal heights, you ask 15 midwives to measure the fundal height of a 2nd trimester mother. You obtain the results shown in Table 5.10.

1. Draw (a) a histogram, (b) a bar graph and (c) a frequency polygon to show these results.
2. In order to identify trends in the results, reduce the units along the horizontal axis and re-draw the frequency polygon.

Table 5.10 Number of midwives recording a particular fundal height

Fundal height (cm)	No of midwives recording a particular score
18–19	0
20–21	1
22–23	3
24–25	5
26–27	4
28–29	1
30–31	1
32+	0

MEASURES OF CENTRAL TENDENCY

As has already been stated, any results from a piece of research must be presented in a way that can be clearly understood by the reader. Besides making tables of the results and drawing graphs, the data can be presented in terms of *measures of central tendency*.

Measures of central tendency involve describing a set of data in terms of the most typical scores within it. This approach may be valuable to the midwife in three ways:

1. A comparison of some characteristic of a group of women with an established norm or standard for that characteristic. For instance you may wish to compare the volume of amniotic fluid of a group of women with polyhydramnios with the normal or average amount of amniotic fluid for women of a comparable gestational stage.

2. Establishing a standard or norm not previously known, e.g. if a new piece of highly sensitive equipment was introduced which you thought might be useful to monitor fetal heart rate. You want to use it in the early identification of fetuses with heart problems; therefore, you would need to use this equipment to monitor fetuses with known heart problems and compare these results with the heart rates derived from fetuses with no known heart problems. In this way you could establish a set of norms for this piece of equipment and any deviation from this would aid the early identification of problems.

3. Comparing different treatment techniques or different groups of women or babies, e.g. does complementary feeding lead to a higher incidence of infant colic than bottle feeding?

In order to answer the questions three measures of central tendency can be used: the *arithmetic mean*, the *median* and the *mode*.

Arithmetic mean

This is the average of a set of scores and is derived from adding all the scores together and dividing the total by the number of scores. It is usually denoted by the symbol $\bar{x}$. It is an extremely valuable concept in statistics and enables the researcher to appraise a set of results, at a glance.

For example, in the illustrations given above, the mean volume of amniotic fluid for the polyhydramnios group can be compared with the mean volume of amniotic fluid for the normal group to establish the extent of the differences. Similarly, the mean incidence of colic in the complementary feeding group can be compared with that of those babies on formula feeds only, to give an estimate of which produces more problems.

While the arithmetic mean is undoubtedly one of the most useful concepts in statistics, it can be misleading. Supposing you were comparing performance on two modules for a group of midwifery students, to find out which module produced better results. You look at the marks gained by students on each module and find that on Module A students score an average 40%, while on Module B students score 51%. From this information alone you would almost certainly assume that Module B was associated with better marks. But let us suppose you were to look at the original data as shown in Table 5.11.

Although Module A certainly produces, on average, poorer marks, the results are much more consistent than those from Module B; furthermore, with the exception of the three 100% scores, the remaining results from Module B are lower than all the scores in Module A. In other words, the presence of three extreme scores

Table 5.11 Performance on two modules for a group of midwifery students

Module A (%)		Module B (%)	
1	38	1	30
2	42	2	28
3	45	3	100
4	36	4	100
5	40	5	31
6	39	6	33
7	44	7	30
8	46	8	28
9	34	9	30
10	36	10	100
$\bar{x} =$	40	$\bar{x} =$	51

in Module B has distorted the mean and could have been misleading had you not looked at the original data. Having examined the raw data, you would probably now believe that Module A was associated with better performance. However, if you were conducting a large scale survey, you might have thousands of data points and consequently it would be impossible to inspect the raw data thoroughly. Therefore, the arithmetic mean, while an essential component to statistics, is insufficient in itself to provide the necessary information about a set of results and other forms of descriptive statistics are required as well.

Median

The median is simply the mid-score in a set of results, such that there are as many scores above it as below it. To compute the median, arrange the scores in order of magnitude; then if there is an odd number of scores, the middle score becomes the median. So, for example, if you had five scores:

14   9   28   5   11

you would arrange them in order of magnitude:

28   14   11   9   5

and the median becomes the third score from the end, i.e. 11. On the other hand, if there is an even number of scores, the median is the average of the two middle scores. So, if you had:

14   9   28   5   11   18

you would arrange these in order of magnitude:

28   18   14   11   9   5

and the median is the average of the two middle scores, i.e.

$$\frac{14 + 11}{2} = 12.5$$

While the median obviously tells you the middle score out of a set of results, it tells you nothing about the range of the scores. For example, in the following sets of scores, the median in both cases is 10:

13   12   11   10   9   8   7
42   41   40   10   3   2   1

However, the nature of the sets of scores is quite different and the pattern of a set of scores may have important implications for their interpretation. For instance, if the first set of figures above referred to the number of weeks gestation of women brought in with a particular problem, you may well think that the problem is one of the first trimester. You would not be inclined to think this if presented with the second set of figures. Thus, the nature of the scores is important in research if they are to be accurately interpreted. So, the median alone gives insufficient information about the nature of a set of data. If it is used in conjunction with the mean, then more information can be derived about the total set of scores. For example, the more similar the mean and median, the smaller the range of scores. This can be illustrated with the above sets of figures. The first set has a mean and a median of 10 and the scores are all within a small range (13–7); however the second set of figures also has a median of 10 but a mean of 19.9 and a range of scores from 42–1.

While the median is not as useful as the mean, if both techniques are used together they can be more useful in describing a set of data, especially where there are extreme scores.

Mode

The mode is the most commonly occurring score in a set of data. So, in the following two sets of scores, 15 is the mode:

15	15	14	10	15	18	15
15	15	3	2	1	4	5

However, within any set of scores, you may have more than one mode. Its value lies primarily in its ability to answer the question 'Which one event occurs most often?' So, for example, you might want to ask: 'what is the commonest stage of pregnancy for pre-eclampsia to develop?'

To answer this question you would simply look at the number of weeks gestation at which the women first presented with the symptoms of the condition and identify which was the most frequently occurring gestational stage.

A comparison of the mean, mode and median

Comparing the value of the arithmetic mean, the median and the mode, the mean is the most commonly used statistic and provides more information about a set of scores than the median and the mode. This is due to the fact that the computation of the mean depends on the exact value of every score in a set of data and alteration of even one score will alter the mean. This is not necessarily the case for the median and the mode, as illustrated by the following set of data:

3	14	10	19	8	5	15	20	3

The mean of these data is 10.8, the median is 10, and the mode is 3. If we alter the 20 to 40, the mean becomes 13, but the median and the mode stay the same.

In addition, the median and the mode may be totally unaffected by altering a large number of scores in a set of data. If the above set of figures is changed to:

3	34	10	39	2	1	45	17	3

although six out of nine figures have been radically altered, the median remains 10 and the mode 3. Conversely, the median and the mode may be drastically altered just by changing one figure. To take the above set of figures, if the first 3 is changed to 34, the median becomes 17 and the mode 34. In other words the median and the mode are less reliable than the mean when providing information about a set of scores because

they may not be altered by radical changes to a lot of scores or they may be changed by altering just one score. The mean on the other hand will alter if any score is changed, however minimally.

However, as already pointed out, the mean may be less useful than the median or mode if there are extreme scores in a set of data, because it is easily distorted by the presence of very large or small scores. Nonetheless, although all three concepts can be used in descriptive statistics to provide information about a set of data, it is advisable always to calculate the mean, and then to decide whether the median and the mode will provide you with relevant information about your particular set of data.

KEY CONCEPTS

Measures of *central tendency* are a form of descriptive statistics and allow the researcher to highlight features of a set of results in terms of the 'most typical values'. The three most commonly used measures of central tendency are:

- the *arithmetic mean* — the average of a set of scores
- the *median* — the mid score in a set of results, such that there are as many scores above it as below
- the *mode* — the most commonly occurring score in a set of data.

Activity 5.2   (Answers on page 235)

1. Calculate the mean, median and the mode for the following sets of figures:

   (i)   91 87 90 76 51 48 72 76 80 44 89
   (ii) 25 39 17 41 24 17 37 31 27
   (iii) 44 43 51 54 60 71 39 41 55 43

2. Just by comparing the means and the medians, find out which set of data has (a) the largest range and (b) the smallest range of scores.

MEASURES OF DISPERSION

If you look back at the measures of central tendency, you will see that it is possible to obtain the same or very similar means for sets of scores which are quite different. For instance, the mean of the following two sets of figures is 10:

9	11	12	8	10	11	12	12	8	7
1	2	3	3	2	1	40	3	15	30

However, the scores in the first set are all quite

similar to each other in that they only range from 7 to 12; the scores in the second set, however, range from 1 to 40. Just knowing the mean of a set of scores, then, can be quite misleading — we need to know how variable the scores are as well, in other words, what the spread of the data is. The statistics which describe the variability of scores are called *measures of dispersion* and are valuable to the midwife for the same reasons as the measures of central tendency. If you look back to page 37, you will see that the first reason given is that the researcher can compare a group of patients with an established standard to discover how far their capacity, or problems, or whatever, resemble the norm. This can be carried out just using means, medians, and modes, but we have already seen that similar means can be obtained from two totally different sets of scores. So, if we use the example on page 37, you might find that four out of five of your polyhydramnios women had extremely large quantities of amniotic fluid, while one had much less than the others. If you simply combine the amniotic fluid volumes of these five women and take the mean you may well find that due to the one lower volume woman, the mean is not much different from that of the non-polydramnios group and yet four of the patients had excessive fluid. In other words you need to know what the spread of scores is.

Similarly if you wish to establish norms for a new piece of apparatus, it is insufficient just to use measures of central tendency, because they can be misleading unless you know how consistent the scores are. Obviously a piece of equipment which produces uniform results will be much more use than one which produces erratic results from poor to excellent even though the mean performances may be similar.

In addition, measures of dispersion can identify people who respond particularly well or particularly poorly. This information may be useful when selecting treatments. And similarly, when comparing two or more treatment types, the treatment which produces homogeneous results, i.e. where the range of scores is small, will be regarded quite differently from the treatment which produces erratic results which cover an enormous range. So, in descriptive statistics, not only do you need to use measures of central tendency, you also need to describe the results in terms of how variable they are and to do this you use techniques called measures of dispersion. There are three measures of dispersion which are valuable to the midwife: (i) *the range*, (ii) *deviation and variance* and (iii) *the standard deviation*.

Range

The range is quite simply the difference between lowest and highest scores in a set of data. To compute it, simply find the smallest score in the set of data and subtract it from the highest score, thus:

$$14 \quad 22 \quad 5 \quad 11 \quad 12 \quad 19 \quad 31 \quad 27$$

the range is:

$$31 - 5 = 26$$

Obviously, when used in conjunction with measures of central tendency, it can provide useful additional information, in the way already outlined. However, the information produced by the range gives a limited picture since a range of $45 - 3$ may describe a set of scores such as:

$$45 \quad 44 \quad 43 \quad 42 \quad 7 \quad 6 \quad 5 \quad 4 \quad 3$$

or

$$45 \quad 40 \quad 35 \quad 30 \quad 30 \quad 15 \quad 10 \quad 5 \quad 3$$

In other words, the range provides no insight into *how* the scores are distributed. One way of getting round this problem is to use deviation and variance measures.

Deviation and variance

One method of overcoming the problem of presenting a picture of the distribution of scores is by expressing the scores in terms of how far each one deviates from the mean. In this way the researcher can present a description of the spread of scores, which, as we have seen, is important in understanding the implications of a set of data.

In order to calculate the deviation of a set of

scores, the mean is subtracted from each score. Thus, for the following set of scores:

10   15   21   8   11   12   14   5

the mean is 12 and the deviation of each score is:

$$10 - 12 = -2$$
$$15 - 12 = +3$$
$$21 - 12 = +9$$
$$8 - 12 = -4$$
$$11 - 12 = -1$$
$$12 - 12 = 0$$
$$14 - 12 = +2$$
$$5 - 12 = -7$$

In subtracting the mean from each score, you can find the position of each score relative to the mean. So, for example, the score of 15 is + 3 deviation points above the mean.

However, as you can probably see, expressing each score as a deviation from the mean is just as long-winded as setting out all your scores and the mean. What is needed is some short-hand method of expressing how varied and dispersed the scores are. While many students assume that the obvious way would be to add together all the deviation scores, the answer is always 0 (try it for yourself and see) so this clearly tells us nothing. So, one way of getting round this problem is to square each deviation score (this obviously gets rid of all the plus and minus signs), add these squared deviation scores up and then take their average. The resulting mean is called the variance.

If we compute the variance for the set of scores above, we get:

$$\frac{(-2^2) + (3^2) + (9^2) + (-4^2) + (-1^2) + (0^2) + (2^2) + (-7^2)}{8}$$

$$= \frac{4 + 9 + 81 + 16 + 1 + 0 + 4 + 49}{8}$$

$$= \frac{164}{8}$$

$$= 20.5$$

The variance of a set of scores tells us by definition how dispersed or varied the scores are. Obviously, the smaller the variance, the more similar the scores, while the greater the variance, the more disparate the scores. If you look back to the example on page 37 about module perform-ance, you can see that knowledge of the spread of scores would be a very useful piece of informa-tion here, since the smaller the variance the more reliable and consistent the placement experience.

Standard deviation

Although the variance score gives you the total degree of variability in a set of scores, it has been obtained, obviously, by adding together such varied squared deviations as 81 and 0 (see the previous set of figures). Sometimes you may want to find out what the average or standard degree of deviation is for a set of scores, rather than the variation. To do this you need a very use-ful statistic called, not unreasonably, the *standard deviation* (or SD).

To calculate it, you simply take the variance figure (i.e. the mean of the squared deviation scores; in the above case 20.5) and then take the square root of this, to give you the standard de-viation of the scores from the mean. The formula then is:

$$SD = \sqrt{\frac{\Sigma(x - \bar{x})^2}{N}}$$

where $\sqrt{}$ = square root of all the calculations under this symbol
x = the individual score
$\bar{x}$ = the mean score
Σ = total, or sum, of every calculation to the right
N = the total number of scores.

(You may have realized that $\Sigma (x - \bar{x})^2$ is the variance score.) So, for the figures above, the standard deviation is

$$\sqrt{\frac{164}{8}}$$

$$= 4.528$$

Sometimes you will find the SD formula given as:

$$\sqrt{\frac{\Sigma(x - \bar{x})^2}{N - 1}}$$

The $N - 1$ is used if you want to infer the standard deviation of the population from which your sample is drawn, whereas just N describes the standard deviation of the sample only. However, in practice, this variation makes very little difference, so do not worry unduly about it.

This means that the standard degree of deviation of this set of scores from the mean is 4.528. Such information gives you a picture of how dispersed or variable a set of scores is in a single figure, which as we have already pointed out, is particularly useful in determining the consistency of a set of figures.

All of this may seem rather confusing to you when deciding how to describe a set of data. As a rule of thumb, I would recommend that you always calculate the mean, range and standard deviation of a set of scores and then decide which of the other measures provides you with information which is relevant to the aims of that particular piece of research.

KEY CONCEPTS

Measures of dispersion are a branch of descriptive statistics which allow the researcher to describe a set of data in terms of how variable the scores are.

The measures of dispersion which are of particular importance to the midwife are:

- the *range* — the difference between the lowest and highest scores in a set of data
- the *deviation* — provides information about the extent to which each score deviates from the mean, and is calculated by subtracting the mean from each score.
- the *variance* — the average amount that a set of scores deviates from the mean and is calculated by squaring each deviation score, adding the results and then dividing by the number of deviation scores to obtain the average.
- the *standard deviation* (SD) is the average amount of deviation and is computed by dividing the variance by the total number of scores and taking the square root of this result.

Activity 5.3   (Answers on page 235)

1. Find the range, deviation, variance and standard deviation of the following sets of scores:
   (i) 14   9   21   23   18   17   33   28   12
   (ii) 71   50   48   64   80   81   79
2. You are concerned about one of the scales in use in the delivery suite, since you are not sure how reliable it is. How might you assess its reliability using descriptive statistics?

Normal distribution

It was pointed out earlier that there are a number of frequency distribution shapes which occur commonly in statistics. The most common of all these is the so-called normal distribution curve (sometimes known as the Gaussian distribution, after Gauss, the astronomer and mathematician who investigated it). The normal distribution curve is a symmetrical bell-shaped distribution (Fig. 5.14).

It possesses a number of important mathematical properties:

1. It is symmetrical.
2. The mean, median and mode all have the same value.
3. The curve descends rapidly at first from its central point, but the descent slows down as the tails of the curve are reached.
4. No matter how far you continue the tails of the curve, they never reach the horizontal axis.
5. The normal distribution curve occurs in data drawn from a wide range of disciplines — mathematics, physics, engineering, psychology etc. For example, height, IQ, and the life of electric light bulbs all have normal distributions. In other words, if we collected, for example, height data from a large number of people randomly drawn from the population and drew a frequency distribution of it, we would end up with something that resembled a normal curve.
6. If the mean and standard deviation of a normally distributed set of data are known, then we can draw the normal distribution curve. The reason this can be done results from the relationship between the standard deviation and the normal distribution curve. This relationship

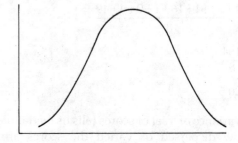

Figure 5.14   Normal distribution curve.

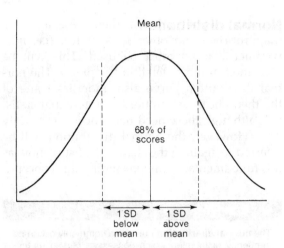

Figure 5.15 Structure of normal distribution curve.

means that a fixed percentage of the scores always falls in a given area under the curve. Therefore, if we take the central point of the curve and move one standard deviation above and below the mean, then 68% of the scores will *always* fall within this range (Fig. 5.15). This is a constant fact of the normal distribution, i.e. that 34% of scores fall within one standard deviation *above* the mean, and 34% of scores fall one standard deviation *below*.

If we move on, we find that a further 13.5% of the scores fall between standard deviations 1 and 2 *above* the mean, and 13.5% fall between standard deviations 1 and 2 *below* the mean. Thus, the two standard deviations either side of the mean account for a total of 95% of the scores (13.5 + 34 + 34 + 13.5). Going on to standard deviations 2–3 above and below the mean, we find that 2.36% of scores fall within each category, thereby allowing a total of 99.73% of the scores to be accounted for by 3 standard deviations above and below the mean (2.36 + 13.5 + 34 + 34 + 13.5 + 2.36 = 99.72, represented normally as 99.73 as a result of calculating further decimal places).

So, to take an example, if we know that the mean IQ of the population is 100 and the standard deviation is 20, then 68% of the population have IQs between 80 and 120, 95% have IQs between 60 and 140, and 99.73% have IQs between 40 and 160. We can see this more clearly in the normal curve below (Fig. 5.16).

The value of the normal distribution is two-fold. Firstly, it allows the researcher to describe a set of data and to predict (from knowledge of the properties of the normal curve) what proportions of people possess certain characteristics.

For example, if we know that the *average* maternal heart rate is 72, with a standard deviation of 5, and that during the third trimester heart

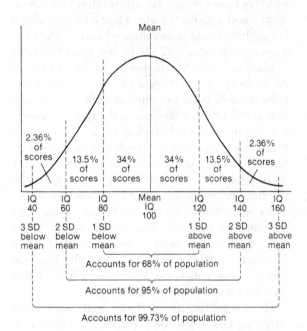

Figure 5.16 Hypothetical normal distribution curve for IQ.

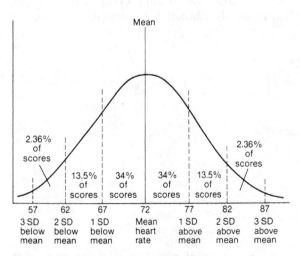

Figure 5.17 Hypothetical normal distribution curve for maternal heart rate during the third trimester.

rate is normally distributed, we can draw the curve presented in Figure 5.17.

Now, because we know that 68% of women are accounted for by scores within 1 standard deviation either side of the mean, we know that 68% of the population of women in the third trimester must have heart rates between 67 and 77 beats per minute. Furthermore, we know a further 13.5% of these women fall within standard deviations 1 and 2 above the mean and a further 13.5% fall within standard deviations 1 and 2 below the mean. This means 13.5% of the population of women in the third trimester have heart rates of 77–82 beats per minute and 13.5% have heart rates of 62–67 beats per minute. Finally, we know that 2.36% of these women in the third trimester fall within standard deviations 2–3 above the mean and a further 2.36% within standard deviations 2–3 below the mean. This means 2.36% of these women have heart rates of 82–87 beats per minute and 2.36% have heart rates of 57–62 beats per minute. This information also allows us to 'work backwards'; if a woman in the third trimester presents with a heart rate of 86, then you can ascertain just how statistically unusual this is, since you know that only 2.36% of this population come within this range.

The second function of the normal distribution curve relates to its role in inferential statistics. Many of the tests used in inferential statistics require that the results being analysed are normally distributed (see section on *parametric*

statistics); it they are not, then these tests are inappropriate and other sorts of test (i.e. *non-parametric tests*) must be used. This will be explained in more detail in Chapter 9. The normal distribution curve also underlies some of the theoretical assumptions of inferential statistics, although these need not concern us unduly here. However, the normal distribution will be referred to again in the chapter on Estimation, as it is fundamental to understanding this concept.

KEY CONCEPTS

The **normal distribution curve** is a commonly occurring frequency distribution which possesses certain mathematical properties:

- If the mean and the standard deviation of a set of scores are known, then the researcher is able to predict what proportion of the population has scores within a certain range. This is possible because a fixed proportion of the population will fall within a certain score range, as long as those scores are normally distributed.
- The normal curve is of fundamental importance in the theory behind inferential statistics.

Activity 5.4   (Answers on page 235)

If we know that heart rate during weeks 10–20 of pregnancy is normally distributed, with a mean of 82 and a standard deviation of 8, then:
1. What percentage of patients will have heart rates between 66 and 98?
2. What percentage of patients will show heart rates of 99–106?
3. If a patient presents with a heart rate of 57, how common is this in terms of percentage?

6

Testing hypotheses

We have briefly covered the topic of descriptive statistics, which provide the researcher with one method of presenting data. However, this approach is typically used to make sense of data derived from some form of survey and is not always appropriate for analysing results from an experiment, where an hypothesis has been tested. What is needed here, is a second branch of statistics known as *inferential statistics*.

There will be many occasions when you do not want simply to collect a mound of general information about a broad topic area but wish, instead, to test out an idea; for instance, comparing the effectiveness of two types of analgesia, or monitoring the progress of a specific group of premature babies. In such cases, you would carry out an experiment and analyse the results from this using a statistical test. This sort of analysis is called inferential statistics, and is so-called because it allows you to infer that the results you obtained from your experiment using a small sample of people may also apply to the larger population from which the sample was drawn. Look back to pages 11–13 to refresh your memory on this.

However, before you can reasonably start inferring anything from the results of an experiment, it is essential that the experiment is properly designed and set up, otherwise false inferences may be made. This chapter and the next are concerned with outlining the principles of good experimental techniques.

When carrying out any research which involves testing an idea or hypothesis, the following steps have to be taken:

- A hypothesis must be devised and stated clearly.
- A research project must be designed which will test the hypothesis.
- Results from the research have to be analysed using an appropriate statistical test.
- A report must be prepared on the research for future reference.

We shall deal with each of these stages in turn. The present chapter will be concerned with the principles involved in devising hypotheses and some basic concepts about research design.

EXPERIMENTAL HYPOTHESIS

The starting point of any research is an idea known as the *experimental* or *research hypothesis*, sometimes referred to as H_1. This is usually based on some theory or observations that the researcher has made. You may, for instance, have noticed in the course of your work, that certain patients seem to respond better to particular types of treatment. An observation of this type would form the basis of an experimental hypothesis. Examples of experimental hypotheses include such ideas as the following:

1. Male premature babies make slower progress than female premature babies.
2. Infected cervical erosions respond better to treatment by pessaries than by cream.
3. Job satisfaction is greater among community midwives than hospital-based midwives.

You probably have a number of such ideas that you are interested in looking at, and it would be useful to write them down at this stage.

If we look at the above hypotheses, we can see that what the experimental hypothesis does is to predict a relationship between two or more things, which are known as *variables**. Therefore,

---

* Throughout the course of this book, we shall deal with hypotheses and experiments that predict a relationship between only two variables. If the reader wants to find out about hypotheses which deal with a predicted relationship between more than two variables then the following books are recommended: Greene & D'Oliviera (1982) and Ferguson (1976).

the first hypothesis predicts a relationship between *gender* of the premature babies (male or female), and *progress*. The two variables here, then, are gender of the baby and progress. The second hypothesis predicts a relationship between *type of treatment* (pessary or cream), and *improvement or response*. The two variables here are type of treatment and improvement. The third hypothesis predicts a relationship between degree of *job satisfaction* and *type of midwife* (community or hospital). The two variables, then, are job satisfaction and type of midwife.

The relationship predicted in the experimental hypothesis is assumed to be a consistent and reliable one. So, if we take the second of the hypotheses above, the underlying assumption is that infected cervical erosions will typically respond better to pessaries than to cream. What we do *not* anticipate is a rather unpredictable outcome, such that sometimes pessaries are better, but sometimes they are not.

> **KEY CONCEPT**
>
> The *experimental hypothesis* is the starting point of any research and predicts a relationship between two or more variables.

Activity 6.1 (Answers on page 236)

Look at the following hypotheses and write down what the two variables are in each case.

1. Placenta praevia is less common in first pregnancies than in subsequent pregnancies.
2. Use of alkaline preparations in the treatment of heartburn during pregnancy increases the chance of developing anaemia.
3. Women from Social Class II are more likely to breast feed over the first 3 months, than are women from Social Class V.
4. Costal margin pain is less common in women over 5' 8" tall than in those under 5' 4".
5. Increasing the intake of calcium-rich foods reduces the incidence of cramp during the third trimester.

Now think about the research project you would like to carry out. State the experimental hypothesis, making sure it predicts a relationship between the two variables. Write down what the variables are.

When formulating your experimental hypothesis, there are some points which would be useful to bear in mind. Firstly, your hypothesis should be *testable*. As an extreme example, you might have predicted that premature babies experience less discomfort when temperatures are taken orally rather than rectally. How would you assess the level of discomfort? It would be a very difficult task to complete without taking instrusive measures which would upset the baby further. Consequently the hypothesis would not be easily testable. Secondly, your hypothesis should be *realistic* in its aims. This means you should not be over ambitious and try to compare the entire population of elderly primigravidas with young primigravidas for placenta praevia. A project of that size would be not only unnecessary, but beyond the scope of any individual researcher or even of a robust cohort of researchers. Consequently, the aims of your experiment should be confined to something more do-able. And thirdly, you must define what your variables *mean*. In the above example, 'premature' is a very loose concept. How premature are the babies? Why are they premature? What is their medical condition? You must be able to clarify exactly what your terms mean. Finally, few researchers push back the frontiers of science with their projects. Most people for whatever reason, have to undertake small scale studies, but this does not necessarily imply that their value is limited. Many such projects can have far reaching implications for health care policy and practice and contribute a great deal to our knowledge base.

The next step is to find out whether the relationship predicted in your hypothesis does, in fact, exist, which means you must design and carry out a suitable project to test your hypothesis. Any results you get from the research are then analysed using the appropriate statistical test. But, before we move on to talk about how you proceed, one very important point must be made.

THE NULL HYPOTHESIS

It must be logically possible for the relationship predicted in your experimental hypothesis to be wrong, otherwise there is no point in wasting your time carrying out any research. For example, anyone who hypothesized that all midwives who were born in 1940 are older than those born in 1945 and then spent 3 days amongst the record books trying to support her hypothesis would be indulging in a pointless exercise, since there would be absolutely no possibility that her prediction would be wrong. Therefore, to make any research project worthwhile, there has to be a chance that the predicted relationship does not exist. To show that there is a possibility that the experimental hypothesis is incorrect, we have to state an alternative hypothesis called the null hypothesis. This is sometimes referred to as H_0. So, while the experimental hypothesis predicts that there *is* a relationship between two variables, the null hypothesis says there is *no* relationship and that any results you get from your research project are due to chance and not to any real and reliable relationship between the variables. Let us take an example. Supposing in the course of your work you have noticed that women are more likely to follow oral rather than written instructions for pelvic floor exercises following delivery. You decide to carry out some research to see if your hunch is right. The first step is to state the experimental hypothesis clearly, i.e. 'Women are more likely to comply with oral instructions than written instructions for pelvic floor exercise following delivery.' So, you are predicting a relationship between the type of instructions given and degree of compliance. But because it is possible that your observations are wrong, you must also state the null hypothesis that there is *no relationship* between the type of instructions and degree of compliance. The null hypothesis also implies that should any differences in degree of compliance be found then these are simply due to chance fluctuations and not to any real and consistent relationship. The usual way of stating the null hypothesis is simply to predict no relationship between the two variables. Therefore, here, your null hypothesis would be: 'There is no relationship between type of instructions and degree of compliance.'

If you ever get stuck when formulating the null hypothesis, the easy way to get round the problem is by:

1. Firstly identifying the relationship in the experimental hypothesis, by stating: 'There is a relationship between a and b' (a and b being the two variables).
2. Changing the first part to: 'There is no relationship between a and b'. This gives you your null hypothesis.

It is very important to note that the null hypothesis predicts *no* relationship; it does not predict the opposite of the experimental hypothesis. Many students get confused over this and in the example just given would assume that the null hypothesis says the reverse of the experimental hypothesis i.e. that written instructions are more likely to be followed than are oral ones. (Just refresh your memory and check that this is the opposite of our original hypothesis.) This assumption is incorrect, because if we look at it, a relationship is still being predicted between type of instructions and compliance. So, the null hypothesis says there is *no* relationship between the two variables — in this case type of instruction and degree of compliance.

Activity 6.2   (Answers on page 236)

To see whether you are happy with this concept, look at the experimental hypotheses on page 46 and write down what the null hypothesis is for each one. State the null hypothesis for the research project you would like to carry out.

Why do we need to state the null hypothesis at all? Could we not just assume that there is a chance that our experimental hypothesis may be wrong without having to spell it out? The answer to this lies in a convention, which has its roots in the philosophy of scientific method. (For further details on this the reader is referred to Chalmers (1983).)

Essentially this convention states that when we carry out any research we do not set out to find direct support for our experimental hypothesis (or at least we should not!) but, rather perversely, to *falsify the null hypothesis*. In other words, we still hope to find the relationship we predicted in the experimental hypothesis, but we do this by stating the null hypothesis and setting out to reject it. It should be noted here that the words 'prove' and 'disprove' in relation to the hypo-

theses are not being used. This is because we cannot really ever prove or disprove anything in midwifery, nursing, psychology or whatever — all we can do is find evidence that supports or fails to support our prediction. The intending researcher need not worry unduly about all this, since it is sufficient simply to state the experimental and null hypotheses at the outset of any experiment. The relevance of the null hypothesis will be discussed further in different parts of the book.

KEY CONCEPTS

The null hypothesis states that the relationship predicted in the experimental hypothesis does *not* exist and implies that any results found from the research are simply due to chance factors and not to any real and consistent relationship between the two variables. In any research project, the experimenter sets out to support his/her prediction by rejecting the null hypothesis.

BASIC TYPES OF DESIGN

Once you have sorted out the experimental and null hypotheses for your research project, you then have to decide on the best way to find out whether your predicted relationship actually exists. In other words you have to design a suitable research project. It should be noted that there are often a number of designs that can be used to test an hypothesis, and it is up to the researcher to select the most appropriate one. The concept that there is usually no single correct way of testing an hypothesis means that the researcher must take into account a number of design considerations, and it is with these that this chapter and the following one are concerned.

There are two basic sorts of research designs: *experimental designs* and *correlational designs*. Both designs start off with an experimental hypothesis which predicts a relationship between two or more variables, but the aims and methods of each approach are different. These differences can be best illustrated by an example. Let us take the hypothesis that the professional grade of the midwife affects the degree of job satisfaction that is experienced. The relationship that is being suggested is between professional grading of the midwife and degree of job satisfaction. Let us see how experimental and correlational designs would each approach the problem of trying to find out whether this relationship does, in fact, exist.

Experimental designs: an introduction

The experimental design would take a group of say 10 Grade G midwives and a group of 10 Grade D midwives, measure the reported job satisfaction expressed by each group and compare the two groups to see if there was any *difference* between them.

We would have the following design:

Group 1
10 Grade G midwives

Group 2
10 Grade D midwives

Compared on expressed job satisfaction for differences between the groups

Correlational designs: an introduction

The correlational design, on the other hand, would select a number of midwives who represented the whole range of professional status from Grade D through to Grade G and measure their reported job satisfaction to see if there is any *similarity or association* between professional level and degree of job satisfaction, such that, for instance, the higher the status, the higher the corresponding job satisfaction.

Table 6.1 A correlational design investigating job satisfaction and professional level

Subject	Grade of midwife	Job satisfaction scores (on a 10-point scale)
1	Grade H	9
2	Grade G	8
3	Grade F	5
4	Grade E	4
5	Grade D	4

The correlational design would look as shown in Table 6.1.

The data on both status and job satisfaction would be examined to see if there is any pattern or association between them.

Experimental and correlational designs will be discussed more fully in the next two sections. It should be stressed, however, that for the hypothesis we are looking at, either design would be appropriate. This illustrates the idea that was mentioned earlier: that for any hypothesis there may be a number of suitable designs to test it, and it is up to the researcher to think carefully about the aims, objectives and the relevant design considerations of the research and to devise the most appropriate method of testing the hypothesis.

> **KEY CONCEPTS**
>
> - *Experimental* designs look for *differences* between sets of results.
> - *Correlational* designs look for *patterns* in sets of results. Therefore, each approach has a different objective and will consequently use a different method to test the hypothesis.

We will deal with the basic principles involved in each design separately, starting with experimental designs.

EXPERIMENTAL DESIGNS

We have already noted that the experimental hypothesis predicts a relationship between two variables. The simplest way to find out whether this relationship actually exists is to alter one of these variables to see what difference it makes to the other. This is the basis of experimental design. This alteration is known as *manipulation of variables*, and is actually something we do in everyday life, often without being aware of it. This can be illustrated by a mundane example. Suppose you were baby-sitting for a friend and had decided to watch the television. You turn it on and discover that the sound is too low. Because you are not familiar with the controls on this set you are not sure how to adjust the volume, but you think it might be the knob on the front right of the set. Unwittingly, you have formulated an hypothesis — that there is a relationship between the knob and the volume. In order to test this hypothesis, you have to manipulate one of the variables; in other words, you alter the knob to see what effect it has on the sound. You have just performed a very simple experiment, which involved hypothesizing a relationship between two variables and manipulating one to see what difference it made to the other. This is the basis of experimental design.

These variables have names. The variable which is manipulated is called the *independent variable* or IV. The variable which is observed for any changes in it resulting from that manipulation is called the *dependent variable* or DV. People sometimes get confused about which variable is which. The easiest way to identify the IV and the DV is to ask the question 'which variable depends on which?' In the above example with the DV the question is: Does the knob depend on the volume or does the volume depend on the knob? Clearly in this case the volume depends on the knob, and thus the volume is the dependent variable. The knob is therefore the independent variable. Some important points emerge out of this. If, after turning the knob, the volume did increase, you might have concluded, (though perhaps not consciously) that twiddling the knob *caused* the volume to increase, and therefore the increase in volume could be seen as the *effect* of twiddling the knob. In this way, the IV can be thought of as the *cause* and the DV as the *effect*. In addition, any changes that you note in the dependent variable which result from manipulating the independent variable, constitute your *data* in an experiment.

Just to clarify this idea, let us return to the hypothesis that cervical erosions improve more quickly with pessaries than with cream. The two variables are: (i) type of treatment and (ii) speed of recovery. Which variable is which? Does the type of treatment depend on speed of recovery? Or does speed of recovery depend on type of treatment? Clearly, the second suggestion is

correct. Type of treatment is the independent variable and speed of recovery is the dependent variable because how quickly a woman recovers depends on the treatment received. What is meant here, then, when we talk about manipulating the independent variable is simply assigning some women to pessaries and some to cream. Their progress is then compared. However, the problem is not always quite as simple as this. Supposing we hypothesized that there is a difference between male and female neonates in Apgar scores. Here the dependent variable is the Apgar score, so the independent variable must be the gender of the neonate. But how does the experimenter manipulate the gender of the neonate? Obviously in the previous example, it was easy (at least theoretically) for the experimenter to decide which treatment a cervical erosion patient should receive, but in the latter case we cannot possibly take a group of neonates and decide what gender they should be! In this case the experimenter would simply select two groups of neonates, one male and one female, and compare their Apgar scores. The independent variable is still being manipulated but in a slightly different way. Obviously, this sort of manipulation is essential when the independent variable is of a 'fixed' nature, such as race, age, type of patient etc. This point will be referred to again later.

One final point before moving on to discuss some basic principles of design. There may be many changes in your dependent variable that you wish to measure. For example, if we look at the hypothesis above we predicted that there was a relationship between type of treatment for cervical erosions (IV) and the speed of improvement (DV). Speed of improvement can be measured in several ways: how long it takes before the woman reports a complete absence of discharge or bleeding, or how yellow the discharge is after 3 days of treatment, or how irritating the discharge is. It would be legitimate to use any or all of these measures as your dependent variable. In other words, you may have a *number* of outcome measures you wish to take; you do not have to confine yourself to just one.

Activity 6.3 (Answers on page 236)

Look at the following hypotheses and decide which is the independent variable, and which is the dependent variable. When you have done that, decide how you would manipulate the independent variable. If you find that you are having difficulty deciding which variable is which, just ask yourself which variable depends on which.

1. There is a higher incidence of UTI following water births than following normal deliveries.
2. Local application of heat is effective in reducing round ligament pain.
3. Raised blood pressure is more likely to be recorded following a wait of more than 2 hours at an ante-natal clinic.
4. Induction by artificial rupture of the membranes has a better outcome for the neonate than induction by prostaglandin pessaries.
5. Delivery by caesarean section is more likely following electronic fetal monitoring.

KEY CONCEPTS

Experimental designs involve manipulating the *independent variable* and measuring the effect of this on the *dependent variable*. The independent variable can be thought of as *cause* and the dependent variable as *effect*.

So far we have assumed that all experimental hypotheses have just one independent variable. However, as we mentioned earlier, this is not always the case and some more complex hypotheses may predict a relationship between more than two independent variables and the dependent variable. An example of this sort of hypothesis would be a predicted relationship between the age of a woman and her response to one or more analgesias, e.g. that there is a difference in reported pain by women over 35 years of age and under 25 years of age according to whether they have had TENS or inhalation analgesia during labour. Here the dependent variable is reported pain, and the independent variables are the age of the woman and the type of analgesia she receives. This hypothesis requires a rather more complicated design, which is outside the scope of this book, but the reader is referred to Greene & D'Oliviera (1982) or Ferguson (1976) for more details on experimental designs with more than one independent variable. In this book we shall deal only with experiments which test hypotheses with just one independent variable.

Some basic principles involved in designing experiments with one independent variable

To recap, experimental designs require the experimenter to manipulate or alter the independent variable and to measure the effect of this on the dependent variable. In other words, you alter one variable and measure the *difference* it makes to the other. Hence experimental designs are said to look for differences. It is important to note that this applies only to experimental designs and not to correlational designs which we shall look at in the next section.

So, having formulated your experimental hypothesis and null hypothesis, the next task is to design a suitable experiment to find out whether the relationship predicted in your hypothesis exists. The basic concepts involved in this are best explained by an example. Suppose you wanted to test the hypothesis that midwives who did a psychology course run by the local college became more tolerant in their attitudes to their clients. The independent variable is attendance on a course and the dependent variable is attitude change. To test this hypothesis you decide to give those midwives who have completed a psychology course an attitude questionnaire. Therefore you would have the design shown in Table 6.2.

What could you conclude from the replies to the questionnaire? Could you assume that the midwives' attitudes had changed or not? You have probably quite correctly decided that we cannot conclude anything from this study since we do not know what the midwives' attitudes were in the first place. So an essential feature of an experiment is a pre-test measure of the dependent variable. Let us revise our design to include this (Table 6.3).

Table 6.2

Independent variable	Dependent variable
Attendance on course	Measurement of attitudes

Table 6.3

1. Pre-test measure of DV (attitudes)	2. Attendance on course (IV)	3. Post-test measure DV (attitudes)

What could you conclude from this experiment now? You could certainly decide on the basis of some statistical analysis of the pre-test and post-test scores whether there had been a significant attitude change but you could not ascribe it necessarily to course attendance, since it is quite possible that there are other explanations for the change. In other words, course attendance is not necessarily the *cause* of any observed change in attitudes.

Activity 6.4 (Answers on page 236)

Can you think of any possible alternative reasons for these results?

Certainly, it is conceivable that these midwives might have become more tolerant anyway, simply because they were just a bit older, and a bit more experienced. They might also have changed jobs, obtained promotion or had any one of a number of experiences which might account for their attitude change. How, then, can we ever be sure that the results in our experiment are due to the independent variable? The only way to do this is to select *another* group of midwives, which does not receive the independent variable, that is, does *not* attend the course. We then have to make sure that the *only* difference between the groups is whether or not they experience the independent variable. So, going back to our example, we would select two groups of midwives, of which just one group had attended a psychology course and we would compare their post-test attitudes. Our revised design looks as shown in Table 6.4.

These two groups are given names: the group who receives the independent variable (in this case, attends a psychology course) is called the *experimental group* or experimental condition. The group who does not receive the independent variable (in this case, does not attend a psychology course) is called the *control group* or control condition. The control group is therefore a 'no-

Table 6.4

Group 1 Midwives who attend a psychology course		
Pre-test measure of DV (attitudes)	Attendance on course (IV)	Post-test measure of DV (attitudes)

Group 2 Midwives who have not attended a psychology course		
Pre-test measure of DV (attitudes)	No attendance on course (no IV)	Post-test measure of DV (attitudes)

treatment' group. The pre-test and post-test scores from the two conditions are then compared using a statistical test to find out if there are any significant *differences* between them. Therefore, if the only difference between the two groups is the fact that one group experienced the IV and the other did not, any differences at the end of the study in the attitudes of the groups *must* have been caused by the IV.

Placebos

Sometimes a control group is used slightly differently. While the proper definition of a control group is a 'no-treatment' group, there may be occasions when it is more appropriate to give this group some 'pretend' treatment. Let us take an example. Imagine a situation where post-natal community midwifery services for first time mothers are being audited. A question arises as to whether there is any evidence to suggest that midwifery services have any benefit for these women, or whether this particular service could be carried out by care assistants or the local baby clinic in order to reduce costs. One way of testing this (as long as the ethics were acceptable), would be to have an experimental group receiving midwifery services and a control group having no such services. However, it occurs to you that one of the factors which may contribute to any benefits that might derive from the midwife's visit is the woman's *expectation* that she will get help or good advice during the visit. In other words, any value the woman reports may be the result not of the midwife herself, but rather of the power of expectation and auto-suggestion. In order to establish whether or not this is the case, you decide to give the control group some dummy treatment which involves the same amount of one-to-one attention by someone who does not have the same level of training or qualification as the midwife. If at the end of the study you found that the experimental group reported greater satisfaction than the controls, then you could conclude that the midwife's visits were beneficial to these women and the audit commission's question would have been answered. The dummy treatment is called a *placebo*. This technique is used a lot in drug trials, where some patients are given the real drug and other patients are given a useless salt or sugar tablet. However, so great is the power of the mind and the patient's expectations that the group on the placebo usually shows a marked improvement, which is known as the *placebo effect*.

KEY CONCEPTS

The subjects in the *experimental condition* are subjected to the independent variable. The experimental condition can therefore be thought of as the 'treatment condition'.

The *control condition* subjects are not subjected to the independent variable. The control condition can therefore be thought of as the 'no-treatment' group.

Sometimes the control group is given a dummy treatment called a *placebo*.

There are still many flaws in our design but we will talk about ways of eliminating them and refining an experiment in the next chapter. Nonetheless, the KEY CONCEPTS that have been outlined should give you an idea about some of the fundamental issues involved in experimental designs.

Ethical issues

By now you might be wanting to raise some moral issues. The above sort of design is fine when we want to look at something like the effects of a psychology course on attitudes. In this instance, there is no real moral dilemma about not giving midwives a psychology course. But supposing your hypothesis was that premature

babies would improve significantly on a new treatment regime. The IV here is the treatment and the DV is the improvement. You select your two groups of babies, and you give the experimental group your new treatment, but according to the above principles of experimental design, the other group of premature babies should receive no treatment. Is this ethical? Surely we cannot possibly leave a group of babies with no treatment while we are busily testing out our ideas? In cases such as this, you would compare *two* experimental groups rather than *one* experimental group and *one* control group. So, instead of comparing your new treatment with no treatment, you would compare it with the conventional treatment or another form of treatment.

Our design would look as shown in Table 6.5.

In this case, both groups are subjected to the independent variable (treatment) and their progress compared, to find out whether there are any differences between the groups.

Activity 6.5   (Answers on page 236)

Look at the following hypotheses and set out the experimental design you would use in each case, using the sort of format and headings shown above:

Hypotheses
1. Women who are given information about the value of an iron supplement during the first trimester are more likely to take the supplements than are women who receive no information.
2. Midwives who have had miscarriages themselves are more sympathetic to women with threatened miscarriage than are midwives who have not had a miscarriage.
3. Midwives who have qualified in the last 5 years are more motivated to do research than those who have been qualified for more than 10 years.

The sort of design we have been looking at is the most simple experimental design of all — a pre-test measure of the dependent variable,

Table 6.5

Experimental condition 1		
Pre-test measure of DV (baby's health)	New treatment regime (IV)	Post-test measure of DV (baby's health)
Experimental condition 2		
Pre-test measure of DV (baby's health)	Conventional treatment	Post-test measure of DV (baby's health)

manipulation of the independent variable and a post-test measure of the dependent variable. Two groups are used, of which one may be a control condition or alternatively, both groups may be experimental conditions. However, you may become a bit more ambitious and decide that you would like to look at something more complex than this. If we take a modification of an earlier hypothesis, that reported pain levels during labour are less with TENS than with inhalation analgesia, we have used a design which involves the comparison of two experimental groups. But you could, if you wished, add further conditions to this design. If you managed to resolve any ethical problem in your mind, you might decide to add a control condition as well, and so your design would look as shown in Table 6.6.

So you still have two experimental *conditions*, or *levels* of the independent variable, but you now have a control condition as well. Alternatively, you might feel that it would be useful to compare three types of pain relief instead of two, perhaps adding narcotics as an additional condition. Therefore, your hypothesis would be something like 'TENS, inhalation, analgesia and narcotics are differentially effective for pain relief in labour.' The dependent variable is the level of pain and the independent variable is still type of pain relief, but this time we have got *three* types of pain relief. Therefore, the independent variable has three experimental conditions or levels — TENS, inhalation and narcotics. Our design would look as shown in Table 6.7.

Table 6.6

Experimental condition 1		
Pre-test measure of DV (pain level)	TENS (IV)	Post-test measure of DV (pain level)
Experimental condition 2		
Pre-test measure of DV (pain level)	Inhalation analgesia treatment (IV)	Post-test measure of DV (pain level)
Control condition		
Pre-test measure of DV (pain level)	No treatment (no IV)	Post-test measure of DV (pain level)

Table 6.7

Experimental condition 1		
Pre-test measure of DV (pain level)	TENS (IV)	Post-test measure of DV (pain level)
Experimental condition 2		
Pre-test measure of DV (pain level)	Inhalation analgesia (IV)	Post-test measure of DV (pain level)
Experimental condition 3		
Pre-test measure of DV (pain level)	Narcotics (IV)	Post-test measure of DV (pain level)

You could extend this further and add a control condition thus:

Experimental condition 1
Experimental condition 2
Experimental condition 3
Control condition

⎫ Compared on the dependent variable to assess whether there are any differences between the conditions ⎬

Or you could go on adding experimental conditions involving different forms of treatment.

In all these cases we still have only one independent variable, i.e. type of treatment, but we have varying numbers of experimental conditions or levels of it.

So, it should be clear by now that hypotheses which predict a relationship between one independent variable and a dependent variable may be tested by comparing:

1. One experimental condition and one control condition.
2. Two experimental conditions.
3. Two experimental conditions and one control condition.
4. Three experimental conditions.
5. Three experimental conditions and one control condition.
6. More than three experimental conditions etc.

These designs require a different statistical test to analyse the results, since unfortunately, there is no multi-purpose test for all experiments. Matching the design with the appropriate statistical test is something that we shall look at in Chapter 9.

CORRELATIONAL DESIGNS

Not all research has to take the form of manipulating an independent variable to see what effect it has on the dependent variable. Sometimes a researcher is not interested in looking for differences between groups or conditions in this way, but instead is concerned to find out whether two variables are associated or related (look back to p. 49 to refresh your memory on the distinctions between experimental and correlational designs). Let us suppose we are interested in finding out whether there is a relationship between students' grades on clinical assessments and performance in theory exams since we have noticed that students who get high grades on one tend to get high grades on the other. Our hypothesis might be that: 'There is a relationship between performance on clinical assessments and performance in theory exams, high marks on one being associated with high marks on the other.' The two variables are clinical assessment and theory exam performance.

However, one of the major differences in the research design needed to test this hypothesis is that the experimenter does *not* manipulate one of the variables, but simply takes a whole range of measures on one of the variables and assesses whether they show a pattern or relationship of some sort with a whole range of measures on the other variable. The correlational designs and analyses which will be covered in this book are only concerned with ordinal and interval/ratio data, since these levels of measurements provide a range or dimension for our data. It is possible to do a correlation with just nominal data, but such analyses are not always very informative and so they have been omitted from this text. In our example, then, we might take a group of direct entry midwifery students and collect their clinical assessments and their theory exam marks to see if the two sets of scores are linked, e.g. high marks on one variable being associated with high marks on the other. Because the experimenter does not manipulate one variable, the concepts of independent and dependent variable are not appropriate in correlational designs. Furthermore, because there is no manipulation of

one variable and hence no measurement of the effect this has on the other variable, we cannot say in a correlational design which variable is cause and which effect. So returning to our example, we do not know whether clinical performance affects theory exam performance or vice versa. For instance, it may be that students who are good at clinical practice use their experience to answer their theory paper. Or it is possible that students who do well in theory use their knowledge in the clinical context. Alternatively, clinical performance and theory exam performance may both be related to a third variable. For example, good marks on both may be due to an 'easy' marker. Therefore, from any results we got from this study we do not actually know if:

practice affects theory

or

theory affects practice

or

another variable affects both theory and practice.

You can see from this that because we cannot ascertain which variable is having an effect on the other, there cannot be an independent or dependent variable or an identifiable cause and effect. Even in correlational studies where we feel we could make an educated guess as to which variable is cause and which effect, we still cannot draw causal conclusions. For instance, a parent might observe that their child's eczema got worse when the child's behaviour got worse. However, while there might indeed be a pattern in the data such that the severity of the child's eczema and naughtiness seemed to go together, it could not be ascertained from this study whether:

- the eczema caused the bad behaviour
- the bad behaviour caused the eczema
  or
- both were caused by a third, unknown factor, such as problems at school.

Because of this inability to state categorically which variable is cause and which is effect in a correlational design, many researchers prefer the certainty of experimental designs. However, because the experimenter is not involved in manipulating anything (such as types of treatment), the correlational design is often thought to be more acceptable ethically. Because causal conclusions are often wrongly drawn from correlational studies this point will be explored again at the end of the next section.

KEY CONCEPTS

- Experimental designs covered by this book have two variables in the hypothesis, one Independent and one dependent. The independent variable is manipulated by the experimenter and the difference or effect this has on the dependent variable is measured. Thus in experimental designs we can ascertain cause and effect.
- Correlational designs also have two variables in the hypothesis but neither is manipulated. Therefore, there is no independent and no dependent variable. As a result, it cannot be ascertained which variable is having an effect on the other. All that can be established is whether or not the scores on the two variables are linked in some way.

Note that correlational designs are not confined to seeing how far just two sets of data are related; they can also be used to look at the degree of similarity between three or more sets of data. Let us imagine you want to assess a student midwife on a number of activities, such as communication, diagnosis, competence with equipment, etc. If you observe the midwife just *once*, how will you know whether what you see is typical of what she can do? Would it not be better to observe her on a number of occasions in order to see whether there is a significant similarity in observed ability? This would mean that you need to assess the midwife on all the aspects of behaviour in which you are interested on several occasions. If you then analysed your data according to the principles of a correlational design, you would find out whether the observations were similar or not and from this you could get some reliable assessments of the midwife's capabilities. This sort of 'self-checking' is useful in midwifery and is called an *intra-observer reliability measure*.

Let us take this idea a step further. Suppose you are a midwifery tutor and have been a particular student's personal tutor for 2 years and you like her a lot. This could bias your observations of her capabilities. Would it be useful,

therefore, to have a number of independent midwifery tutors (say five) observing the student according to your checklist of activities to see if they were in agreement? If you then analysed their scores using a test for correlational designs and found that the ratings given by the independent midwifery tutors were significantly similar, you would have a better and more reliable basis for making your statements about the student's capabilities. This form of 'other-checking' is called *inter-observer reliability*, and again is a valuable tool for the midwife.

The correlation coefficient

It should be noted here that the degree to which each variable is associated in a correlational design is determined using an appropriate statistical test. We will deal with these tests in more detail in Chapter 9 but it is important to look at the underlying concepts here. To do this, let us return to our hypothesis and imagine that we have collected the students' clinical and theory exam marks; the next step is to find out whether there is a significant relationship between them, so we use the correct statistical test (see Ch. 9). When we have finished the calculations involved in this test, we will end up with a number somewhere on a range from −1.0 through 0 to +1.0.

This figure is known as a *correlation coefficient*. The size of the correlation coefficient indicates the closeness of the relationship between the two variables. The closer the figure is to −1 or +1, the closer the relationship, while the closer it is to 0 the weaker the relationship. This concept is illustrated by the continuum below (Fig. 6.1).

Let us explore this idea a bit further, using the hypothesis about the link between clinical assessments and theory exam marks. Supposing you had collected the clinical assessments and theory exam marks from 30 students (so you would have two scores for each student) you could plot

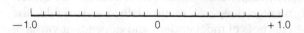

Figure 6.1 The value of the correlation coefficient lies somewhere on a range from −1 to +1.

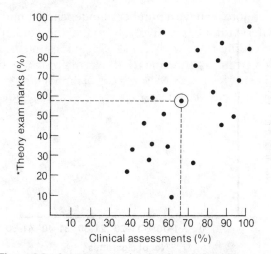

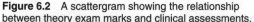

Figure 6.2 A scattergram showing the relationship between theory exam marks and clinical assessments.
* In plotting a correlational graph, it does not matter which variable is plotted against the vertical axis and which against the horizontal one. However, should you ever wish to plot the data from an experimental design it is a convention that the independent variable scores are plotted along the horizontal axis and those from the dependent variable along the vertical axis.

Table 6.8 Number of weeks gestation and neonatal birth weight

Subject	No. of weeks gestation	Neonatal birth weight (kg)
1	36	2.5
2	33	2.4
3	37	2.5
4	39	3.5
5	37	3.3
6	41	4.0
7	35	3.0
8	34	3.2
9	30	2.0
10	40	4.1

their scores on a graph, known as a *scattergram*, to see if there is any association between the marks. You might end up with a scattergram which looks like Figure 6.2.

In order to construct a scattergram, you would need to take each student's pair of scores (say, for the dot ringed in Figure 6.2, 58% on the theory exam and 66% on the clinical assessment) and move along each relevant axis until you had located her score. You would make a mark at the intersection point.

Activity 6.6 (Answers on page 236)

To practise doing this, plot the scores in Table 6.8 as a scattergram. The hypothesis is that there is a relationship between the number of weeks gestation and neonatal birth weight.

When you have plotted a scattergram, you can see whether there appears to be a relationship between the two variables by the nature of the pattern of dots. If the dots show a general upward or downward slope, it is likely that there is a relationship between the two variables. So in

the example about theory and practice marks, it seems that there *is* a relationship, because the pattern of dots shows a general upward slope. This is known as a *positive correlation*.

A positive correlation means that *high* scores on one variable are associated with *high* scores on the other and hence *low* scores on one variable are linked with *low* scores on the other. For example, suppose there is a positive correlation between weight gain and hypertension, such that the greater the weight gain the higher the hypertension. So a scattergram pattern which shows a general upward slope as shown in Figure 6.3 indicates a positive correlation.

It should be noted that the perfectly smooth upward slope on the graph below (Fig. 6.3) shows a perfect positive correlation (i.e. there is a one-to-one relationship between high scores on

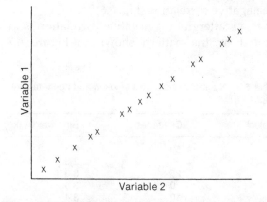

Figure 6.3 The upward slope in this scattergram indicates a positive correlation between variable 1 and variable 2.

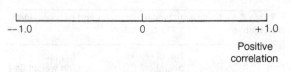

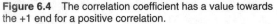

Figure 6.4 The correlation coefficient has a value towards the +1 end for a positive correlation.

one variable and high scores on the other). However, perfect correlations are extremely rare, if they exist at all. But, the smoother and straighter the upward slope, the stronger the positive correlation between the two variables. A *positive* correlation would be represented on our continuum somewhere around the +1.0 end, as in Figure 6.4.

This figure would have been derived from a statistical analysis and the nearer to +1, the stronger the relationship. This, however, is not the only sort of correlation that can occur. Sometimes it is possible that *high* scores on one variable are associated with *low* scores on the other. For example we might hypothesize a relationship between number of cigarettes smoked and neonatal birth weight, such that the greater the number of cigarettes smoked, the lower the birth weight. Our data may look like Table 6.9.

Plotting these results on a scattergram, we end up with the pattern in Figure 6.5.

There is a general downward slope in the pattern of dots. When this sort of pattern emerges, it suggests that high scores on one variable are associated with low scores on the other. This is known as a negative correlation and would be represented on our correlation coefficient near the −1 end; the closer to −1, the stronger the negative correlation (Fig. 6.6).

On a scattergram, a negative correlation is indicated by the pattern shown in Figure 6.7.

Table 6.9 Number of cigarettes smoked and neonatal birth weight

Subject	Cigarettes	Birth weight (kg)
1	50	2.5
2	40	2.8
3	25	3.0
4	0	3.5
5	10	3.4
6	15	3.2

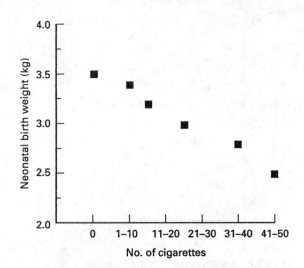

Figure 6.5 Scattergram showing relationship between number of cigarettes smoked and neonatal birth weight.

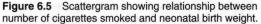

Figure 6.6 A scattergram pattern indicating a negative correlation.

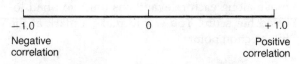

Figure 6.7 A correlation coefficient value near to −1 indicates a strong negative correlation.

(Again this shows a perfect negative correlation, which is very unlikely ever to occur.)

It is very important to note that a negative correlation does *not* mean *no* correlation. This is a point that confuses some students. A *negative* correlation indicates a relationship between *high* scores on one variable and *low* scores on the other, while no correlation means that there is no relationship at all between the two variables.

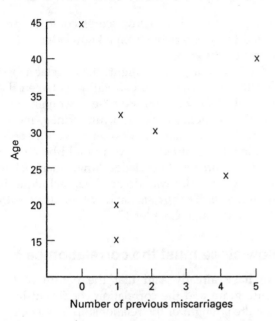

Figure 6.8 Number of previous miscarriages plotted against age.

Table 6.10 Age of mother and number of previous miscarriages

Subject	Age	No. of previous miscarriages
1	19	1
2	30	2
3	43	0
4	41	5
5	25	4
6	32	1

The following data demonstrate this concept of 'no correlation':

Hypothesis: There is a relationship between the age of mother and the number of previous miscarriages.

The data obtained are shown in Table 6.10.

Plotting these on a scattergram we get the picture shown in Figure 6.8.

This shows a fairly random scattering of dots, suggesting there is no link between the variables of age and the number of previous miscarriages.

In this case, the correlation coefficient score from our statistical analysis would be around 0 (Fig. 6.9).

```
|--------------------|--------------------|
-1.0                  0                 + 1.0
Negative          No correlation        Positive
correlation                            correlation
```

Figure 6.9 A correlation coefficient value around 0 indicates little or no relationship between the two variables.

KEY CONCEPTS

- Positive correlations indicate that high scores on one variable are associated with high scores on the other and therefore, low scores on one variable are associated with low scores on the other:
  - they are represented by an upward slope on a scattergram
  - they have a correlation coefficient near +1, with the closer the coefficient to +1, the stronger the positive correlation.
- Negative correlations indicate that high scores on one variable are associated with low scores on the other:
  - they are represented by a downward slope on a scattergram
  - they have a correlation coefficient of around −1, with the nearer the coefficient to −1, the stronger the negative correlation.
- No correlation indicates that there is no relationship between the scores on the two variables:
  - they are represented by random clusterings on a scattergram with no obvious direction to the pattern
  - they have a correlation coefficient of around 0, with the closer the coefficient to 0, the weaker the relationship between the two variables.

Activity 6.7 (Answers on page 237)

1. Look at the following hypotheses and state whether they suggest positive or negative correlations between the variables. Also state how they would be represented on a scattergram and where on a scale of −1 to +1 the correlation coefficient would be.
   (i) The older the woman, the longer the length of labour.
   (ii) The further from an ante-natal clinic a woman lives, the less the likelihood of keeping an appointment.
   (iii) The lower the 'GCSE' level results of direct entry midwifery students, the lower the exam mark in the final year.
   (iv) The higher the intake of dietary fibre, the lower the incidence of constipation during the third trimester.
2. Look at the following correlation coefficients and rank them from the *strongest* relationship to the *weakest*:
   −0.73 −0.42 +0.61 +0.21 −0.17 +0.09

A word of warning

It should be reiterated that even if you do find a strong positive or negative correlation, you still cannot conclude that the variables are *causally* related. However, many people do make this error. For example, when the AIDS problem started to reach public awareness a few years ago, one politician asked whether the condition was caused by Greek yoghurt, since he had noted that the amount of yoghurt appearing in supermarkets had risen alongside the number of reported AIDS cases. Almost certainly, had the data been analysed using the appropriate test, a positive correlation would have been found, but there is clearly no way in which Greek yoghurt was *causing* the epidemic. Similarly, over the past year, a Sunday newspaper has been making a deliberate play out of 'casual' correlations. For example, it reported that over the previous few years the number of divorces had risen. Furthermore, it was noted that there had been an increase in the lofts that were being insulated. The paper concluded, tongue-in-cheek, that insulating lofts causes divorce. I am sure you can see from this that just because data are correlated, does not mean that they are also *causally* related.

Making predictions

However, if you do find that the two variables are correlated together, you can make predictions about one variable from information about the other. Therefore, if you found that two variables were negatively correlated, you could predict high scores on one variable from knowledge of low scores on the other and vice versa. Equally, if you found that two variables were positively correlated, you could predict high scores on one variable from a knowledge of high scores on the other or low scores could be predicted for one variable from a knowledge of low scores on the other.

For example, you might have established that there is a negative correlation between the amount of pelvic floor exercise a woman does and the frequency of post-partum urinary incontinence. If a woman then presents with a specified incidence of leakage, you would be able to predict from this knowledge how much pelvic floor exercise she was doing. This technique is known as *linear regression* and will be dealt with in more detail in Chapter 17.

How close must the correlation be?

We have already said that the nature of the scattergram and the correlation coefficient indicate the strength of the relationship between the two variables and that there is no such thing as a perfect correlation. Therefore how smooth must the scattergram slope be and how close must the correlation coefficient be to +1 or −1 before we decide that there is a relationship? Will +0.63 do? or −0.54? Because we cannot make an arbitrary decision like this, after we have calculated the correlation coefficient using a statistical test, we use a set of statistical tables to see whether the correlation coefficient is sufficiently big to indicate that the relationship between the two variables is significant. This will also depend on how many subjects you have used in your project. We will deal with these concepts in more detail in Chapter 17.

7

Designing your study

SOME BASIC CONCEPTS

When you carry out any research you will almost certainly recruit people to take part in it. The people who take part in research are called *subjects*, sometimes referred to as *Ss*. You will always have to decide what sort of subjects you need in your research, for instance, pre-registration midwives, premature babies, women who have had a termination etc. and these participants must be defined carefully and clearly. It is insufficient, for example, just to state 'premature babies' since the term covers a range of gestational ages. So you must be clear as to the precise nature of your subjects. But whoever you decide to use, there is a very important point to note — you do not want your results to apply only to the small group or sample of people you used in your experiment, as you need to be able to *generalize* your results. This is a crucial feature of research and central to the topic of inferential statistics. For example, supposing you had compared two interventions for rotating breech presentation fetuses. To one group of 20 mothers a specially prepared exercise regime was given, while the other group had external cephalic version (ECV). The version rate and psychological stress level of the two groups of women were compared. Let us suppose that the results at the end of the study showed that the success rate for rotation was comparable for both groups, but that the exercise group suffered significantly *less* stress than the ECV group. This would suggest that exercises would be a preferable way of treating known breech presentations in future. However, you can only make this assumption if the results you obtained from your study do not apply *only* to those mothers who participated, but rather would be likely to apply to other breech presentations. The point here is that if your results can be generalized in this way, then *predictions* can be made, and this is an essential feature of research. So, when you find at an ante-natal visit that one of your mothers has a breech presentation fetus you can predict with some confidence that exercises are more likely to be effective than ECV on the basis of the generalizability of the results from your research, and consequently this knowledge informs your recommended treatment.

However, short of carrying out your experiment on huge numbers of mothers with breech presentations, how can you ascertain that your results *are* generalizable? We have already touched on this issue when the topic of inferential statistics was introduced; if you recall, inferential statistics allow the researcher to use a small sample of people in an experiment, and from the results of these experiments to infer that the same findings would apply to the larger population from which the sample comes. Now in order to be able to make this assumption, you must ensure that the sample you selected for study is:

1. Sufficiently large to ensure that it reflects the larger group or population from which it is derived. Let us consider the situation whereby the Director of Midwifery Services in a large maternity unit is thinking about altering the number of hours in the day shift. If she asks one midwife out of the 100 in the unit, then it is less likely that she will receive a view which reflects the opinion of the whole group (or *population*) than if she asks 15 or 30. In other words the number of subjects you select for study must be sufficiently large for you to be able to generalize the results from your experiment. What does this mean in practice? Well, although opinions on this vary, it is usually considered that 12 to 15 subjects per group or condition is the absolute minimum number required. Of course, if you are dealing with hydatidiform moles it will be un-

likely that you will get as many as 12, and you may want to consider a single case study instead. There are also situations where more subjects are required. Where this is the case, it will be pointed out in the relevant chapter. (In some of the illustrations quoted in later chapters, fewer than 12 subjects are used. This has been done simply for ease of calculation.)

2. Representative of the population from which they come and so are fairly typical. The easiest way to ensure reasonable typicality is to select your subjects randomly, for instance putting the names of all the breech presentation mothers you might have access to in a hat and randomly selecting 20. This point was covered in more detail in Chapter 3 and will be referred to again later in this chapter. Before moving on though, it is important to recognize that you cannot always select your subjects randomly because there are insufficient numbers of particular patient/client types and you may just have to use everyone you find. If this is the case, then you must be aware of the limitations of generalizing the results from such a study.

TREATMENT OF YOUR SUBJECTS

Before moving on to discuss how your subjects can be used to test your hypothesis, a very important point should be noted concerning how you treat your subjects. You should *never* do anything to your subjects which would harm or upset them in any way. It is important that you treat your subjects well, that you do not deceive them or use your position to pressurize them to take part. It is important that your subjects know what they are letting themselves in for before they agree to participate — in other words they give their informed consent. Midwife researchers are particularly likely to use as their subjects very vulnerable members of the population — the fetus, the neonate, distressed parents etc. — who may not be able to give rational and informed consent to participation. It is therefore essential that any intending researcher considers carefully the ethical aspects of her research design, paying close attention to issues which might compromise or disadvantage the subjects.

A great deal has been written on ethics in health research, but the reader might like to look at Hicks' (1996) chapter on Ethics in Midwifery Research. In all events, your research project should be referred to the ethical committee for consideration before you begin. Failure to observe these guidelines would undoubtedly tarnish a researcher's reputation and may damage the participants physically or psychologically.

TYPES OF EXPERIMENTAL DESIGN

Whatever sort of subjects are involved in your study, you will need to decide how to use them in the research design and this decision is a crucial one when designing a piece of research.

For example, if you look back to the hypothesis given on page 51 where it was predicted that midwives who attended a psychology course developed more tolerant attitudes than those who did not attend, you will see that to test this hypothesis it was suggested that two groups of midwives were selected, one of which attended the course, and the other of which did not. In other words, two *different* groups of midwives were used, one in the control condition and one in the experimental condition. However, not all hypotheses are best tested by comparing different groups of subjects in this way; sometimes it is more appropriate to use just *one* group of subjects and to measure them on two or more occasions.

When two or more different groups of subjects are used and compared in a project, it is called an *unrelated, between* or *different subject design*. When just one group of subjects is used in all conditions it is called a *related, within* or *same subject design*. We will look at each of these more closely.

(1) Different subject designs (also known as unrelated subject or between subject designs)

It was said earlier that hypotheses could often be tested in different ways, using different types of experimental designs, and that it was the job of the experimenter to decide on the most suitable

Group of midwives	*Condition 1* (Experimental Condition) Attendance on course	Groups compared for differences in attitude
Group of midwives	*Condition 2* (Control Condition) No attendance on course	

Figure 7.1 A different subject design.

design for a particular hypothesis. However, for some hypotheses there is really only one obvious way to test them. If you look again at the hypothesis about midwives' attendance on a psychology course, two different groups of midwives were used, one as a control condition and one as an experimental condition.

The design looked like Figure 7.1.

At the end of the experiment the attitude change of the two groups would be compared to see if, in fact, the group who had attended the course became more tolerant.

This is a typical example of the sort of hypothesis which requires a different subject design since it would have been totally inappropriate to use just one group for both conditions. If we think about this idea a bit more closely, it becomes clear that if we *had* selected just one group of midwives, to be both the control (no course) condition and the experimental (attendance on course) condition, all sorts of problems emerge. Let us explore this a bit further. There are two possible ways of carrying out this experiment, using just one group of subjects. You could either send your group of midwives:

(a) on a course for 3 months (experimental condition)
followed by
'no course' for 3 months (control condition)

or

(b) on 'no course' for 3 months (control condition)
followed by
a course for 3 months (experimental condition).

You can see from this that although there are

control and experimental conditions in each design, the results from the second condition would always be contaminated by the results from the first because the group had done *both* conditions. For example, in the first design, if we did find that there was a significant attitude change after going on a course for 3 months and that there was no further change after the 'no course' condition what could we really conclude about the control condition? It may be that the control condition had no effect because the group's attitudes had changed as far as they could by the end of the course or because the control condition was a time for consolidating the attitude change already experienced. Alternatively, if we found that there was a change during the control condition this may be due to the continued effect of the course, or the effects of 3 months more time and experience; but we would not know which.

In the second design, any change in attitude found after doing the course might simply be due to the combined effects of the control and experimental conditions or the passage of time on the experience, opinions and attitudes of these subjects and not to the course. In other words, whatever the order these designs adopt, any results obtained would have more than one explanation because we have contaminated the outcome by subjecting the subjects to both conditions. This is known as an *order effect* and will be discussed in more detail in the next chapter. Therefore, an hypothesis like this one requires a different subject design in order to eliminate the confounding effects of participating in both conditions. It is important to note here that in this context, 'different' simply means 'separate'. In other words, in the previous example, while all the subjects were midwives and were therefore the same in this respect, they were split into two separate or different groups.

There are many other hypotheses in midwifery research which necessitate using two or more different groups of subjects. The example given earlier comparing two intervention approaches for mothers known to have a breech presentation fetus used two different groups of mothers, one group receiving exercises and the other ECV. Any comparisons of different races, ages, sexes, type of patient etc. all mean that different subjects have to be used. For example, if you wanted to compare Apgar scores of Asian and African Caribbean neonates, you would have to use one group of Asian neonates and another group of African Caribbean neonates. One subject group is quite obviously inappropriate here, since it is impossible for a baby to be of both discrete racial origins. In other words, if the manipulation of the independent variable simply involves the comparison of two or more inherently different groups of subjects (old vs. young primigravida, male vs. female neonate, forceps vs. ventouse deliveries etc.) you *must* use a different subject design. Remember that you do not need to confine yourself to the comparison of just two different or separate groups. It is perfectly acceptable to compare three or more groups, although the type of analysis will be different.

While it is sometimes essential to use different groups of subjects in your experiment, there is a major disadvantage in the design: that of individual differences among the subjects. If we look at the example regarding differences in Apgar scores between Asian and African Caribbean neonates, it is quite possible that some neonates are inherently less active, or that some had been more or less affected by maternal analgesia, or that there were differences in the way in which the baby was handled immediately after delivery etc. All these factors may influence how a neonate reacts and so will affect the results. For example, a baby who had been adversely affected by pethidine may register a lower Apgar score. This score may therefore not be a true reflection of the neonate's condition but rather of its idiosyncratic reaction to the analgesia. While these individual differences may be evenly distributed among all the groups thereby cancelling the effects out, it is also possible that more of the individual differences that affect the results may occur in only one of the groups and thus will artificially distort the results.

The problem of individual differences can be partly overcome by ensuring that the subjects are randomly selected and used. Randomization can mean one of two things in different subject designs. Firstly, it can mean selecting a group of subjects (e.g. mothers with known breech presentations) and randomly allocating half of them to one treatment (ECV) and half to the other (exercises), in order to compare the effects. Obviously, this cannot be done in our example about Apgar scores, since it would not be possible to select a group of neonates and randomly allocate them to being Asian or African Caribbean. Here randomness means something different — that the subjects in each group should be a random, and therefore reasonably typical, selection of the group they represent. In other words, the neonates in the Asian group should be reasonably typical of Asian neonates as a whole, and not particularly weak, premature, distressed, or anything else. The same should be true of the neonates in the African Caribbean group. The ways in which random selection can be achieved are outlined in Chapter 3 and also throughout this chapter.

KEY CONCEPTS

When two or more different groups of subjects are used in an experiment it is called:

an *unrelated subject* design
or
a *between subject* design
or
a *different subject* design.

The advantages of this design are that it can overcome any problems associated with the order of conditions and it is also essential when 'fixed' differences such as race, sex, ages, types of patient are being compared. However, its major disadvantage is that individual differences among the subjects may distort the results. This can be partially overcome by *randomly* selecting the subjects and then *randomly* allocating them to conditions where possible.

---

(2) Same subject designs (also known as related subject or within subject designs)

Some hypotheses, however, are not suited to using designs with different subjects in each condition. Some hypotheses are more suited to being tested by designs which use only one

group of subjects, but this group is measured under all the conditions and its performance in each condition is compared.

For example, you might be interested in looking at the issue of the 'named midwife'. In particular, you want to ascertain whether midwives operating as 'named' professionals felt that the quality of care they delivered was better than when they operated on the traditional random allocation system. To test this out, you would select one group of midwives and compare the evaluations of their service delivery under two conditions; one as a named midwife and the other as a randomly allocated midwife. The design would look like Figure 7.2.

Thus, one group of subjects is tested under both conditions and the two sets of ratings are compared to see if there is any difference between them. It would be inappropriate here to use two groups of midwives, one to rate the 'named' midwife condition and the other to rate the random allocation condition, because the groups may differ inherently in a number of ways which would affect the outcome of the results. For example, one group may be generally more competent and self confident anyway, may be more unrealistic about their own performance, or may try to gain praise and recognition for their clinical skills by inflating their ratings etc. and we would not know this because we have nothing against which to measure their ratings. Hence, there may be basic individual differences between the two groups which might affect the results and which would prevent us from establishing any baseline for comparison. However, if we use just one group of midwives then whatever their idiosyncrasies and personal

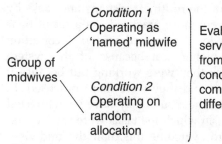

Figure 7.2 A same subject design.

characteristics, they will at least be constant over both ratings. Therefore, one important advantage of a same subject design is the fact that it overcomes the problem of individual differences inherent in different subject designs. Because of this, it is especially useful in 'before and after' type experiments, where the researcher wants to look at the effects of a treatment procedure on a group of subjects. A common example of this is the television advertisement for washing powder, showing viewers the dirty washing *before* being washed in the product and the same linen *after* being washed. The same clothes are used when the *before* and *after* assessments are made and thus constitute a same subject design.

However, this design too has its snags. If we look at the example concerning midwives' self-ratings under two conditions, supposing we gave all the midwives the random allocation condition first, and the named midwife condition second. Let us suppose further that for the first half of a selected ante-natal shift, the midwives had to operate on the traditional basis of just dealing with any woman who attended, while for the second half of the shift, they had to initiate the introductory routine necessary for the 'named midwife' service. It is quite possible that the self-evaluations the group recorded for the random-allocation condition were higher simply because it was the beginning of the shift. They were fresher, more enthusiastic and more alert. Consequently, their clinical skills were better, not necessarily because the midwives functioned in a superior way under the traditional system, but simply because this condition was first. An alternative scenario might be one where the midwives performed better during the second half of the shift, because they had already carried out many of the routines, systems and tasks by then and were more practised. As a result their self-ratings for the 'named midwife' condition would be higher, not because of the system under which they were working but because it came second and they were more practised. In other words, the results may have been affected by the *order* in which the tasks were carried out. Therefore to overcome this, half the midwives should do Condition 1 first, followed by Condi-

tion 2, while for the remaining midwives, the order would be reversed. This is called *counterbalancing* and is discussed more fully later in the chapter. It should also be noted that one group of subjects can be tested on more than two occasions. For example, you might wish to look at the pain levels experienced by a group of women in the first stage of labour using TENS. To do this, you decide to select one group of say, 20 women and you assess their pain levels before using TENS, 1 hour after using TENS, 2 hours after using TENS and 3 hours after using TENS. Your design would look like Figure 7.3.

You have here a same subject design, with the subjects being measured under four conditions, to establish whether the use of TENS makes any difference to their pain levels.

KEY CONCEPT

When one group of subjects is tested or measured on all the conditions and their performance compared, it is known as a

related subject design
or
same subject design
or
within subject design.

The advantage of this design is that it eliminates the distorting effects of individual subject differences. However, it has two disadvantages: firstly, it cannot be used when 'fixed' differences such as sex, race, type of problem are being compared and secondly, any effects deriving from the order of the conditions may have to be counterbalanced.

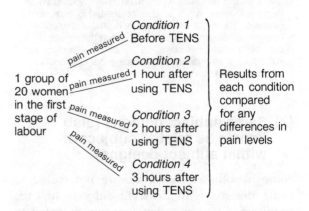

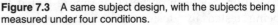

Figure 7.3 A same subject design, with the subjects being measured under four conditions.

(3) Matched subject designs

One way of overcoming all the disadvantages of both different and same subject designs is to use two or more groups of subjects who are matched on a number of characteristics. Let us take an example. Suppose you wanted to compare the maternal and fetal outcomes following episiotomies or tears. You obviously cannot use a same subject design because the mother must have had either an episiotomy or a tear in order to compare the effects. If you used women who experienced both during the same labour, you would not be able to identify which event caused which maternal or fetal effect. Alternatively, if you used a different subject design there may be so many individual differences in physical and psychological reactions both in the mother and the neonate that it might be difficult to ascertain whether it was these rather than the type of perineal wound which was responsible for any outcomes. For example, tendency to complain about pain, individual healing capacity, personal hygiene etc. may all impact upon the mother's reaction to the perineal damage, but if all these factors just happened to be more prevalent in the episiotomy group as opposed to the tear group then it would be difficult to draw any definitive conclusions about perineal wounds from the study. In such cases, then, it is necessary to try to identify the characteristics which may bias the results of the experiment and to ensure that the groups are matched on these factors.

The way in which the matching is carried out involves firstly, identifying all the possible characteristics which may influence the results, and then selecting a subject (for example, an episiotomy mother) and assessing how she rates on each factor. Therefore, the points you might have identified as having a potential influence on the study's outcomes might be:

Age
Height
Parity
Gestational weeks
Length of labour
Known fetal problems
Neonatal size

Presentation
Type of analgesia used
Type of delivery etc.

You will undoubtedly be able to add to this list, but the factors identified above will suffice for the purpose of illustration. The first episiotomy mother has to be assessed on each factor thus:

32
5' 3"
Primip
38.5 weeks
14.2 hours
No known fetal problems
Suspected large baby
Cephalic presentation
Entonox + Pethidine
Normal vaginal.

You must now find a mother who has had a tear who rates the same as the first episiotomy mother on all the identified factors. You then need to find another set of 'twins'. These pairs of women do not need to be identical to the first pair selected, but they must be the same as each other. Therefore, in terms of the characteristics which are likely to influence the results from the experiment, each pair of subjects is like identical twins, with the only difference between them being the type of perineal wound experienced. Thus, for every subject in one group, there is an 'identical twin' in the other. However, the matching should not stop there. You would also need to ensure that the quality, type and extent of treatment were also the same for each patient, together with any other factors which were likely to influence the study's outcomes.

When you are involved in comparing 'non-fixed' groups, e.g. the effects of the different treatments, you can match up a pair of subjects first and then randomly allocate one subject to one treatment and the 'twin' to the other treatment. Because of the similarity of the subjects, matched designs are treated like same subject designs for the purposes of statistical analysis. Similarly, as with same subject designs, the matched design overcomes the problem of individual differences, because of the 'twinning' of the subjects. Yet the matched design has all the advantages of a different subject design, since 'fixed' groups can be compared and there need be no order effects.

So why do we not always use matched designs if they are so good? I am sure you will have realized already that it is often extremely difficult to match pairs of subjects in this way, usually because there are limited numbers of suitable subjects to choose from. Even if we allow ourselves a little leeway, say by matching an episiotomy mother aged 30 with a tear mother aged 28, there may still be many important differences between the subject pair that we either cannot identify or cannot match for, e.g. histology of perineal tissue that affects healing rates. Thus, while these designs are theoretically very desirable, in practical terms they are extremely difficult to implement properly. It must be stressed that it is not adequate simply to select 20 women with episiotomies and 20 with tears, all of whom are between 5' and 5' 6" and under 40 and say that you have matched them. For every subject in one group, there must be a 'twinned' subject in the other, matched on all the relevant variables which may influence the outcome of the experiment. Therefore, because of the difficulties involved in matching people, caused largely through our lack of knowledge of which factors are relevant, it is usually desirable to use a same subject design in preference to a matched subject design. As one statistician says:

A matching design is only as good as the Experimenter's ability to determine how to match the pairs, and this ability is frequently very limited.

Sidney Siegel (1956)

While matched subject designs *can* be used with more than two groups of subjects, because of the problems outlined above, it is very unlikely that you will ever be able to match subjects up in 'triplets' or 'quadruplets', and so may be better avoided.

REVIEW

Let us recap on the essential guidelines involved

> **KEY CONCEPT**
>
> Matched designs involve selecting pairs of subjects, matched on any variable which may influence the outcome of the experiment, and allocating one of the pair to one condition and one to the other. This design has all the advantages of same and different subject designs, but has the major disadvantage that it is very difficult to match subjects in this way because firstly it is not always possible to find subjects who are sufficiently similar, and secondly, you can never be sure that you have matched pairs of subjects on all the factors that may influence the results.

in designing a piece of research that have been covered so far:

1. Have you formulated an experimental hypothesis which clearly predicts a relationship between two variables? Have you stated your null (no relationship) hypothesis?

2. Are you going to test this hypothesis using a correlational design (i.e., are you predicting that as scores on one variable go up, so scores on the other variable go up or down accordingly)? Or are you going to use an experimental design which will test for differences between conditions or subject groups? If you are going to use a correlational design, go on to Chapter 11.

3. If you are going to use an experimental design, have you sorted out *what* you are going to measure (i.e. what is the DV?) Have you decided *when* you will take the pre-test measures of the DV and the post-test measures? What *level* of measurement are you using?

4. Will you be using a control group? Is this ethically acceptable? If you are not, how many experimental conditions have you decided upon?

5. Who are your subjects going to be? Can you select them randomly? How many will you need?

6. Are you going to use a different, same or matched subject design? Are you sure that this is the most appropriate design for your hypothesis? Why? If you are going to use a matched subject design, have you identified the critical variables on which the Ss have to be matched?

7. Is there any need to counterbalance the conditions to overcome order effects?

8. Have you controlled for experimenter bias?

8

Sources of error in research

There are a number of potential sources of bias or error which can creep into the design of an experiment which may distort your results and therefore must be controlled for. We will look at each of these separately.

ORDER EFFECTS

When a piece of research is carried out which follows an experimental design the experimenter manipulates the independent variable and measures the effect of this on the dependent variable, in the hope that altering the IV will have a significant effect on the DV. Changes in the DV are called the experimental effect and constitute the data in your study. Let us take an example. Suppose you are a midwifery tutor responsible for pre-registration training. Looking back at the academic record over the past 10 years, you notice that physiology examination results appear to be substantially worse than results on the psychology examination. Clearly if your observations are correct then this may have implications both for the teaching of the physiology course and for clinical preparation. To test out your hunch you compare the previous year's physiology examination marks with the psychology examination marks. You therefore have the design shown in Figure 8.1.

This is a same subject design, with one group of students being measured on two occasions and their performances on both examinations compared (using the appropriate statistical test) to see if they differ. Let us assume that you did in

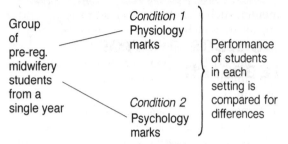

Figure 8.1 A same subject design, with one group of subjects being measured on two occasions.

fact find that students seem to do better on the psychology examination; can we conclude that the results are the effect of some inherent difficulty associated with physiology or how it is taught? Or might there be some other explanations?

One obvious alternative explanation that we have already touched on and you have probably thought of, relates to the sequence of the examinations. If the examination timetable has been arranged so that the psychology examination takes place on a Monday morning, while the physiology examination has been timetabled for Friday afternoon, then, it is conceivable that their poor performance on the physiology examination may be due simply to the fact that it came last on a Friday afternoon. In other words, the students may do worse on any second examination (regardless of its nature) because they are more tired, more fed-up, more burnt out with examinations — they are *fatigued*. Hence, this is known as a *fatigue effect*. It is, of course, possible that students do better on their second examination because they are more practised, more elated because the examinations are almost at an end, more skilled at examination techniques — this is known as a *practice effect*.

Regardless of which argument you favour, the general issue is the same: that order effects, rather than the subject of the examination itself, could be affecting students' performance. Order effects are a common problem in experiments where one group of subjects is compared on two or more conditions i.e. same subject designs. In order to get round this problem, a technique called *counterbalancing* is used, where half the subjects do activity A first, followed by activity B,

while the other half do activity B first, followed by activity A. In our example, then, for the coming year, the examination timetable would be altered, so that the physiology examination now came on a Monday morning and the psychology examination on a Friday afternoon. The results obtained from each of these examinations would be combined with those from the previous year and compared for differences. Sometimes a study's design and topic allow you to select by random allocation which subjects complete the tasks in a particular order. The random allocation can be achieved by a number of methods: selecting the first ten subjects alphabetically; the first ten names pulled out of a hat; alternate names alphabetically. While it does not really matter which method you use, do try to ensure that the subjects are *randomly* allocated. The section on random selection (pp 21–22) may clarify this point further.

So, by counterbalancing in this way, any bias in the results due to order effects is cancelled out. One point is important here: we cannot eliminate order effects totally, because one activity must precede the other in designs like this. All we can do is to balance out the order effects as far as possible.

KEY CONCEPTS

If one group of subjects has to be measured in all the conditions then the order in which they do these conditions may influence the results. For example, they may perform better on the last activity because of *practice effects*, or they may perform worse on the last activity because of *fatigue effects*. In order to eliminate these sources of bias, the order in which the subjects carry out the activities should be counterbalanced, such that half the subjects does activity A first, followed by B, while for the remainder, the order is reversed.

So, one explanation for the results from this experiment is the possible influence of order effects. However, even if you had counterbalanced these, there are still other variables which could account for your results.

EXPERIMENTER BIAS EFFECTS

Suppose, like all experimenters, you are very

committed to your research and are very keen that your hypothesis will be supported. It is conceivable that in your anxiety and enthusiasm to obtain the predicted outcome, you will unwittingly influence the results. I do not mean by this that you will cook the books, but that unawares, you may use a slightly different method of collecting your data, or you may over-focus on some results, whilst paying less attention to those which did not support your hypothesis. In other words, you may have a set of expectations about the outcome of the experiment which will influence what you perceive, how you behave etc. Alternatively, you may unconsciously influence your subjects' responses by using a set of non-verbal cues. If we return to the hypothetical project comparing midwives' self-evaluations of clinical performance under two conditions, the 'named midwife' and the traditional random allocation, let us suppose that you as the researcher are very enthusiastic about the named midwife initiative and therefore would be delighted if your sample reported that their service delivery was better under this condition. You interview your first midwife who begins by saying how relatively incompetent and de-skilled she felt under the traditional regime. This is exactly what you want to hear because it supports your hypothesis! And when we hear something we like we automatically respond with a set of non-verbal cues which the other person quickly picks up; for instance, we might smile, nod our head, lean forward into the conversation and this encourages the other person to go on saying similar things. When we hear something we do not like, we might frown or lean out of the discussion and this has the effect of discouraging further comments of that type. In addition, the subjects may take a dislike to the experimenter and so deliberately say things they know will not support the hypothesis or they may like the experimenter and distort their responses to help him/her. In all cases, there is the potential for bias, particularly where the data involve subjective report. Such influences are very common and are known as *experimenter bias effects*. Other sources of experimenter bias include the personal characteristics of the experi-

menter, such as status, sex, class, race, age and so on, all of which may have some effect on the subjects and their performance.

It should be emphasized that normally such experimenter influences are quite unintentional and unconscious, but there is a great deal of documented evidence to show that they exist. How can we get round this problem? The usual solution is to operate a *blind procedure*, whereby you ask someone who does not know what your hypothesis is to collect your data — in this case, to interview the midwives. Because she is not aware of what you have predicted, she will also not know how the subjects are meant to behave in each condition and so their responses during the interview should be much more objective. Blind procedures may be of two sorts — *single blind* procedures where either the subjects or the person collecting the data is unaware of the hypothesis being tested. Alternatively, *double blind* procedures can be used where neither party knows what the aims of the study are. This sort of double blind procedure is very common in medical research, particularly when carrying out drug trials. In these cases, one group of patients is given the drug, while another group is given a placebo. But neither the doctors assessing the outcome nor the patients themselves know who has been given which. In this way, the results cannot be biased by expectations, or deliberate or unintentional manipulation.

KEY CONCEPTS

Sometimes experimenters unwittingly influence the outcome of their experiment by the way in which they behave, appear or interact with the subjects. This is known as *experimenter bias*. Subjects sometimes distort their responses too. To overcome this sort of problem in your research, you should use a *blind* procedure, whereby you ask someone who is absolutely unaware of what your hypothesis is to collect your data from subjects who are also unaware of your hypothesis. In this way, any bias due to expectations and predictions will be eliminated.

However, there are still other variables which may influence our results, besides the manipulation of the IV even if we control for order and experimenter bias effects. These are called *con-*

stant errors and *random errors*. Let us look at constant errors first.

CONSTANT ERRORS

Constant errors are all the possible sources of bias and influence that will affect the results in a constant and predictable way. If we go back to our example of comparing midwives' self-evaluations of clinical performance under two conditions, we can identify a number of potential sources of constant error. Suppose that the circumstances were such that the mothers who were treated under the traditional random allocation system spoke no English and consequently communication was difficult; they were all primigravidas, and so were all extremely tense making the internal examination almost impossible to carry out properly. In addition, the clinic was well attended that shift but was also short staffed with the result that all the appointments were very late and very rushed. Under these conditions it would be hardly surprising if the midwives' clinical skills were worse because of workload and client characteristics. Thus any low self-evaluations may be the result of these other influences rather than of the random allocation model.

On the other hand, under the 'named midwife' condition, the mothers all spoke English, were multips and so were not particularly tense, the backlog of appointments had been cleared because more staff had transferred from another part of the hospital to cope with the workload. Under such improved circumstances it would be entirely likely that clinical performance would be enhanced irrespective of the nature of the care model. Note that each of these factors can be called a constant error because of the predictable way in which they would distort the results. For example, poor client/staff ratios are more likely to depress clinical performance than improve it and so the effect of this variable is constant; inability to communicate will also depress, not improve, clinical performance, as will difficulties in carrying out routine checks because of maternal tension. Thus, each of these factors will have a similar effect on the clinical skills of the mid-

Table 8.1 Control or elimination of constant errors

Constant error	Solution
1. Amount of English spoken	Ensure that clients in both conditions speak similar amounts of English
2. Tension levels due to parity	Ensure that parity is comparable for both conditions
3. Staff/client ratios	Ensure workload is similar under each condition

wives and so will distort the results in a constant, predictable way.

It is your job as a researcher to try to identify all the possible sources of constant error in your experiment and either eliminate or control them. If you leave any constant error uncontrolled then your results may be explained by that, rather than by the manipulation of the IV. Taking the constant errors quoted as examples here, we can eliminate or control them in the following way (Table 8.1).

In other words, you must standardize all relevant aspects of the experimental situation in each condition.

Thus, when designing an experiment you must try to highlight all the factors which will bias your results in a constant and predictable way and then make attempts to eliminate or control them by standardizing the situation and procedures in each condition.

RANDOM ERRORS

Random errors are not as easy to deal with. As their name suggests, they are random; randomly occurring, randomly distributed and with a random and unpredictable impact on the results. If we look back to our example, we identified some factors that would influence our results in a very predictable way, but there are other factors — the random errors which will obscure our results in a totally variable or chance way.

In the above example, the moods of the mothers and midwives will all have an effect on clinical performance. If all the random allocation mothers were in a bad mood and all the 'named midwife' mothers were in a good mood then moods would influence the results in a predictable way and so would be classified as constant errors. But moods are not like that — they fluctuate up and down and interact with other people's behaviour, mood and attitudes. As a result they cannot be eliminated or controlled. Transitory changes in health states among the clients and midwifery staff, their personalities, attitudes, beliefs, motivations etc. are all examples of random error factors which will obscure the results in an unpredictable, chance way and about which we can do very little.

The only real precaution that we can take against random errors is to ensure as far as possible that the people involved in our research are drawn randomly from the population they represent. Therefore, our midwives should be fairly typical of midwives as a whole and not particularly deviant, disturbed, problematic, good, able or anything else. The mothers in the random allocation group should be fairly typical of pregnant women as a whole and not particularly unusual, ill, well, independent, dependent, irascible, helpful etc., and similarly with the mothers in the named midwife group. In this way the random errors should be fairly evenly distributed across both the conditions, and therefore should (at least theoretically) affect the midwives' performance in each setting in a similar, if random, way.

One other point is important here: if your subjects can be randomly allocated to conditions (e.g. to different treatments, or in this case, allocating mothers to a particular care model) so much the better, because the random errors should then be evenly distributed, again at least theoretically.

KEY CONCEPTS

- *Constant errors* are those factors that distort the results in a constant or predictable way. They can be eliminated or controlled by ensuring the procedures, conditions and other essential factors are similar.
- *Random errors* are those factors which obscure the results in a random or unpredictable way. They cannot be eliminated, although random selection and allocation of subjects will distribute them evenly across conditions (at least theoretically).

Activity 8.1   (Answers on page 237)

Look at the following hypotheses and identify the sources of constant and random error and their solutions:

H_1: Premature babies nursed on sheepskins gain weight more quickly than those nursed on cotton sheeting.

H_1: Mothers who drink more than 14 units of alcohol per week while pregnant are more likely to deliver pre-term than are those women who abstain from alcohol during pregnancy.

PROBABILITIES

If we cannot get rid of random errors, how can we be sure that the results from our experiment are due to some real and significant relationship between the variables, as predicted in the hypothesis, and not to the obscuring effect of random errors? The answer to this lies in the use of statistical tests. At a general level, when we use a statistical test to analyse a set of results, we end up with a numerical value. This value is looked up in a set of probability tables, to give us a probability or *p value*, which is expressed either as a decimal (e.g. 0.01) or as a percentage (e.g. 1%). *This p value tells us how probable it is that the results from our experiment are due to random errors.* It is very important to understand and remember this, as it is the basis of all statistical analyses.

Because this *p* value tells us how likely it is that the results from the experiment are due to random error (and *not* to the real and consistent relationship predicted in your hypothesis) then the smaller the *p* value, the *smaller* the possibility that random error or chance factors can account for your results. Therefore, by implication, the smaller the possibility that your results are due to random error, then the *greater* the possibility that they are due to the relationship you predicted in your hypothesis. Thus, the smaller the *p* value, the greater the implied support for your experimental hypothesis. Do bear in mind that it is highly unlikely that you will ever get 100% support for your hypothesis, and so *p* will always have a value greater than 0. If your *p* value is very low, then you can reject the null (no relationship) hypothesis, and conclude the experimental hypothesis has been supported. (Remember! When we carry out an experiment we do not set out to support our experimental hypothesis directly, but instead, we try to reject the null (no relationship) hypothesis).

Probability values, as was noted earlier, can be expressed either as a percentage or as a decimal. Therefore, if our p value was 5% (or 0.05) then we could say that there is a 5% chance that the results are due to random error. A p value of 3% means that there is a 3/100 chance that your results are due to the effects of chance or random error factors. Put crudely, then, the smaller the p value you obtain for your results the less the probability that random error can explain your findings and consequently, the better it is for your hypothesis.

Activity 8.2   (Answers on page 237)

Look at the following p values and order them in terms of greatest support for your experimental hypothesis. (Greatest support on the left, to least support on the right.)

$p = 5\%$ $p = 19\%$ $p = 7\%$ $p = 0.01\%$ $p = 15\%$ $p = 3\%$

When you have done this, convert each p value to a decimal.

KEY CONCEPTS

When you carry out a statistical analysis, you end up with a numerical value which you look up in a set of probability tables to give you a p value. The p value tells you how likely it is that the results from your experiment are due to random error or chance. The smaller the p value, the stronger the support for your hypothesis. P values are expressed as percentages or decimals.

Activity 8.3   (Answers on page 237)

Suppose you saw the following p values in a midwifery article, what do they mean in terms of the possibility of chance or random factors being responsible for the results?

p value	% probability that the results are due to chance
$p = 0.01$	
$p = 0.07$	
$p = 0.03$	
$p = 0.05$	
$p = 0.50$	

SIGNIFICANCE LEVELS

It was said earlier that if your p value was very small you could reject the null (no relationship)

hypothesis and conclude that your experimental hypothesis had been supported by the results. When the null hypothesis is rejected in this way, the results are said to be *significant*. But how small must your p value be before you can conclude that your results are significant? There is no simple answer to this as it depends upon the nature of the experiment you have carried out.

For example, suppose you had hypothesized that a new tactile-kinaesthetic programme was valuable in enhancing the progress of babies born at less than 28 weeks' gestation. To test this out, you give a group of premature babies the new programme and compare their progress with a group of comparable babies who did not receive the intervention. The results are analysed using the appropriate statistical test. Let us assume the resulting p value is 5%, which means that if you treated 100 very premature babies with the new programme, 95 are likely to improve as a result of the treatment but five would not (or if they did, it would be due to chance and not to the effects of the treatment). If nothing too awful happened to these five babies when they failed to respond to treatment, you would probably be quite happy to treat all very premature babies with the new treatment, since there is only a 5% potential for error. However, supposing that the new treatment, when it did not work, proved fatal, and killed the five babies instead. With this outcome you would probably require a much smaller error margin in your results — perhaps 1 error in every 1000 or 10 000 — before you recommended the new treatment. In other words, the effect of the random errors determines how small your p value must be before you can conclude your results are significant. We could compare this to placing a bet on Grand National Day. Supposing you have looked at the horses, and you have decided to place a bet on a particular horse; you have unwittingly formulated a hypothesis that there is a relationship between this horse and final placing. If you are only going to put 10p on this horse, you will not mind a fairly high significance level (or p value) because losing 10p is not too disastrous. However, if you have placed all your life-savings and assets on this horse, then you want to be very sure that it's going to win. In other words, you will want to ensure a small chance that random error will influence the outcome before you bet, since if you are wrong, the effects will be devastating.

The *p* value you decide upon in an experiment is called the *level of significance*. It is so-called because when you look up the results of your statistical analysis in a set of probability tables, you will find the *p* value for your results and if this *p* value is equal to or smaller than the significance level you have selected as being appropriate for your research, then your results are said to be *significant*. This means that you can reject the null (no relationship) hypothesis and accept that your experimental hypothesis has been supported. If the *p* value is larger than the significance level you have selected, your results are classed as not significant, which means you cannot reject the null hypothesis.

Therefore, it is up to you, the experimenter, to state what significance level you think is appropriate for a particular piece of research and the significance level you finally select will reflect the nature of your experiment. All this seems to leave the field wide open for you. However, a good rule-of-thumb if you are not doing anything that may have a disastrous outcome if you are wrong, is to use a cut-off point or significance level of 5%. So if you obtain a *p* value of 5% or less, then you can conclude that your results are significant and that your experimental hypothesis has been supported.

This point will be referred to again later.

MAKING ERRORS IN YOUR CONCLUSIONS REGARDING SIGNIFICANCE

When you have analysed your results and looked these up in the probability tables, you will obtain a probability or *p* value which is a statement of how likely it is that your results are due to random error. Usually, if this *p* value is 5% or less, the results are said to be significant and therefore support your experimental hypothesis. On the basis of such a conclusion, you would be in a position to make predictions and recommendations based on your findings.

However, it is possible to draw the wrong conclusions from your study and these errors are known as Type I and Type II errors.

Type I errors

These refer to those situations when we conclude our experimental hypothesis has been supported when, in fact, it has not. Such errors can be avoided by two safeguards:

1. Ensuring that the selected significance level is appropriate; in other words, do not use a significance level of more than 5% for most research, and reduce this to 1% in cases where any errors in your conclusions could be disastrous (see previous section).
2. Replication of the study and its findings by independent researchers adds credibility to the original conclusions.

Type II errors

These refer to situations when the experimental hypothesis is rejected in favour of the null (no relationship) hypothesis, when the data do, in reality, support the experimental hypothesis.

The chances of making this mistake can be reduced by:

1. Increasing the size of the sample.
2. Using a less stringent significance level.

It is essential when selecting a significance level that all the implications of any errors deriving from decisions about the results are considered. If they are not, then patient well-being could be at risk.

STATISTICAL AND CLINICAL SIGNIFICANCE OF RESEARCH FINDINGS

It should also be pointed out that results are sometimes statistically significant but yet have very little clinical meaning. For example, you might conduct a study of the relative strength of the pelvic floor muscles post-partum dependent on the type of exercise regime the women undertook. One group of women might exercise for 30 minutes per day and the other group for 60 minutes. Let us imagine at the end of the study that this latter group was found to have pelvic floor muscles which were significantly stronger statistically, but yet they still suffered a high level of stress incontinence. It could be said that these results were statistically significant but were clinically meaningless. Therefore, while significance levels are essential guides to deciding whether or not your data support your hypothesis, it is important to remember that these results should be considered in conjunction with their clinical implications.

KEY CONCEPTS

The *p value* states the probability of your results being due to chance or random error. If the *p* value is very small you can conclude that your results are significant. This means you can reject the null (no difference) hypothesis and conclude that your experimental hypothesis has been supported. The experimenter decides upon how small the error margin must be before the results are said to be significant. The size of the error margin is called the significance level. The decision about the size of the significance level is based on the effects of the error. If the error is likely to be disastrous, then the significance level is reduced. If the effects are not likely to be terrible, then the significance level can be increased. A good rule-of-thumb is to use a 5% significance level as long as you are not doing anything dangerous.

9

Matching the research design to the statistical test

DECIDING WHICH STATISTICAL TEST TO USE

The previous chapters have all been concerned with how to design a piece of research to test a hypothesis. Once you have designed and carried out your research, you need to analyse your data to find out whether the results do, in fact, support your hypothesis. The analysis involves using statistical tests. Essentially, what this means is that you apply a particular formula to your data and then work through the formula to get the answer. This answer is then looked up in the probability tables to see whether it supports your hypothesis. However, there is no single all purpose test which you can use to analyse your results, since each experimental design has an appropriate statistical test. Therefore, one of your tasks as a researcher is to match up the appropriate statistical test with your research design. If you select the wrong test to analyse your data, then your conclusions will be vitiated — it is as critical as that. Unfortunately, many people become very worried about this matching task, but as long as you ask yourself some basic questions about your design, you shouldn't have too much trouble. A word of warning first, though: when you are planning your research project, do ensure that you know which statistical test you will be using. All too often people carry out their experiment without doing this first and then find that they do not know how to analyse the results, or that they need a complicated computer programme to which they do not have access. So, make sure at the planning stage that you know which statistical test you will need for your design.

KEY CONCEPT

Each experimental design has its own statistical test which must be used when analysing the results. Thus, a key feature when planning your research is to match up the design with the appropriate statistical test.

Therefore, to decide on which statistical test to use with an experimental design, the following questions must be asked:

(1) Have you got an experimental or a correlational design?

To answer this, it is usually easier to look back at your hypothesis and decide whether you were predicting differences in your results (for example, between patient groups, types of treatment, elderly primigravidas vs. young primigravidas, or whether you were predicting patterns between sets of data. If you were predicting differences, you will have used an experimental design, while if you were predicting patterns, you will have used a correlational design. Since this is often a focus of confusion for some people, it may be useful to go over the concepts again.

If you look back to Chapter 2, you will see that in an experimental design, we manipulate one variable (the independent variable) and measure the effect of this on the other variable (the dependent variable). So, if you were hypothesizing that water births result in higher neonatal Apgar scores than do ordinary deliveries, your IV would be the type of delivery and the DV would be the Apgar scores. Typically you would design a study whereby you randomly selected a group of women having water births and a second group having normal land deliveries (manipulation of the IV) and you would compare the Apgar scores of babies (DV) delivered by each group to see if there was any difference between them. In other words you would be assessing the effect on the DV of manipulating the IV. Here then you are looking for differences in Apgar scores between the two groups dependent upon mode of delivery.

On the other hand, in some hypotheses you may predict patterns or similarities between the two variables; look back to page 59. These require a correlational design. In these hypotheses you are predicting either:

(a) that as scores on one variable go up, so the scores on the other variable will also go up (positive correlation)

or

(b) that as scores on one variable go up, so the scores on the other variable will go down (negative correlation).

For example, if you hypothesized that direct-entry midwifery students who do well on theory exams also do well on their practical assessments, you would take a group of students and look at their performance in both situations, on the assumption that the higher the theory mark, the higher the corresponding practical grade. This is called a *positive correlation*.

Alternatively, you may predict a link between the number of cigarettes a woman smokes during pregnancy and neonatal birth weight, such that the higher the number of cigarettes smoked, the lower the neonatal birth weight. This is called a *negative correlation*.

In these correlational designs you do not manipulate one variable to see what effect it has on the other; instead you take a whole range of scores on one variable and see whether they are related to a whole range of scores on the other variable. If you are still unclear about the differences between experimental and correlational designs, re-read Chapter 6.

(2) How many conditions are there?

If you have a correlational design, you need to ask whether you are comparing two sets of results, or more than two sets. Once you have answered this, you need only ask yourself about the levels of measurement you have on each variable. This point is dealt with in Chapter 17, which covers analysis of data deriving from correlational designs.

If you have an experimental design, however, you need to decide how many conditions you have (see page 54) since designs with only two conditions in total require a different type of statistical test from those with more than two conditions. For example, if you compared two groups of women, one of whom had received some treatment (experimental condition) and the other of whom had received no treatment (control condition), then you would have two conditions. If you had compared two types of treatment (i.e. two experimental conditions) you would again have two conditions. On the other hand, if you had compared the effectiveness of three treatment procedures, you would have three conditions. Look back to page 54 to refresh your memory on this.

(3) If you have an experimental design, is it a same, matched or different subject design?

The next question is concerned with whether you used the same, matched or different subjects in your experimental design. For example, did you use just one group of subjects for all conditions (e.g. comparing the attitudes of one group of midwives towards women with AIDS vs. women without AIDS). Or did you use two or more totally different groups of subjects and compare them in some way (e.g. a comparison of attendance levels at an ante-natal clinic of women from social class I vs. women from social class V?). Or did you use two or more groups of subjects who were matched on certain key features (e.g. a comparison of the quality of newly qualified midwives from three different colleges, which would necessitate matching the subjects on such variables as 'A'-level grades, attendance levels etc.) (see Ch. 7).

Remember, for the purposes of statistical analysis, matched and same subject designs are treated alike, so you only have to decide between:

same/matched subject design
or
different subject design.

These questions can be set out as decision charts like those in Figures 9.1 and 9.2. Note that the

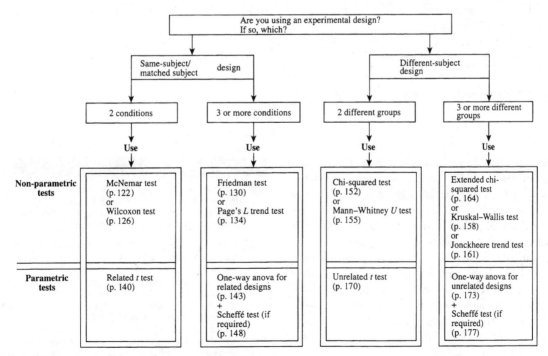

Figure 9.1 Choosing the correct test for an experimental design.

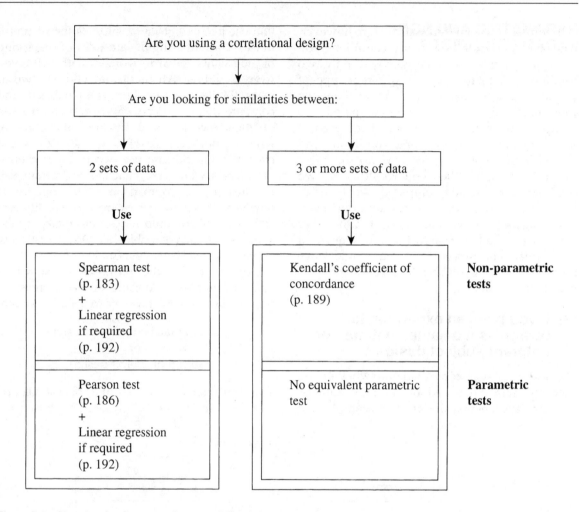

Figure 9.2 Choosing the correct test for a correlational design.

names of the appropriate statistical tests are given in the boxes on the charts. You can see from those charts that sometimes the names of two or three tests are given. This does not mean that any one of them can be selected but that instead each requires slightly different conditions for use, for example, a different level of measurement. These differences are outlined in the relevant chapter. You will also notice that you are given the choice of *non-parametric* or *parametric* tests. The differences between these will be outlined before proceeding to the decision charts for selecting your statistical test.

KEY CONCEPTS

Each experimental design has its own statistical test(s) which must be used to analyse the data. In order to select the appropriate statistical test for your own design you must ask yourself a number of questions:

1. Were you looking for differences (i.e. an experimental design) or patterns/similarities (i.e. a correlational design).
2. If you had a correlational design, you must also ask 'how many sets of data did I have?'
3. If you had an experimental design, then you must ask: How many conditions were there? (Two or more than two)
4. Did you use the same or matched subjects in each condition? Or did you use different subjects in each condition?

PARAMETRIC AND NON-PARAMETRIC TESTS

You will notice that in the boxes with the names of the statistical tests in Figures 9.1 and 9.2, there are the headings 'Parametric test' and 'Non-parametric test'. Essentially, for most of the designs you are likely to use, you have a choice of using a parametric test or a non-parametric test. What is the difference?

Basically, a parametric test is a much more sensitive tool of statistical analysis. If, for example, you are comparing responses to two different kinds of treatment, and there are differences in responsiveness, the parametric test is more likely to find them than is the non-parametric test. Perhaps the point can be clarified by an analogy. Supposing you were making a cake and you wanted to weigh out the ingredients. You have two weighing machines in the house, the bathroom scales and the kitchen scales. You could use your bathroom scales to weigh out your 8 oz of sugar, but they will give you a less accurate and less sensitive reading than your kitchen scales. The non-parametric test is like the bathroom scales as it will analyse your results, but it will not be as fine or as sensitive as the analysis of the parametric test (the kitchen scales).

If parametric tests are so good, then why do we bother with non-parametric tests at all? Like most things that are good, there are prices to pay and conditions to fulfil, and so it is with parametric tests. Before you can use one to analyse your results, four conditions have to be satisfied. The first of these is critical: your data must be of an interval/ratio level of measurement, since parametric tests cannot be used on nominal or ordinal data. *This condition cannot ever be violated.* The other three conditions are not quite as important, and may be waived to some degree. The first of these is that your subjects should be randomly selected from the population they represent. Second, your data should be normally distributed. As you will probably remember from Chapter 5, a normal distribution looks like an inverted U shape and you can plot your data on a graph to find out whether it is (more or less) normally distributed. Third, the variation in the results from each condition should be roughly the same. This means that the range of scores in each condition should be more or less similar. If, for instance, the scores in one condition ranged from 20–120, while for the other they ranged from 60–80, the degree of variation in each condition's scores would be too dissimilar for a parametric test to be used. On the other hand if they ranged from 50–100 in one condition and 60–90 in the other, this would be acceptable. To each of these three conditions we would add the caveat 'within reason', because parametric tests are said to be 'robust'. Essentially, what this means is that it does not matter too much if you cannot fulfil the last three conditions; as long as your data is of an interval/ratio level, and there are no glaring deviations with respect to the other three conditions, you can use a parametric test.

Table 9.1 may help to clarify this point.

If you are ever in doubt as to whether you have satisfied the conditions adequately, then use a non-parametric test. *So, when in doubt, use the non-parametric test.*

KEY CONCEPTS

The results from any research design may usually be analysed either by a parametric or a non-parametric test. A parametric test is much more sensitive and will identify significant results more readily than a non-parametric test. However, before you can use a parametric test, four conditions must be fulfilled:

- the data must be of an interval/ratio level
- the subjects should have been randomly selected
- the data should be normally distributed
- the variance in the results from each condition should be similar.

The first condition is essential.
The other three can be waived to some extent.
Non-parametric tests do not require these conditions to be fulfilled and can be used with any level of measurement.

Table 9.1 Levels of measurement for parametric and non-parametric tests

Level of measurement	Type of test which can be used
Nominal	Non-parametric
Ordinal	Non-parametric
Interval	Parametric and non-parametric
Ratio	Parametric and non-parametric

ANOTHER WAY OF DECIDING WHICH TEST TO USE

Alternatively, some students prefer to make this decision by using diagrammatic representations of the design. These are set out in Tables 9.2–9.6. You should note that in Examples 2, 4 and 6 you can use more than three groups or conditions and still apply the same test.

Experimental designs

Table 9.2   Same-subject designs

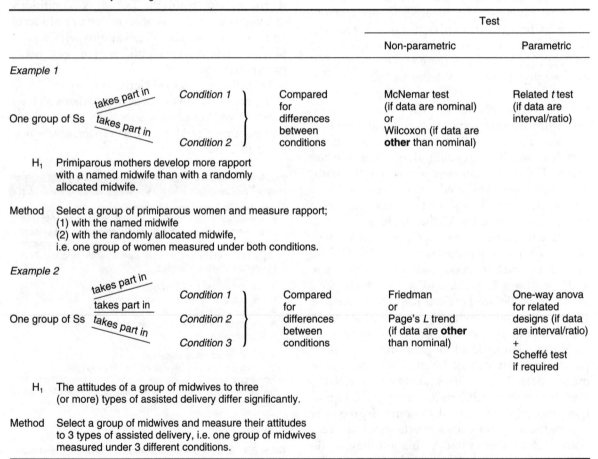

| | | Test | |
		Non-parametric	Parametric
Example 1			
One group of Ss takes part in Condition 1 / takes part in Condition 2	Compared for differences between conditions	McNemar test (if data are nominal) or Wilcoxon (if data are **other** than nominal)	Related *t* test (if data are interval/ratio)

H₁   Primiparous mothers develop more rapport with a named midwife than with a randomly allocated midwife.

Method   Select a group of primiparous women and measure rapport;
(1) with the named midwife
(2) with the randomly allocated midwife,
i.e. one group of women measured under both conditions.

Example 2			
One group of Ss takes part in Condition 1 / takes part in Condition 2 / takes part in Condition 3	Compared for differences between conditions	Friedman or Page's *L* trend (if data are **other** than nominal)	One-way anova for related designs (if data are interval/ratio) + Scheffé test if required

H₁   The attitudes of a group of midwives to three (or more) types of assisted delivery differ significantly.

Method   Select a group of midwives and measure their attitudes to 3 types of assisted delivery, i.e. one group of midwives measured under 3 different conditions.

Table 9.3   Different-subject designs

				Test	
				Non-parametric	Parametric
Example 3 Subject group 1	takes part in	*Condition 1*	⎫ ⎬ Compared ⎭ for differences between conditions	Chi-squared test (if data are nominal) or Mann-Whitney *U* test (if data are **other** than nominal)	Unrelated *t* test (if data are interval/ratio)
Subject group 2	takes part in	*Condition 2*			

H₁   Male premature babies are more likely to suffer respiratory
      complications following delivery than are female premature babies.

Method   Select a group of male premature babies and a group of female
          premature babies and compare the degree of respiratory complication.

Example 4 Subject group 1	takes part in	*Condition 1*	⎫ ⎬ Compared ⎭ for differences between conditions	Extended Chi-squared test (if data are nominal) or Kruskal-Wallis or Jonckheere trend (if data are **other** than nominal)	One-way anova for unrelated designs (if data are interval/ ratio) + Scheffé test if required
Subject group 2	takes part in	*Condition 2*			
Subject group 3	takes part in	*Condition 3*			

H₁   There is a difference in responsiveness to
      pelvic floor exercises in women with no children,
      2 children or 4 + children.

Method   Select 3 groups of women: 1 with no children,
          1 with 2 children and 1 with 4 or more children and
          compare their responsiveness to treatment,
          i.e. 3 different groups of Ss compared
(This is an extension of Example 3.)

Table 9.4 Matched subject designs

				Test	
				Non-parametric	Parametric

Example 5
Subjects **matched**
on key
variables

Subject group 1	_takes part in_	*Condition 1*	⎫ Compared for differences between conditions	McNemar (if data are nominal) or Wilcoxon (if data are **other** than nominal)	Related *t* test (if data are interval/ratio)
Subject group 2	_takes part in_	*Condition 2*	⎭		

H₁   TENS is more effective than inhalation
analgesia during the first stage of labour for controlling pain.

Method   Take two groups of women, matched on certain key factors,
e.g. age, parity, fetal position etc, of which one group has received
TENS and the other inhalation analgesia. Compare reported pain
levels, i.e. two groups matched on certain critical factors and compared.

Example 6
Subjects **matched**
on key
variables

	takes part in				
Subject group 1	_takes part in_	*Condition 1*	⎫ Compared for differences between conditions	Friedman or Page's *L* trend (if data are **other** than nominal)	One-way anova for related designs (if data are interval/ratio) + Scheffé test if required
Subject group 2	_takes part in_	*Condition 2*	⎬		
Subject group 3		*Condition 3*	⎭		

H₁   To extend the hypothesis in Example 5, you add a
further group of women, on narcotics.

Method   You select a further group of women, matched with groups
1 and 2 on the same critical factors and compare the reported pain levels,
i.e. 3 groups of Ss matched on certain critical factors and compared.

Correlational designs

Table 9.5 A correlational design where two sets of scores are involved

	Test	
	Non-parametric	Parametric
Example 7 These may predict: a. positive correlation, i.e. high scores on one variable are associated with high scores on the other (Fig. 9.3).	Spearman (if data are **other** than nominal) + Linear regression if required	Pearson (if data are interval/ratio) + Linear regression if required

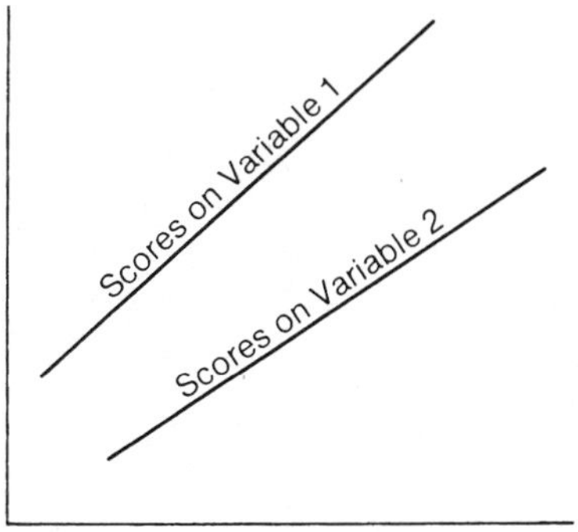

Figure 9.3

H₁   There is a correlation between the age of the mother and the length of the first stage of labour, such that the older the mother, the longer the first stage.

Method   Select a whole range of primiparous mothers and note the length of the first stage of labour.

b. negative correlation i.e. high scores on one variable are related to low scores on the other (Fig. 9.4).	Spearman (if data are **other** than nominal) + Linear regression if required	Pearson (if data are interval/ratio) + Linear regression if required

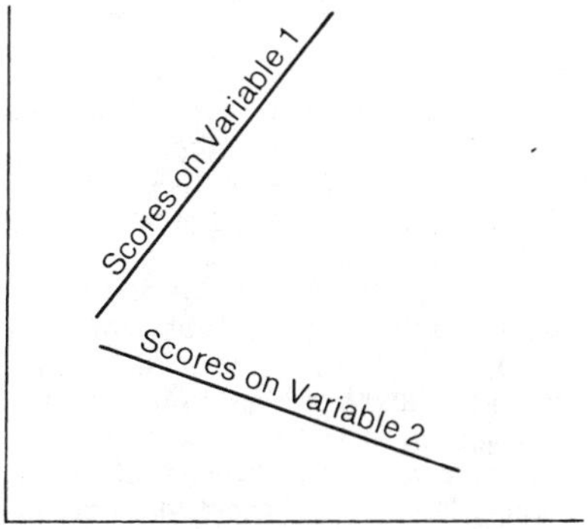

Figure 9.4

H₁   There is a correlation between the number of cigarettes smoked during pregnancy and neonatal birth weight, with high numbers of cigarettes being associated with low birth weights.

Method   Select a whole range of smoking mothers (e.g. non-smokers to 60 + per day and measure the birth weights of their babies).

Table 9.6 A correlational design where more than two sets of scores are involved

	Test	
	Non-parametric	Parametric

Example 8
Where you are looking for the degree of similarity between 3 or more sets of scores (Fig. 9.5).

Kendall coefficient of concordance (if data are **other** than nominal)

There is no parametric test

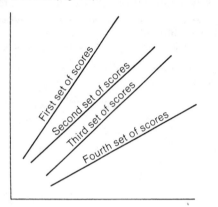

Figure 9.5

(Here you can only predict a positive correlation; see Ch. 17 for the reason why).

H₁ There is a positive correlation among midwives' judgements of the health outcomes of 6 premature babies.

Method Select 4 midwives and ask them to rank order 6 premature babies for their assumed health outcomes (i.e. how likely a full recovery will be made).

Activity 9.1 (Answers on page 238)

Using the decision guidelines presented earlier, look at the following brief descriptions of some research projects, and decide which statistical tests you should use. (Quote both the parametric and non parametric alternatives where relevant, since at this stage you would not know whether your data would allow you to use a parametric test.)

1. In order to compare the working preferences of a group of newly qualified midwives and a group of midwives with at least 10 years' experience, you select two groups each of 30 midwives and ask them to indicate whether they prefer community based work or hospital based work.
2. To compare the fetal movements of male vs. female fetuses, you select two groups of 15 women, post amniocentesis, one group of which has known male fetuses and the other group female fetuses. The two groups are matched on certain key factors, such as gestational stage, maternal age and well-being, parity etc. and the average numbers of fetal movements are compared over a 4 week period.
3. On the assumption that fundal height is related to gestational stage, such that the greater the height, the greater the gestational stage, you select a number of women covering a range of fundal heights and you then find out their gestational stage.
4. To find out whether satisfaction with care is greater in trust as opposed to non-trust status maternity units, you randomly select 25 women who have just delivered in each unit and ask them to rate on a 5-point scale their satisfaction with care.
5. To compare the effectiveness of three types of pain relief during labour, you select three groups of primips who have received either TENS, Entonox or Pethidine and who are matched on certain key variables, such as age, health, gestational stage, etc. Within 30 minutes of parturition you ask the women to rate on a visual analogue pain scale how much pain they experienced.
6. In order to compare the birth experience of women delivered at home, in a GP unit and a consultant unit, you select 15 women from each context and ask them to rate their satisfaction with their experience on a 5-point scale.

LOOKING UP THE RESULTS OF YOUR ANALYSIS IN THE PROBABILITY TABLES

Let us suppose you have designed and carried out your experiments and have analysed the results using the correct statistical test. As you will remember, it was stated earlier that a statistical test will give you a result which you look up in a set of probability tables in order to find out whether your results are significant and support your hypothesis. This process will be described more fully in the chapters which deal with the particular statistical tests, but an outline of the general principles will be given here.

When you have worked through the appropriate statistical test or formula, you will end up with a number which you look up in a set of probability tables for that particular test. It is important to note that each statistical test has its own set of probability tables, which you will find at the back of this book. Thus, the Mann-Whitney *U*-test will provide you with a numerical value which is looked up in the probability tables for the Mann-Whitney test (see Tables A2.7a–d). The Wilcoxon test provides you with a numerical value which is looked up in the probability tables for the Wilcoxon test, and so on. More details on this will be given with the description for each statistical test.

However, before you can look up that numerical value, some tests require an additional numerical value — either the number of Ss you used or a number called the *degrees of freedom* (*d.f.*). This concept which is quite a complex one to understand refers to the degree of potential variability in the data. (The reader is referred to Ferguson (1976) for a discussion of this.) However, although the concept is hard to understand, the d.f. is very easy to calculate. The details of how to do this will be given in the description of the tests which require the d.f. However, before you can conclude whether your numerical value represents a significant result from your experiment, you require one further piece of information, namely, whether you have a one- or two-tailed hypothesis.

ONE- AND TWO-TAILED HYPOTHESES

The way in which you state your hypothesis has implications for how you look up your numerical value in the probability tables. Some hypotheses are stated very specifically in that they predict precisely what the outcomes will be. For example, if we hypothesized that women who drink more than 14 units of alcohol per week will be more likely to have low-birth weight babies than will women who are teetotal during pregnancy, we are predicting a very precise outcome, in that we are expecting lower birth weights for women who drink 14+ units of alcohol. Again, if we hypothesized that IVF treatment caused more psychological distress than GIFT, we are making a very precise prediction that IVF will create more distress than GIFT. These are known as *one-tailed hypotheses or tests* because the results are expected to go in one particular direction. The following are all examples of one-tailed hypotheses:

1. Women who are shaved prior to delivery experience a higher incidence of infection than do those who are not shaved.
2. Women who have their first child after the age of 35 are more likely to breast feed.
3. Male neonates are more likely to experience jaundice during the first week than are female neonates.
4. Deep vein thrombosis is more likely to occur following caesarean section than a vaginal delivery.
5. Women who have had previous caesarean sections are more likely to experience uterine rupture than are those who have had vaginal deliveries.

However, hypotheses can be stated much more vaguely, without any precise predictions. For example, it might have been hypothesized that there is a difference in the birth weights of babies born to women who have been either teetotal during pregnancy or who have consumed 14+ units of alcohol per week. In contrast to the one-tailed hypothesis which predicted that the birth weights would be lower in women who had consumed large quantities of alcohol, this revised hypothesis allows for the possibility that birth weight could be higher either for the tee-total group or for the high alcohol group. The hypothesis simply predicts differences in the birth weight without specifying which group would have the larger babies. Similarly, we could restate the IVF/GIFT hypothesis such that we predict differences in psychological distress according to the fertility treatment undergone. Here we are not saying which group will experience greater distress but simply that there will be a difference in distress between the two groups. It could, therefore, be that the IVF group records more distress or that the GIFT group records more. These hypotheses are known as *two-tailed hypotheses or tests* because the results could go in either of two directions. The following are examples of two-tailed hypotheses:

1. There is a difference in the length of the first stage of labour depending on whether the membranes rupture spontaneously or artificially.
2. There is a difference in the incidence of post-partum psychosis among women who have had fertility problems and those who have not.
3. There is a difference in clinical skills amongst direct-entry midwives and those who have completed an 18-month post-registration training.
4. There is a difference in the healing rate of perineal wounds among women who have either saline, or plain water baths.
5. There is a difference in the amount of amniotic fluid present at 30 weeks' gestation according to whether the mother is over 35 or under 30 at conception.

Activity 9.2 (Answers on page 238)

Look at the following hypotheses and identify which are one-tailed and which are two-tailed:

1. Parentcraft classes are more effective when both partners attend rather than the mother only.
2. Forceps deliveries and ventouse extractions have different effects on maternal well-being.
3. Women who are more than 10% overweight at conception are more likely to have an operative delivery than are those who are of normal weight.
4. There is a difference in the length of the second stage of labour according to ethnic origin.
5. Pre-conceptual counselling leads to a greater take-up of ante-natal services.

Look back at the examples of one-tailed hypotheses and convert them to two-tailed hypotheses.
Then look at the examples of two-tailed hypotheses and convert them to one-tailed hypotheses. (It does not matter in which direction you predict the results will go.)

Why is choosing a one-tailed or two-tailed hypothesis important? Supposing you had stated a one-tailed hypothesis, (i.e. that your results will go in one specific direction) and having done your experiment and statistics, had ended up with a p value of 1%. This means that there is a 1% chance that your results are due to random error. However, had your hypothesis been two-tailed instead, you would be predicting that your results could go in either of two directions. Therefore, because your results could go in either of two directions there will be twice the possibility that random error could account for your results and so for exactly the same data your p value would be doubled to 2%, i.e. a 2% chance that your results are due to random error. Let us illustrate this with an example.

Suppose you had hypothesized that exercise is more effective than external cephalic version (ECV) for rotating breech presentations (i.e. you have stated a one-tailed hypothesis), you would probably have selected two groups of women, one of which received exercise and the other ECV. You would expect a greater likelihood of rotation of the fetuses of the exercise group following treatment. Suppose again, that your results suggest this is the case, and you end up with a p value of 5%. This means that there is a 5/100 chance that your results are due to error, and that for every 100 women treated in this way, five would not improve significantly as a result of treatment. However, had you simply hypothesized that ECV and exercise are differentially effective in rotating a breech presentation fetus then you would expect either the exercise group or the ECV group to do better. This is now a 2-tailed hypothesis, because you have allowed for the possibility that the results could go in either of two directions. You carry out exactly the same study and achieve exactly the same results, but your *p* value would now be 10% (i.e. doubled) because if your results are expected to go in either of two directions, there must be twice the possibility that random error can account for the results. Let us see how this works in practice by turning to Table A2.2 (Wilcoxon).

At the top of the table you will see two headings: 'Level of significance for one-tailed tests' and 'Level of significance for two-tailed tests'. You can see that every level of significance for a two-tailed test is twice the corresponding level for a one-tailed test, i.e. 0.10 is twice 0.05; 0.05 is twice 0.025; 0.02 is twice 0.01; 0.01 is twice 0.005.

Many students ask how they should decide on whether a hypothesis should be one or two-tailed. The answer to this lies in the background theory associated with the research you are carrying out. For example, if you are concerned with the relationship between smoking and respiratory problems in the neonate, the background reading that you will have done prior to embarking on this research will probably have revealed that:

- smoking is related to low birth weight babies
- prematurity is associated with respiratory problems
- ultrasound evidence suggests that fetal breathing patterns are disturbed by both maternal active and passive smoking.

Therefore, it would be reasonable to predict that babies born to women who smoke are more likely to have respiratory complications (i.e. a specific one-tailed prediction). Thus, the existing research and literature will guide your prediction here.

If, however, you were interested in looking at the effects of having a named midwife on mothers' experiences, you may well have found background literature which suggests that some women are more comfortable with anonymity of health care, especially during delivery, while others prefer that the intimacy of the birth experience is shared with someone they already know. Thus, because the background research is less clear cut here, you would probably not wish to make a specific prediction about women's atti-

tudes to the named midwife, and would therefore formulate a two-tailed hypothesis. In other words, existing research knowledge and theory should guide you when making predictions in the hypothesis.

KEY CONCEPTS

When you use a statistical test to analyse the results from your research you will end up with a numerical value.

This value is looked up in the set of probability tables which are specific to the statistical test you have used. In order to look up the value you will also need to know either the d.f. value or the number of subjects who participated in the experiment — each statistical test requires one or the other. Additionally, you must decide whether your hypothesis is *one-tailed* (predicts that the results will go in *one* direction only) or *two-tailed* (predicts that the results will go in either of *two* directions). Hypotheses which are two-tailed have *twice* the probability that random error can account for the results, and so will affect the *p* value for your data.

Using these two values, you will end up with a *p* value, i.e. a decimal or percentage probability that your results are due to random error. According to the size of the *p* value you can either claim your results are significant (i.e. support your hypothesis) or not significant (do not support your hypothesis.)

A CHECKLIST OF STAGES INVOLVED IN SETTING UP YOUR RESEARCH PROJECT

Let us recap on the essential guidelines involved in designing a piece of research that have been covered so far. Please note that this checklist only applies to studies which are involved in hypothesis testing.

1. Have you formulated an experimental hypothesis which clearly predicts a relationship between two variables? Have you stated your null (no relationship) hypothesis?
2. Are you going to test this hypothesis using a correlational design (i.e., are you predicting that as scores on one variable go up, so scores on the other variable go up or down accordingly)? Or are you going to use an experimental design which will test for differences between conditions or subject groups? If you are going to use a correlational design, go on to Chapter 17.

3. If you are using a correlational design, what level of data do you have on each variable?

4. If you are going to use an experimental design, have you sorted out what you are going to measure (i.e. what is the DV?) Have you decided when you will take the pretest measures of the DV and the post-test measures? What level of measurement are you using?

5. Will you be using a control group? Is this ethically acceptable? If you are not, how many experimental conditions have you decided upon?

6. Who are your subjects going to be? Can you select them randomly? How many will you need?

7. Are you going to use a different, same or matched subject design? Are you sure that this is the most appropriate design for your hypothesis? Why? If you are going to use a matched subject design, have you identified the critical variables on which the Ss have to be matched?

8. Is there any need to counterbalance the conditions to overcome order effects?

9. Have you controlled for experimenter bias?

10. What are the sources of constant error? Have you controlled or eliminated them? Have you taken account of the random errors as far as you are able?

11. Is your experimental hypothesis one or two-tailed?

12. What test will you need to analyse your results?

10

Putting the theory into practice

Everything that has been said so far is theory. To carry out a piece of research, you need to put this theory into practice. This section is concerned with providing some practical guidelines to help you set up your research project.

PREPARATION FOR RESEARCH

Stating your aims and objectives

It is essential that you clarify in your own mind what the object of your research is to be. All too often students say rather vaguely 'I'd like to do something on birth plans/breast feeding/miscarriage' etc. without having any idea what exactly they want to investigate. While a general topic area like this is a good starting point, since it defines your area of interest, you will need to develop a more precise idea of what you are trying to find out before you start your research. In some cases, this will involve collecting large amounts of data for a survey.

Alternatively, you may wish to test a specific hypothesis at the outset. If this is the case, ensure that the hypothesis conforms to the principles outlined on pages 46–47, in that it makes a clear prediction of a relationship between two variables, and that it is a testable hypothesis. Some topics in which you are interested may simply not be researchable because the necessary skills, techniques, procedures etc. are not available or ethically acceptable, or because the project would involve major policy changes, which are out of the control of the researcher or would take too long or involve too many people. So do ask yourself whether the hypothesis is testable and feasible.

Furthermore, do *define* the terms in your hypothesis clearly and unambiguously. Using terms like 'safe practice', or 'effective' or 'improvement' are too vague as they stand and you must have a clear idea of what they mean in *real* terms.

Alternatively, if you are interested in a particular area and simply want to explore it fully without formulating any hypothesis (i.e. some form of survey technique) you will still need to clarify your aims and terms so that you can define precisely the area to be studied.

Reviewing the background research

Once you have formulated your hypothesis or defined your survey area, you will have to review all the relevant literature relating to the area you want to investigate. The purposes of this activity are to:

1. Acquaint yourself fully with the theoretical background to the topic, so that you have a full understanding of the issue.
2. Familiarize yourself with all the existing research that has been carried out in the area, firstly to ensure that your own project has not been conducted before, and secondly to provide a context for your experiment. These points are particularly important if you want to write up your research project for publication in a journal.
3. Consider the possible methods and techniques of conducting your research.

However, having just said that one of the purposes of reviewing the research literature is to ensure that your intended study has not been carried out before (i.e. it is an original piece of work), there will be occasions when you simply want to replicate someone else's experiment in order to see whether their results apply to your own professional setting. In such a case, the process is slightly different, in that your aim or hypothesis will be identical to that of the study you wish to replicate, and the entire experimen-

tal procedure will also be the same. You will still need to acquaint yourself with the background literature so that you are familiar with the theories and related studies, but its purpose is obviously not to ensure the originality of your project.

It should be pointed out that it is perfectly acceptable to replicate an existing study as long as this is your real intention and not just the result of your not being aware of what has already been done in the area!

Do not underestimate the importance of a really thorough search of the literature — there is nothing more infuriating than to carry out a superb (!) piece of research with earth-shattering results, only to be told by a colleague that Bloggs et al. performed an identical piece of research a year ago. A full search of the literature will prevent time wastage and disappointment. That having been said, there are a number of useful sources of midwifery research information:

MIDIRS (Midwifery digest)

An extremely informative quarterly journal containing information from 460 journals. The journals are scanned and the most interesting information is presented in the digest. The journal contains information on study days and conferences, book reviews, specially commissioned papers on current key issues, together with a synopsis of relevant research in midwifery. There is an index of subjects covered at the back of each issue. Also offered is a very good, competitively priced literature search service. For example, a UK subscriber to MIDIRS can obtain a search on a range of standard topics for £3.95, while a non-subscriber can obtain this service for £8.00. Further details can be obtained from MIDIRS, 9 Elmdale Road, Clifton, Bristol BS8 1SL. Telephone 01179–251791.

Nursing Research Abstracts

This is a quarterly publication of nursing, midwifery and health visiting research which has been carried out in the UK. The Index contains information about books, articles and other reports, as well as details of unpublished research studies currently in progress. The Index is organized under major subject headings, within which synopses of articles are included. There are also alphabetical lists of both the specific topic areas covered as well as the authors. The Index is an information system only and does not undertake to supply copies of articles. The Index is also available on a computerized database of the DH/DSS library — DHSS-DATA. Further information can be obtained from:

Debra Jessop and Kerry Hanson,
Department of Health,
Index of Nursing Research,
5E05 Quarry House,
Quarry Hill,
Leeds LS2 7UE.
(01132–545561/2).

Nursing Bibliography

This is a monthly publication, listing current articles in nursing and allied health care areas. The Bibliography is a selection of new material received in the Royal College of Nursing Library each month and consists of articles, books and dissertations. The Bibliography is divided into two sections, the first of which covers journal articles and the second, books and theses. The journal section is organized alphabetically by subject headings and under each subject heading the authors are arranged alphabetically. Cross referencing is included if an article has more than one principal topic. The second section on books and theses is also organized alphabetically by author. Photocopies of articles contained in the bibliography can be obtained from the Royal College of Nursing Library, 20 Cavendish Square, London, W1M 0AB, telephone 0171–409–3333. The cost of the photocopying depends on the length of the article and whether or not the person requesting the photocopy is a member of the RCN.

American Journal of Nursing International Nursing Index

This is a quarterly publication, indexing over 270 international nursing journals as well as all nursing articles published in allied journals currently indexed by Index Medicus (see below). It also lists all new nursing and allied books. The Index is arranged in two sections, an alphabetical subject section and an alphabetical author section. The subject section gives full reference details of each article, but no summary of its content. The information in the Index is also on a computer database Medline. Further information can be obtained from:

International Nursing Index,
555 West 57th Street,
New York,
10019–2961, USA.

Popular Medical Index

Provides indexes of medical articles from over 60 journals, from popular magazines e.g. 'Woman' and 'Good Housekeeping' to more academic journals like the British Medical Journal. It also lists new books in the health care field. Its coverage is primarily topics of popular interest.

Index is by subject area which is cross referenced to other articles written in the area. Most items referenced can be obtained from the British Library, Lending Division. For further information contact Sally Knight, Norton Mede, 77 Norton Road, Letchworth, Herts, SG6 1AD.

NMI

NMI is a monthly index of articles relevant to nursing, midwifery and community care. It is based on journals received in a selection of hospitals based in the south of England, as well as those kept by Bournemouth University. The Index is arranged alphabetically by subject headings, which provide full references for all articles published on that topic. No synopsis of the article's content is provided. Within each subject heading, the authors are listed in alphabetical order. Details are available from:

College Library Network Publications,
c/o Bournemouth University Library,
Bournemouth University,

Dorset House,
Talbot Campus,
Fern Barrow,
Poole,
Dorset BH12 5BB.

Index Medicus

Index Medicus is, as it suggests, a medical index citing all the medical research which has been published in over 3000 journals. However, it should be pointed out that it does not cover nursing or midwifery journals. It is produced monthly, and a cumulative volume is issued annually. There are two stages to using Index Medicus. The first stage involves using a volume called MeSH (Medical Subject Headings) which contains all the official subject headings under which articles are classified in Index Medicus itself. It is essential to consult MeSH before proceeding, for two reasons:

1. You could waste a considerable amount of time searching through Index Medicus for a topic heading which is not officially used. For example, you might be interested in hemicrania. Thus you would look this up in MeSH. You would find the following: 'Hemicrania *see* Migraine'.

This tells you that hemicrania is classified as migraine in Index Medicus and that you should refer to this heading instead.

2. MeSH provides a list of related topics in which you might be interested, e.g.

Mental Health Services
see related   Halfway Houses
                 Hospital Psychiatric Departments
                 Hospitals, Psychiatric

Once you have identified all the subject areas which may be relevant to you, move on to Index Medicus itself. The first half of the Index Medicus volume has an alphabetical list of research topics, which is followed by titles of articles published in the area, the author(s) and a reference to the journal where the article was originally published. The second half has an alphabetical list of researchers followed by what they have published and where the article can be located.

Thus, if you just want to find out what has been done on placenta praevia over the last decade, you simply find out the official listing of this topic in MeSH and then look this up in the last ten issues of Index Medicus and make a note of all the relevant articles, so you can go and read them in the original journal. Alternatively, if you know that Payne is famous for her work on analgesia during labour, you would look up Payne in the name section of Index Medicus to find out what she has published recently. You would similarly make a note of where to find the relevant articles and go and read the originals. If when reading the article, it appears to be relevant, make a note of it (see next point) and its content. You might also want to look at the list of references at the end of the article to see if there are any important ones which you have missed.

You will find that the journal title is given in abbreviated form. If you are not sure about the abbreviations, you will find a list of all the journals referred to, together with their shortened form in the January issue of Index Medicus.

In addition, many articles, although having English titles, are written in a foreign language. These articles can be identified by the square brackets which enclose the title. The language of the original paper is provided at the end of this, together with information on whether or not an English abstract is available.

If you are just starting a literature search on an area which is fairly new to you, articles which review subject areas are particularly useful, since they provide you with an excellent résumé of the topic as well as a list of useful references. Review papers are listed at the front of each monthly issue of Index Medicus and in the first volume of the annual publication.

A particularly easy way of carrying out your literature search is an on-line computer facility, which many medical libraries run. Medline is the major computer database and is the CD-ROM version of Index Medicus. It has details of articles from 3000 of the world's most important journals in the areas of nursing, midwifery, medicine and dentistry. Many medical libraries offer courses in how to use Medline fully; alternatively you could seek help from library staff. Computer searches are especially valuable if you are interested in a particularly esoteric topic, such as 'Effectiveness of locally applied compresses in the treatment of thrombosed prolapsed piles during the third trimester'. However, you do have to pay for this facility and the cost will depend on the number of articles produced. Information about the availability of this service should be obtained from your library. (It should be noted that there is an International Nursing Index which works according to the same format, but has the drawback of referring to numerous journals which are not available in this country.)

Health Service Abstracts

This index covers major topic areas in the health services. Entries are made under key topics listed at the start of each index and each entry has a full reference as well as a summary of contents. There is also an alphabetical keyword index and author index. The information is also contained on DATA-STAR. Lending and photocopying services are only available to members of staff of the Departments of Health and Social Security. Further information can be obtained from:

Department of Health and Social Security
Library Services,
Skipton House,
80 London Road,
London SE1 6LW.

Applied Social Sciences Index and Abstracts (ASSIA)

This bi-monthly Index covers information on a range of topics, including health. It indexes professional journals, general interest periodicals and weeklies. It is divided into four sections. The main section provides abstracts of the articles, together with a full reference. The second section is an author index, the third section a subject index and the final section a source index, all arranged alphabetically. Further information can be obtained from:

The Editor, ASSIA,
Bowker-Saur Ltd,
Maypole House,
Maypole Road,
East Grinstead,
W Sussex,
RH19 1HH.

Miscellaneous Indexes

All the following Indexes have a self-explanatory topic coverage and may be of peripheral interest to the midwife.

Ethnic Minorities Health: A Current Awareness Bulletin
Medical Library,
Field House Teaching Centre,
Bradford Royal Infirmary,
Bradford,
West Yorkshire,
BD9 6RJ,
01274-364130.

Physiotherapy Index
Medical Information Centre,
British Library,
Boston Spa,
Wetherby,
West Yorkshire,
LS23 7BQ,
01937–546039.

Occupational Therapy Index
Address as above.

Social Service Abstracts
Social Service Abstracts,
Room G12,
Wellington House,
133–155 Waterloo Road,
London SE1 8UG,
0171-972-4206.

For those who have computing facilities there is also available an on-line database called AMED (Allied and Alternative Medicine) and a CD-ROM database called CINAHL (Cumulative Index to Nursing and Allied Health) both of which might provide useful information.

These Indexes, while an invaluable source of information on the available literature are by no means exhaustive, since there may be research projects on the fringe of conventional care practices which are not included or which are thought to be more appropriately classified elsewhere. It is a good idea, therefore, to browse through any professional journals which you think may contain salient articles, as well as through textbooks on the topic.

Reference information

Keep a card index of all the references you think are useful. For each relevant reference use one large index card and include, for journal articles:

- the full name of the author
- the date of the journal
- the precise title of the article
- the precise title of the journal where the article appears
- the volume (and part if relevant) of the journal
- the first and last page numbers of the article
- a résumé of the article with all the relevant details.

For chapter references in a book, where the book has an editor, include:

- the full name of the author of the chapter
- the date of publication of the book
- the title of the chapter
- the full name of the editor
- the full title of the book
- where the book was published
- the name of the publisher
- a résumé of the chapter, with all the relevant details.

For references to a book which has an author rather than an editor, include:

- the full name of the author
- the date of publication of the book
- the full title of the book
- where the book was published
- the name of the publisher
- a résumé of the relevant information.

You may think this is rather fussy, but I can assure you that a fully detailed card index file is worth its weight in gold. All too often researchers assume (and I have been amongst them) that if they need a particular reference again, they will know where to find it and so then fail either to make a note of it at all or they make an insufficiently detailed note of it. I can guarantee that by the time you have completed your project and you are ready to write it up, your memory for references will have let you down and you will consequently waste hours in libraries trying to track down a piece of information which you are sure you saw on the top right-hand page of a newish blue book. Shortcutting references really is not worth the time, frustration and energy so do keep a full card index of all relevant references as you go along. And, in addition, if you continue to research a topic, such a fund of references will be used time and again.

Deciding how you will carry out the project

Once you have completed a thorough literature review and made sure that your proposed project has not been carried out before, you must then decide on the best method of proceeding with your research. Are you going to conduct a survey, whereby you collect a large quantity of data and then use some form of descriptive statistics to highlight important features of it (Ch. 5)? Or are you going to use a correlational design whereby you measure two (or more) variables to see whether they co-vary in some predicted way (Ch. 6)? Or is an experiment more appropriate for the particular project, which will involve manipulating one variable to see what effect it has on the other (Ch. 6)?

To re-cap on the salient issues involved in each approach:

Survey methods involve collecting a large quantity of data on a particular subject and using descriptive statistics to highlight the important aspects of the data. Surveys can be used for a number of purposes:

- to describe the topic area, e.g. how many women suffer from some degree of skin pigmentation during pregnancy, their ages, parity, social class, previous health, occupation, weeks' gestation at onset of pigmentation etc.

- to pinpoint problem areas. If, in the above example, you found that women who worked with VDU systems were more likely to develop the butterfly mask of pregnancy, you might want to establish whether or not there is a causal link. This might then give rise to an experimental study where you tested this hypothesis.
- to identify trends, both past and present. Is there, for instance, an increased tendency towards fetal alcohol syndrome over the last decade? If so, it is conceivable that this trend may continue. If it does, then this might point the way towards developing appropriate health education programmes specifically targeted at women of child-bearing age.

Remember, though, that survey techniques are unsuitable for testing specific hypotheses. For this, experimental and correlational designs are needed.

Experimental designs are used to test whether the relationship predicted between the two variables in the hypothesis actually exists. To do this one of the variables must be manipulated and the effects of this on the other variable are then measured. Such an approach has to be carefully designed and controlled, which may involve the researcher in a considerable amount of effort. The results of this approach have to be analyzed using statistical tests (see Chs. 13–17). However, if the experiment has been carried out properly, the results can provide very useful answers, by identifying causes and effects of certain events. The approach can also establish which of a number of treatment procedures is more effective, which types of women respond best to particular analgesias etc. and so may be especially useful in streamlining and systematizing the profession.

However, it does, of course, have its disadvantages. Experiments can be complicated and time-consuming to carry out and they may be entirely unsuitable if any ethical issues are involved. For example, it would be of dubious ethical value to look at the effects of psycho-prophylactic relaxation techniques during childbirth on length of labour by comparing a group who had been trained in the technique with a group who had had no preparation for childbirth at all. In such cases, alternative approaches must be considered. One such is the correlational design.

Correlational designs are used to test hypotheses where it would be unethical to manipulate deliberately the independent variable (in the latter case, relaxation techniques) to see what effect it had on the dependent variable (length of labour). In correlational designs, the researcher simply takes a range of measures on each variable to ascertain whether they vary together in an associated way. For example, are high scores on one variable associated with high scores on the other? Or alternatively, are high scores on one variable associated with low scores on the other? Because the technique does not involve any artificial manipulation of patients or treatments, it is easier to carry out than experimental procedures and can more easily be used in naturalistic settings. However, it is for the same reason that cause and effect cannot be established using a correlational design, and therefore cannot provide the same degree of conclusive evidence.

You must decide which of these approaches is most suited to the topic you wish to research.

Writing a research proposal

Once you have decided on your research topic, carried out a literature review and established which general approach to the project would be most appropriate, it is a good idea to write out a fairly detailed research proposal, so that you can plan the structure and specifics of the project. Many people consider a research proposal to be a waste of time unless they are trying to obtain financial support from some organization, when a proposal is absolutely essential. However, writing up a research proposal has three important functions:

- It helps the researcher to plan the project and to focus attention on all the essential issues, such as aims, methods, analysis and relevance.
- In medical and paramedical research, it is often necessary to check the suitability of a project with ethical and related committees before beginning. For this, a research proposal is

vital, since it not only provides the necessary details of the project so that the ethical issues can be fully evaluated, but also demonstrates the researcher's competence, expertise and understanding of the topic area — an important consideration when someone's health and well-being may be affected.

• On occasions, the research you wish to do will require more time, staff or equipment than is readily available and it may, therefore, be necessary to obtain financial support for your project (see next section). In order to apply for funding you will need to provide the potential sponsors with a fairly detailed research proposal, so that they can assess its value, viability and relevance.

Thus, for these three reasons, it is good practice to prepare a research proposal prior to starting your project. No great detail about writing proposals will be given here, since a lot of the content will be similar to that contained in the next chapter on writing up research for publication. Where this is the case, it will be indicated. Nonetheless, the following information should be included in a proposal in the order given:

1. The title of the research project (see next chapter) which should be clear and succinct.

2. Background theory and the research context for the project (similar to the 'Introduction' in the next chapter).

3. A clear statement of the aim or hypothesis under investigation.

4. The method of conducting the research should be clearly outlined. This is very similar in content to the 'Method' section of an article (see next chapter) and should include a statement of the design of the project, the subjects (type, number etc.) materials, apparatus and actual procedure. In addition, any relevant information about how the public relations aspect will be handled should be included here (i.e. feedback of results to participants, anonymity of the subjects, security of the data, co-operation with other members of the hospital staff etc.)

5. The type of statistical analysis to be used for the results should be included.

6. The implications and relevance of the study must be highlighted, particularly if the proposal is to go to an ethical committee or a funding body. It is pointless just outlining an experiment without pointing out its direct application and worth to the patients/hospital/staff/funding body etc.

7. The estimated length of time required to carry out each section of the research, as well as the overall time involved, should be included, since this will obviously influence the feasibility and finances of the study. Fifty sets of identical triplets conceived with the aid of fertility drugs might be difficult to find in a fortnight! Obviously, you cannot be exact in your time predictions because all sorts of unforeseen circumstances will crop up which will delay the completion. Hence, it is better to be pessimistic rather than optimistic on this one.

If you can draw some sort of chart showing the sequence and timing of the main events, this would be invaluable, both in setting an overall idea of the project and in guiding its execution.

8. If the proposal is to be presented to ethical or funding bodies, then it will be necessary to include details of any personnel (including yourself) who may be involved in the project; either existing personnel or staff recruited specifically for the purpose of the project. There are usually three types of personnel involved in research work:

• *Research supervisor or director*. This is the person who takes overall responsibility for the project's execution, directing and rescuing as necessary. If you are the person generating the ideas and submitting the proposal for consideration by ethical and financial committees, the odds are you will also be the research supervisor.

• *Research workers*. These people carry out the everyday running of the project, collecting data, administering the treatments etc. They usually have some grounding in research methods or at least receive some training prior to the start of the project. Obviously, careful thought needs to be given to the qualifications and skills required of the research staff.

• *Support staff*. These are quite often the lynchpin on which the whole project depends. They include secretarial and clerical staff, computer operators, technicians etc.

In a research proposal, it is a good idea to name the participants involved, together with their qualifications, work and research experience and particular expertise for the job. If you need to recruit anyone specially for the project, you will need to specify the sort of person you want, how long you want them for and what the cost will be. Always remember when you specify the salary range that the appointee will probably only be on a short-term contract and so should be paid slightly more than usual. In addition to the cost of the salary, you will need to add the Employer's National Insurance contributions, superannuation, additional costs and overheads.

Even if you are not applying for any funding it is still a good idea to work out the cost of the project, even if only approximately. You may find that an outcome of limited impact may not justify the expense of new equipment, staff time, computing etc. However, if you are applying for outside money then you should itemize the following costs, overall or per annum, if the project is to last longer than 12 months:

1. Salaries, superannuation, N.I. of all staff to be employed on the project.
2. Any capital outlay on equipment, together with revenue expenditure of any apparatus etc.
3. Travel and subsistence costs; if anybody needs to travel to other hospital departments, patients' homes etc., these costs should be incorporated.
4. Stationery costs, postage, telephone, typing, computing etc. must be estimated. If you are proposing to handle a large amount of data, your computing costs may be fairly high. It is worthwhile having a preliminary chat with the computing centre you intend to use about estimated costs and the types of statistical analysis available.

Two words of caution, though. Firstly, do not forget to build in some allowance for inflation. Too many promising projects have had to be abandoned before completion simply because the money ran out. And secondly, check out the sort of financial information your potential sponsors require and the format they wish to receive it in before you submit your proposal. A familiar layout and content can go a long way towards getting your proposal seriously considered.

Allied to this is the length of the proposal. Many ethical committees and funding agencies have specific criteria for proposal formats and length and it is always wise to find these out and stick to them. Skimpy, underworded proposals look superficial and ill thought out, while excessively verbose ones will inspire boredom and irritation in the readers. Consequently, you should pay close attention to any recommendations laid down by the appropriate body.

Before taking off on your research, do ensure that not only does it have the approval (if necessary) of the ethical committee, but that it has been discussed and given the go-ahead by all the necessary people. This may involve your director of midwifery services, the relevant consultant, senior registrars, colleagues etc. It does little for staff relations for a senior colleague to find suddenly that there is a major research programme starting tomorrow, which will involve a total reorganization of the department. So, do discuss your proposals with all the relevant personnel from the outset. This is a critical stage in any research project and should never be overlooked.

Obtaining financial support

Some research projects can be extremely expensive in both time and money, and you may, therefore, need to apply for financial aid in order to carry out your research. Sources of financial support are many and various and all should be considered as possible sponsors at the outset. Undoubtedly, the easiest avenue through which to apply for (though not necessarily to obtain!) money is your own organization's research fund. Many hospitals, District or Regional Health Authorities have money available for research, although its existence is not always widely known. However, a relevant research programme carried out on home ground, with direct value to the sponsoring institution or organization is often a tempting cause and you may find the money forthcoming.

Beyond this immediate channel, there are outside sources, such as the Medical Research Council, pharmaceutical companies, manufacturers of apparatus or babyfood and the like, all of whom may be suitable targets for your application for money.

In order to decide which of these is likely to be most profitable, it is worth doing some homework. Some agencies obviously favour certain types of research and these inclinations will be indicated by the sort of project they have supported in the past, as well as the nature of their own activities. Obviously, a manufacturer of electronic thermometers is unlikely to sponsor research into the impact of complementary feeding on neonatal development, unless the project has some direct impact on their product. Some funding bodies even lay down specific guidelines as to the sort of project they will consider sponsoring.

Once you have decided who to approach, have an informal discussion with them about your ideas, and if they are interested, get the relevant application forms from them, together with any general information they might provide to guide intending applicants. These must be read thoroughly and completed in accordance with any regulations laid down by the organization.

Some words of advice. The funding bodies are only likely to concern themselves with novel, useful and relevant pieces of work. Projects which are run-of-the-mill or contentious are usually avoided for obvious reasons. Therefore, before applying for money, do think carefully about the nature and implications of your research and how likely it is to fit in with the overall flavour of the sponsor's interests. Also, check the final presentation of your research proposal, ensuring that it is typed, and without errors. Omissions, incorrect spelling and poor syntax will do little to create a favourable impression of your professional competence!

If your proposal is turned down in the end, try to find out why and whether the sponsors would reconsider it if amendments were made. If, on the other hand, it is accepted, then you must keep your sponsor happy. This will involve you in three activities. Firstly, do try to keep within your time and financial budget — funding agencies are rarely pleased with requests for more money or time extensions. Secondly, do send regular progress reports so that they can be satisfied that all is going according to plan (or if it is not that they are informed about the problem and what you are doing about it). And thirdly, do provide a detailed final report on time, with clear conclusions, implications and recommendations. (You might even consider inviting someone from the sponsoring organization to be on a Steering Committee for the project. In that way, the sponsors can be kept fully informed at all stages).

All this may seem like a lot of time and effort which perhaps could be better spent on the actual research project itself. Undoubtedly, there are borderline cases where you are not sure whether it really is worth the trouble to make an application for money. This is something only you and the other researchers can decide. However, if you do decide to apply for funding, remember that the sponsors are being asked to invest a lot of money in you and they will obviously want to assure themselves that it will be money well spent.

Planning the details of the study

If you write a proper research proposal many of the details of the study will have been considered and decided upon. Even if you decide against a research proposal, you must make a detailed outline of your plans and ideas for your own benefit, since when you come to write up the research report (probably a considerable time after the completion of the project) you will be surprised at how difficult it is to remember why you actually decided on one approach rather than another. So keep detailed notes for yourself as you go along as to the reasons for choosing each methodological or design stage of your research.

At this juncture, if you are using an experimental design, you should also decide in detail the following points:

- Any instructions you will be giving to your subjects during the course of the experiment should be prepared verbatim, and typed up.
- Prepare sufficient score sheets on which to record the data; if your subjects are to be asked to make written replies during the experiment, ensure that you prepare enough response sheets for them.
- If you are going to randomize the order of presentation of the experimental conditions, or the order of subjects' participation, make sure this is done in advance.
- If you are keeping the subjects anonymous and just assigning them numbers, do keep a record of any relevant details of all the subjects (age, health, sex, experimental condition) on a separate sheet with the appropriate number attached. This is essential if you are to contact them with the results of the experiment.
- How you will select your subjects and who they will be.
- Prepare for yourself and any other researchers who will be working with you, a worksheet which outlines detailed instructions of what should happen when, and how it should be carried out.
- Make sure that you know how to analyse the data, and, if it requires a computer, where and how you can obtain appropriate computing facilities.
- If you are going to use someone else to run the experiment, because you suspect there will be some experimenter bias if you carry it out, then make absolutely sure that the substitute experimenter has only the relevant details (i.e. exactly *how* to carry out the project) and *not* what the predicted outcome will be, otherwise the possibility of experimenter bias will remain.
- If you have to write to people to ask them to participate as subjects, do enclose a stamped, addressed envelope for their reply, and do check just before the start of the project that they are still able and willing to come.
- Do run a pilot study before carrying out the experiment proper to iron out any problems in advance.

If you are conducting a survey, you must decide:

- How you will collect your data, e.g. by using a questionnaire, by post, in person etc.
- How to design your measuring instrument i.e. your attitude scale or questionnaire. This must be piloted before you run the full survey.
- What instructions for completion you will append to the questionnaire.
- How you are going to select your subjects.
- How you will ensure an adequate response rate if you are using a postal survey.
- How you are going to analyse your data.

Carrying out the study

A number of points are important here:

1. If you are using any apparatus do double-check before you start that it works properly. It is extremely irritating to collect your subject sample from far and wide only to discover when they arrive that the necessary equipment is out of order and they have to go away again. This is the way in which you lose subjects, time, patience and motivation. Also, do make sure you know how to use the equipment properly. While this may seem a ludicrously obvious point to make, it has been known for experimenters to spend a considerable time fiddling about with the apparatus, attempting to find the necessary switches. Trying to convince the subjects of your competence thereafter becomes a major task.

2. Always, always, always run some pilot trials before you begin the experiment proper. Pilot trials simply mean running through the experimental procedure with a few subjects to see whether there are any practical hitches. By doing this, you can establish:

 (i) whether your procedure is appropriate;
 (ii) whether the tasks you have set your subjects are of the right level, if they are too hard or too easy they can be adjusted;
 (iii) whether you have allocated a reasonable amount of time for the tasks;
 (iv) whether your instructions can be clearly understood by the subjects;
 (v) whether there are any practical problems in the project.

If you do find any hitches or difficulties at this

stage, you can iron them out before beginning the real experiment.

3. Do familiarize yourself totally with the experimental procedure, and what should be done when. It does not inspire the confidence of subjects to see the experimenter scrabbling around for scraps of paper or trying to find out what to do next. So make the running of the experiment as smooth and automatic as possible. The pilot trials should help in this.

4. Treat your subjects well. They are the cornerstone of your study and must be looked after. This means keeping them informed (as far as is reasonable) of the purpose of the study and of the outcome. Should it ever be necessary to keep your subjects in the dark over the aim of a study, because their knowledge of this would bias the results, do debrief them when the project is over. Also tell them in advance, if possible, what is required of them and how long it will take. Do *not* do anything which will cause distress or embarrassment. People are understandably apprehensive about any form of research, so it is in their, and your, best interest, to try to achieve some rapport with them and an easy, pleasant atmosphere. Lastly, try to minimize the amount of inconvenience subjects ex-perience during the course of the study. If they have to make lengthy and expensive journeys at unsociable hours of the day or night, they are unlikely to turn up. Quite simply, try to keep your subjects happy, particularly if they are patients when not only their psychological, but also their physical, well-being may be at stake.

Interpreting and disseminating the results of your research

There is no value in simply analysing your results and then forgetting all about them — they must be interpreted fully in terms of their relevance to the profession. What is the meaning of the outcome? How does it relate to current midwifery practice? What are the implications for policy changes / therapeutic procedures? etc.

However, even this is not enough. If only you are aware of the nature and implications of your results then they are of limited value. The information must be disseminated to other members of the profession. And the easiest way to do this is by writing up the research either as an article for publication in a professional journal, or as a report produced within your department for circulation. While the former method will reach a greater audience, both require the same sort of format and approach.

With the increasing emphasis on research based clinical practice within the health care professions, together with reductions in resources, it is essential that the results of sound research projects are published. Without this knowledge clinicians will not be able to make informed decisions, practice will not be accountable on objective grounds and clients' welfare will not be optimized through the best intervention procedures. Publication of results is an essential final stage of research, and is a moral obligation for any midwives who have conducted good research with potentially useful findings. Guidelines for writing up research are given in the next chapter.

And finally, remember that there is no such thing as a perfect piece of applied research. In designing any study involving human subjects, compromises will have to be made in the design. However, these considerations must be informed and well-judged. As long as the researcher can make reasoned, judicious adjustments to her design in order to accommodate the practical problems surrounding her study, the research will still be valid.

11

Writing up the research for publication

Sometimes you will want to carry out a piece of research just for your own satisfaction or to resolve some issue that exists in your own work. However, there will be occasions when your experiment produces such an interesting and useful outcome that you will want to publish it so that the results can be disseminated to other related professionals. Hence you will need to prepare an article for publication in a suitable journal. I would urge you always to consider publishing your research, however, for two main reasons. Firstly, if you have some interesting findings there is a moral obligation to share these with other midwives so that they can integrate them into their practice. And secondly, if patient care is to be improved through the use of research results then it is essential that these are widely disseminated to other practitioners.

A word of caution, though. Good scientific journalese comes with practice. Even if you follow the guidelines provided here you may not be terribly satisfied with your first attempt at writing up a piece of research. I would recommend that you do not despair and throw it in the bin but instead put the first draft away for a week or two and forget about it. When you re-read it afresh you will probably find a number of points that could be expressed more clearly or succinctly. If you are still not satisfied after doing this, repeat the process. You will soon find that you are able to produce a written style which is suitable for scientific journals at the first attempt.

GENERAL GUIDELINES FOR WRITING UP RESEARCH

1. Always bear in mind that the aims of writing up research for publication are to inform readers of (a) the purpose of your study (i.e. the aims or hypothesis) (b) the results (c) how you came by them (i.e. the procedure you adopted for your experiment and (d) what the implications of your results are.

More details of the basic structure of a report are given in the next section.

2. Always write in the third person not in the first or second person. In other words, use phrases such as 'The subjects were required to . . .' rather than 'I asked the subjects to . . . . .' While this is easy enough when describing the experimental procedure, many students find it more difficult when discussing the implications of their results, tending to write phrases such as: 'I think the results can be explained by . . .'

The 'I think' would be better replaced by phrases such as 'it is suggested/posited/hypothesized that the results etc. . . .' or 'One possible explanation for the results is . . .' or 'The results can be explained by . . .' etc. If you have difficulty in writing in the third person, it is often a good idea to take a passage from a book which is written in the first person and simply rewrite it in the third person, for practice.

If all this sounds unnecessarily pedantic, remember that any research should be objective and disinterested. If you start including 'I', 'me', 'my', personally' etc the report begins to look highly subjective and consequently not very scientific. The use of the third person is a much better style for journal articles (and gives you a greater chance of publication!).

3. Keep your sentences clear and simple and try to convey just one idea per sentence. Remember that your report may well be read by people unfamiliar with the field, so confronting them with complex grammar or sentences with several adjectival clauses will keep them unfamiliar with it! Clarity of style is easier to attain if you do not assume your reader had any prior knowledge of the specific area. (However, do not fall into the trap of writing as though the reader is a half-wit!)

And finally, if you are going to use abbreviations, give their meaning in full at the first mention. For example:

'Women of 32+ weeks' gestation and with low levels of Human Placental Lactogen (HPL) were selected for study.' etc.

4. Do not include any anecdotal evidence in the report, however relevant and interesting it may appear. Science is too formal, theoretical and empirical for personal experience to be introduced.

5. Try to make your article clear, logical, succinct and free of irrelevancies. Remember always that the purpose of any article is to provide information. Therefore, if someone unfamiliar with your area of research is to understand the article then it is essential that it is clear and logical. Similarly, in order to get the essential points across to the reader, it is important not to wrap them up in irrelevant information. The colour of the subject's night-dress is rarely apposite, although I have seen it included in one student's report!

6. It is important to quote relevant research in your article for a number of reasons. Firstly, it shows the reader that you are familiar with the research area and that you have a number of important facts at your finger tips. Secondly, it adds weight to any argument you produce: if you simply say that 'Ptyalism is not the result of any physiological changes which occur during pregnancy, but rather of an hysterical nemotic condition which is impossible to treat', the reader may think 'who says?' However, if you quote the source of this information thus 'Swallow and Spitz (1993) found that ptyalism is not the result of any physiological changes . . . . etc.', your argument carries more credibility. (You will note, that I have quoted the surnames of the researchers here, together with the date of their publication on ptyalism. Some journals specify different formats when quoting research — do check what is required by your intended publisher.) And thirdly, you need to refer to some plausible theory when explaining your results. As you might imagine, theories by identifiable authors carry more weight than anonymous theories which cannot be checked out.

7. There is no one correct way of writing up a report, since each journal tends to have its own format and requirements. It is therefore important to look at the journal's specifications (usually inside the front or back cover) and to read a couple of articles produced in it before starting your own. That having been said, the following sub-headings should provide you with a structure for presenting the essential information from your experiment; you can leave out the sub-headings when a particular journal does not use them.

SPECIFIC GUIDELINES FOR STRUCTURING AN ARTICLE

The title

This should convey succinctly to the reader the essential point of your experiment. For an experimental report it is often easier to construct your title from the relationship predicted in your experimental hypothesis.

For example, if your experimental hypothesis had been: 'healing of perineal wounds takes longer in women who were more than 10% overweight pre-pregnancy than in women who were of normal weight', your title could then be:

A Study of Relationship between Pre-Pregnancy Weight and Rate of Healing of Perineal Wounds

To practise producing pithy and clear titles, you could turn back to the hypotheses on page 46 and construct titles from them.

Authors

List the author(s) and their occupation and place of work. It is usually understood that in a multi-authorship article, the first person on the list is the main contributor to the research, in terms of initiating and/or conducting it. The subsequent order of authors should reflect their contribution. Sometimes, however, the person who holds the most senior position will claim the prestigious first authorship place, irrespective of input. Since this may cause ill-feeling, author sequence should be negotiated before the research is even started.

The author in this hypothetical study might be:
Olivia Waite
Midwifery Sister
St. Perineum's Hospital
London.

Abstract or summary

The abstract or summary is a short précis of the experiment or study. Usually around ten lines or 100–150 words long, the abstract includes:

- the aim or hypothesis of the study
- a brief summary of the procedure
- the results, stating their level of significance if appropriate
- a brief, general statement of the implications of the results.

Therefore, the abstract for an experiment testing the previous hypothesis might be:

A study was carried out to investigate the hypothesis that healing of perineal wounds takes longer in women who were more than 10% overweight prior to conception than in women who were of normal weight [Aims and Hypothesis]. Twenty overweight women and twenty normal weight women (pre-pregnancy) who had medio-lateral perineal incisions during the second stage of labour were randomly selected for study. Following delivery, all the subjects were prescribed 'Periheal' baths. After 3 days post partum the degree of healing was assessed using a 5-point ordinal scale [Brief Experimental Procedure]. Using the Mann-Whitney U-Test to analyse the data, the results were found to be significant ($U = 97.5$, $p < 0.005$), suggesting that the healing of perineal wounds takes longer in women who were overweight prior to conception. [Brief Results]. The implications of these results are discussed in terms of pre-conceptual counselling programmes. [Conclusions and Implications].

Obviously, though, you do not include the words in brackets. (You should also note that all the illustrations are fictitious and not derived from any actual research evidence!)

While not all journals require abstracts, they are very useful, not only to the reader who can find out whether the article will be worth reading in full by simply looking at the abstract, but also to the writer who is forced to summarize the critical points of the research in a few lines. This usually focuses the author's mind on the basic structure of the article.

Introduction

The point of the introduction is to put your study into a theoretical context. There are five main topics you should include:

1. It should start off with a general description about the background to the research area. In the above example some reference could be made to any relevant work which has been carried out on perineal wounds or problems of obesity during pregnancy. You might start off by stating something like:

> Over the last few years there has been increasing evidence of problems resulting from episiotomies.

In other words you have defined the topic area.

2. The next stage is to review the relevant literature which relates to this, by briefly quoting appropriate research work. So, you might continue with, for example:

> One particular difficulty relates to the healing of perineal wounds, often because of the heightened risk of infection in that area (Bugg, 1992). Moreover, despite the evidence pertaining to maternal pain and discomfort deriving from the wound, no single method of treatment has been found to be generally effective in the promotion of healing of the episiotomy (Scarr and Heale, 1993). Indeed, average healing time of the perineum following incision has been found to be 9.3 days in the over -30s (Old, 1992), while for the 20–25 age group it has been shown to be 8.7 days (Younger, 1991). A number of factors have been demonstrated to be associated with retarded healing following episiotomies. Besides age (op.cit.) maternal health and smoking behaviour have been shown to be important (Wellman, 1993). A full review of the relevant literature can be found in Midline (1994).

3. The third stage involves providing the reader with some theoretical explanation for these findings. Thus:

> Clearly, what emerges from this literature is the implication that any factor which has the effect of reducing circulation to the perineal area may have an adverse impact on healing rate.

4. The next part of the introduction provides a rationale for your own research, so the previous two stages of the introduction should be structured in such a way as to highlight the need for your study. Most reported research is original; that is to say, the study has usually investigated previously unexplored areas. Therefore, the initial part of your introduction should present any relevant work which has been carried out, and should involve some statement as to where there was a gap in the research. For example, you may find that a particular treatment has not been tried out with a specific client group, or that a variation on a treatment procedure has not been evaluated. This gap provides you with the rationale for your experiment. Therefore, you might conclude the previous section with:

> However, to date no work has been carried out on the effects of pre-pregnancy weight on perineal wound healing and yet obesity might have a cumulative impact on circulation over the duration of pregnancy. This study, therefore, was concerned with looking at the effects of pre-conception obesity on the healing of episiotomies.

5. Finally, you need to state clearly what your experimental hypothesis was, i.e.

> The hypothesis under investigation, then, was that women who were more than 10% overweight prior to conception will experience longer healing times of perineal incisions than will women who were of normal weight before conception.

If you now read just the parts in smaller type, you can get the overall idea of what the introduction should look like.

Bear in mind that the literature you quote in the introduction should be comprehensive, up-to-date and critically evaluated if appropriate. Include any seminal works in the area.

Method

The aim of the method section is to tell the reader exactly how the study was carried out. It has to be sufficiently clear that you could present your method section to anybody and they would be able to replicate your research exactly without having to ask for clarification on any point. It is usually sub-divided into the following sections (but once again, you should check the journal first).

Design

The independent and dependent variables in your experiment are usually defined here (if appropriate), together with a statement of whether you used a same, matched or different subject design (again if appropriate). Furthermore, if you have eliminated any sources of error by counterbalancing, randomizing the allocation of subjects to conditions, using a double-blind procedure etc., you should say so in this section. If you have conducted a survey, you might include here any essential decisions concerning your questionnaire design, how the questionnaires were distributed and why you chose this method. You might state then, for this section:

> The independent variable was pre-pregnancy weight, while the dependent variable was healing rate of perineal incisions. A different subject experimental design was used to compare the two groups of women who differed in pre-pregnancy weight. To eliminate any problems accruing from previous perineal scar tissue, only primigravidas were used. To control for any possible effects of experimenter bias, a midwife who was unaware of the topic under investigation, assessed the healing rate.

Subjects

You should describe your subjects succinctly, giving all the relevant details, e.g. age, sex, medical condition, previous pregnancies, occupation and how they were selected. If you just asked the first 20 women who required episiotomies, say so. However, it is important to specify whether they volunteered, were press-ganged, paid etc., since it makes a difference to the way in which they react. Therefore, in the above example, the Subject section might read:

> Two groups each comprising 20 women were randomly selected from a maternity unit. All were primigravidas, were between 25 and 30 years of age and had no known medical problems (e.g. diabetes, or pelvic inflammatory disease). All had been given medio-lateral incisions during the second stage of labour. However, one of the two

groups was recorded to have been at least 10% overweight at conception (Group 0) while the other group recorded weights within normal limits (Group N). All subjects volunteered to participate.

Apparatus

Any apparatus used should be referred to in sufficient detail so that anyone wanting to replicate your experiment can obtain the same equipment. Thus, manufacturer's name, make and type of apparatus, plus a brief description of its capacities should be included. If the equipment has been made specially for you, it should be described in detail and should be accompanied by a diagram showing its main features.

In the above example, then, no apparatus was used: therefore this section might be:

> No apparatus was used in the study.

Materials

Any non-mechanical equipment used should be included in this section, e.g. score sheets, record cards, etc. If a questionnaire or attitude scale was used, you should describe the measure in detail. In addition, it is often appropriate to include a copy of it in an Appendix at the end of the article. Here, the section would read something like:

> The materials used in the experiment included record cards to record the healing rate of the incision, using a 5-point ordinal scale (1 = no healing, 5 = complete healing).

Procedure

This sub-section of the method is very important and should include a detailed description of what you did when you actually carried out the study. It should be clear and logical and should provide the reader with something akin to the method part of a recipe, i.e. a step-by-step account of what was done in the appropriate order. Remember that although this part, like the rest of the report, should be relevant and succinct, it should also be sufficiently detailed that anyone who reads the procedure could go away and replicate what you did to the letter. The word 'relevant' is important as well – you should only include those details which might have some influence on the outcome of the experiment. For example, the height of a chair a patient sat in to carry out the experiment would not be relevant unless you were carrying out research into an area which related to ergonomics or the ability to get in and out of chairs. It is not always easy at first to include just the right amount of detail, but it is a skill which develops over time.

Details which should be included here are things like order of presentation of tasks, and standardized instructions to the subject (which should be reproduced verbatim), how the dependent variable was measured and at what time intervals, number of treatment sessions etc. Therefore, the procedure section here might be:

All the subjects were given a medio-lateral episiotomy during the second stage of labour to assist delivery. Following delivery, the women were advised to take warm 'Periheal' baths twice daily and to observe scrupulous hygiene of the perineal area. After 3 days, their incisions were assessed for degree of healing by a midwife independent to the study and unaware of the hypothesis under investigation. A five-point ordinal scale was used, with 1 = no healing and 5 = complete healing. The healing rates of the two groups were compared using a Mann-Whitney U-Test.

Results

The actual scores derived from your study do not need to be presented in this section, but may be included in an Appendix, if this is appropriate. However, it is necessary to include the mean scores for each group or condition. If you present a graph, ensure that it conforms to the guidelines outlined on page 35. Perhaps the most important part of this section, though, are the results of the statistical analysis performed on the scores. While it is unnecessary to include the workings-out, you do need to say:

1. What statistical analysis you used.
2. What the result was.
3. What the level of significance was (if inferential techniques were used).
4. A brief statement of what these results actually mean (a point many people forget). It

is insufficient just to say 'The results are significant at the 0.01 level.' You must interpret this for the reader.

So, in the above example, the results section might be (the numbered points refer to the list above):

The mean healing score for Group 0 at 3 days was 1.7, while for Group N, it was 3.4. The data was analysed using a Mann-Whitney U-Test (point 1) and were found to be significant ($U = 97.5$, (point 2) $p < 0.005$ for a 1-tailed test (point 3)). These results suggest that healing of the perineal incision is significantly retarded in the women who were overweight at conception (point 4).

Discussion

1. This section starts off with a re-statement of the outcome of your statistical analysis (usually a variant on the last sentence in the results section), and may add a comment as to whether or not it supports the experimental hypothesis (if this is appropriate). For example:

The results of the present study suggest that healing of perineal incisions takes longer in women who were overweight at conception than in women who were of normal weight, thereby supporting the experimental hypothesis.

2. You should then go on to make some statement about how your results fit in with the findings from other related research. This can incorporate studies which produced contradictory as well as corroborative findings, as long as you provide some plausible explanation for the discrepancy. Here, then you might say:

These results accord with those of Heale (1993) who found that healing of lower limb wounds was slower in overweight patients. Brake (1991) similarly found that lower leg amputations took longer to heal in the obese. However, Langerhan (1992) found no difference between normal and overweight women in the healing of perineal 1st degree tears. This discrepancy could be explained by the lesser severity of the trauma experienced by Langerhan's subjects, as well as by the fact that they all had Type II diabetes, which would retard healing anyway.

3. You must produce a cogent theoretical explanation for your results and also some

comment about their practical implications. For instance.

> The present results could be explained by the circulation problems known to affect many overweight people, which would of necessity influence perineal incision healing. In addition, it is conceivable that the overweight group might have had an increased susceptibility to developing intertrigo in the groin area which might have influenced the condition of the perineal wound. Moreover, it has been well-documented that the overweight take less exercise in the course of the day (Idle, 1989) and if this pertained also to the obese subjects in the study, then any circulatory problems might have been exacerbated.

4. Next you should include any additional analysis which you carried out and which produced some interesting results, together with some comment on these (ideally their theoretical and practical relevance). For example, you might compare male vs. female neonates; older vs. younger primigravidas; social class or occupational groups etc. In the present example:

> Further inspection of the data suggested that those women who had epidurals during delivery experienced slower perineal wound healing than did those women who had alternative forms of analgesia *irrespective of body weight* ($U = 52.5$, $p < 0.02$). Since epidurals inevitably limit immediate post-delivery activity (and consequently circulation) these findings add further support to the suggestion that circulation is a major contributory factor in perineal wound healing.

5. You should then acknowledge any limitations of your study, design flaws, unforeseen practical problems that you encountered (e.g. patients not turning up, apparatus breaking down etc.), variables which you failed to control for etc. While this may look as though it is condemning your experiment to the waste bin, it is not, as long as there are no major methodological flaws which would totally vitiate your results. Most research (especially applied research like midwifery) will have some minor faults since the perfect experiment is all but a fantasy. However, if you acknowledge the problems and recommend ways of overcoming them were the study to be repeated in future, then your work will not be dismissed as nonsense. The researcher who

thinks his/her study is perfect is the one who is more likely to be rejected. For example:

> While this latter finding is interesting, it does, nonetheless, highlight epidural analgesia as an uncontrolled constant error in the study. As epidurals lower both blood pressure and circulation in the lower limbs, the results in the main study could be partly attributable to this rather than to the independent variable of obesity. Additional studies are needed to eliminate this factor as a source of error. Furthermore, it was impossible to ascertain how far each subject complied with the treatment recommendations following delivery. While it is unlikely, it is nevertheless possible, that the obese subjects might have been less punctilious in their use of 'Periheal'. Some check of patient compliance with instructions would have tightened the design.

6. Finally, if your study throws up any ideas for future research, say so. Here you might suggest:

> The results from the present study point the way to future investigations of perineal wound healing such as the impact of massage or gentle lower limb exercise following delivery to stimulate circulation.

You should also clarify the conclusions and the practical implications deriving from your research:

> This study has demonstrated that women who were overweight at conception are more likely to experience retarded healing of perineal incisions than are women who were of normal weight. One possible explanation for the finding highlights circulatory problems. Therefore, what seems to be needed are recommendations for weight reduction programmes at pre conceptual counselling sessions, as well as exercise and diet programmes for those women found to be overweight at booking in.

References

Every researcher you have quoted in your report must be included in the reference section in order that the reader can follow up ideas and theories in the area by going back to the original article or book. Usually, all the names are quoted in alphabetical order and you *must* give the full reference. While many journals have their own formats (which you should check first), there are standard ways of presenting references for books and journal articles. For books, the author's surname is quoted first followed by initials, date of publication, title of the book (underlined), where it was published and by whom. Therefore, the reference would look like:

Midline, A. (1994) Care of the Perineum, Midshire, Gravidas Press.

However, you must check the journal's requirements first, because if the above reference was listed in a book published by Churchill Livingstone, it would appear as follows:

Midline A 1994 Care of the perineum. Gravidas Press, Midshire

For journal articles, the format is similar: surname, initials, date of article, title of article, title of journal (underlined), volume of journal (underlined) and first and last page numbers of the article. Therefore, a journal article would be:

Scarr, I. and Heale, U. (1993) Intervention in perineal trauma.
Journal of Obstetric Trauma 14 (1): 15–19.

In the example quoted throughout this chapter, all the cited research would have to be referenced in alphabetical order, using the correct format. You would therefore have:

Brake, M. (1991) etc.
Bugg, O. (1992) etc.
Idle, W. (1989) etc.
Langerhan, I. (1992) etc.
Midline, A. (1994) etc.

Do note though, that some journals require that authors are referenced not in alphabetical order, but in the order in which they appeared in the report. The cardinal rule is *check the journal's requirements on format of article and reference presentation*. Styles of reference presentation do vary. If you go back and read just the sections in small type you should get an idea about the style and format of a journal article, although I would stress again that prior to writing your research up, you should select a journal which specializes in your research area and check the details of presentation it requires.

Submitting articles for publication

● Do not submit the article to more than one journal at a time. If the journal of your choice turns it down, then send it off to another one, but never submit simultaneously. (Always keep a copy!)

● If you carried out the research with colleagues, then it may be appropriate to include their names as authors. Where there is multiple authorship of an article, the person quoted first is usually assumed either to be the most senior contributor (in terms of professional status) or alternatively to have carried out the bulk of the work. However, there is no fixed precedent for the order of names, and trouble frequently arises when the most senior author has done least work but still wants to take first place. So, sort out the issue in advance.

● Throughout the course of any research project many individuals will have helped either by sponsoring the research or helping with computing. Those people who have made significant contributions should be acknowledged at the end of the article.

● You might consider asking the editor of the journal if your article can be refereed 'blind' since there is some evidence that this produces a fairer and more objective evaluation. Remember that getting research published may be something of a game (if you are interested to know just what sort of game, you might like to read Peters and Ceci, 1982). However, if you observe the rules of the game as outlined above you should be successful in having your article accepted for publication.

Some final morale boosters

● Do not be disheartened if your article is rejected; even the most seasoned of researchers regularly experience rejection. Try to use the referees' comments to improve your article before sending it off to another journal. In other words, use the rejection as a learning exercise.

● Bear in mind that getting something published takes a long time. It may be months before the editor comes back to you with the referees' views and if adjustments have to be made, the referees may need to see the article again, which will add to the time it takes for your report to be accepted formally. Added to this is the time lag before the article appears in print once it *has* been accepted, and this can run into months or sometimes years.

• Seeing your article in print is always gratifying, however many times you have experienced it before. It makes all the effort in its production worthwhile.

• Do not ever lose sight of the fact that a sound piece of research, however small, may have the power to influence patient care radically. You have a moral imperative to put up with the problems of publication, given the potential benefits to midwifery practice at all levels.

12

Reading published research critically

If midwifery practice is to become increasingly research-based, then three essential requirements must be fulfilled. Firstly, midwives must carry out sound research which has the capacity to influence service delivery; secondly, this research must be published, and thirdly, the published reports must be read and evaluated prior to any findings being implemented into clinical practice.

While it is neither appropriate nor realistic to expect that all midwives will become research-active, it is imperative that they become research-minded. By this is meant (a) that well carried out research is universally acknowledged to be of value to the profession as a whole and to the clients it serves and (b) as a consequence of this, that midwives keep themselves up-dated on relevant research findings, with a view to modifying their practice if it is appropriate to do so in the light of those findings. This, of course, means that they should be in a position to assess the quality of the research they read and the validity of its conclusions before implementation into service delivery.

Many midwives express concern at the prospect of evaluating published research, particularly if it has appeared in a reputable journal. Such diffidence may in part be a function of our society's traditional belief that anything which appears in print must be true, but it is often also the result of midwives' lack of confidence about how to go about evaluating published research. Clearly, where clients' physical and psychological well-being may be adversely affected by un-questioningly implementing the results of a poorly conducted study, it is self-evident that midwives should have a working knowledge of how to assess what they read. This will also mean that they will need to be familiar with some of the concepts outlined earlier in this section of the book, since without this information, their judgements may not be fully informed.

This chapter is concerned with providing general guidelines on how to make informed assessments of published research. It may be useful to read Chapter 11 on presenting research for publication prior to reading this one, since it gives a fairly detailed account of what should normally go in a research report.

THE TITLE

When you first look through a journal, you need an at-a-glance knowledge of what the contents are, to see if they have any relevance for you. Consequently, the title of the article will be your first point of contact. Therefore, the title should be a clear statement of what the research project was about, so the first question you need to ask is:

1. Is the title a clear and succinct statement of the research study?

ABSTRACT OR SUMMARY

The abstract is a short statement of the aims, methods, findings and conclusions of a research project. While not all journals use abstracts as a means of providing a summarized overview of the research, where they do, you should ask:

2. Does the abstract provide a clear statement of the aims, methods, results and conclusions/implications of the study?
3. After reading the abstract, am I clear about the nature of the study?

A negative answer to either question may constitute a flaw. Certainly if no clear aim is stated then it may be impossible to evaluate the rest of the abstract, since it would not be obvious whether the method adequately tests the aims, nor whether the results and conclusions support them.

INTRODUCTION

The introduction to a piece of research should give a clear statement of the context and general background to the study since this will give the reader an idea as to the importance and relevance of the project; it should provide a comprehensive and up-to-date critical review of the relevant research literature since this will demonstrate the researcher's knowledge of the topic area and enhance the credibility of the project as a whole; it should provide a rationale for why a further piece of research was necessary and it should plug a gap in existing midwifery knowledge; and it *must* give an unambiguous statement of the aims or hypothesis to be tested. Without this, it will be impossible to assess whether the study is a proper test of the aims. Therefore, the questions concerning the introduction are as follows:

4. Is there an adequate description of the general context for the study?
5. Is the literature reviewed thorough, relevant, recent and properly used to provide a structured argument leading to the reason for conducting the reported piece of research?
6. Is the hypothesis (if appropriate) clearly stated, and the predicted relationship between the variables apparent?
7. If the research does not test a hypothesis, are the aims of the study clear?
8. Are the aims or hypothesis useful to midwifery?
9. Is the project likely to be of value to midwifery?

If the answers to these questions are 'no' then doubt must be cast on the quality of the project.

METHOD

The general format of the method section varies from journal to journal. However, the actual content is usually very similar. The method should tell the reader exactly *what* was done, *how* it was done, the *order* in which it was done, *why* this approach was chosen and with *whom* the project was conducted. After reading this section, you should know all the relevant details and be in a position to replicate the study exactly if you so wished. If you have to ask any questions or you need clarification on anything at all, then this section is not adequate, and the report must be considered flawed.

So the questions concerning the method section are:

10. Has the design of the study been properly described?
11. Has the researcher made it clear *why* this design was chosen?
12. Is the design appropriate for the aims/hypothesis stated in the Introduction?
13. Are sources of error acknowledged and controlled?
14. Is the sample: suitable? of an appropriate size? fully described? properly selected?
15. Were any sources of bias or error evident in the sample and/or in the process by which they were chosen?
16. Would this impact upon the study's outcome?
17. Was any mechanical apparatus used in the study and if so, was it properly described? Was it suitable for the project?
18. Were any other materials used, such as questionnaires, score sheets, attitude scales etc?
19. Were these described fully and/or included in the Appendix, if appropriate?
20. Were any questionnaires or scales which were used properly constructed? Were they adequately tested before using them in the study? Were they suitable for their purpose?
21. Is the description of what was done absolutely clear?
22. Does it state the *order* in which things were done?
23. Does it provide a verbatim report of any instructions given to the subjects? Were the instructions clear?
24. Were the sources of error dealt with appropriately?
25. Was the method of data collection clearly described and appropriate?
26. Were the data a suitable measure of the dependent variable (if the study tested an

hypothesis?) or of the information required by the survey's aims?
27. Were the subjects treated well, their rights and confidentiality protected?
28. Was the study ethical?
29. Could you repeat this study to the letter, if it was considered necessary?

If the answer to this last question in particular was 'no' then the method section does not fulfil its purpose. Other negative answers in this section would also suggest not only a *report* beset by omissions and obscurities, but might also reflect a poorly conducted piece of research.

RESULTS

The results section should summarize what was actually found in the project. While it does not typically include raw data or the workings-out of any statistical analysis both these elements can be summarized. Raw data can be presented by tabulating means, standard deviations, etc., and the results of any statistical analysis by the numerical value obtained as a result of calculating the correct statistical test. This should be accompanied by a p value and an interpretation of this. Whatever the nature of the study, the meaning of the results should be made clear to the reader. The questions relating to this section then are:

30. Are the graphs (if provided) clear, self-explanatory and useful?
31. Are the tables (if used) clearly labelled and constructed and with an obvious relevance to the study?
32. Are the statistical tests used the correct ones for the project's design?
33. Is the selected level of significance appropriate for the topic area?
34. Is the p-value clearly stated and correct for the hypothesis as stated (i.e. one or two-tailed)?

If the analysis at any level is incorrect this will invalidate the study and conclusions. Therefore, positive answers to every question in this section are critical.

DISCUSSION

The discussion section of a research report should do just as it says; it should discuss the findings from the project in relation to other research work in the area, thus providing a broader context for the project's results. In addition, some theoretical explanation for the results should be provided, as theory and practice should go together. Sometimes results do not tie in with findings of existing research and some convincing reason for this discrepancy must be put forward, otherwise doubts must inevitably be cast on the methodology and analysis used in the study.

The conclusions drawn in the discussion should reflect the results. They should not be extravagant and extend beyond what was actually found. Neither should the conclusions be incomplete and refer only to those parts of the data which confirm the researcher's original aims, while ignoring results which oppose those aims. Such selective discussion has the potential to be every bit as misleading as incorrect analysis and interpretation.

In addition, the discussion section offers the researcher an opportunity to acknowledge flaws in the study, together with suggestions for how these may be rectified in the future. Unconditional acceptance of the design of a research project may mean that the results are given more credence than they are due. Field research is never perfect and it is essential that the researcher recognizes that, in order that the results can be interpreted with due caution. And lastly, a good research project should spawn ideas for other studies. If it does not, then it is possible that the original project was too narrow and limited to be of much real value.

So the questions relating to this section are:

35. Are the results and conclusions clearly stated?
36. Are they related to other studies in the area, thereby putting them into a broader research framework?
37. Is a cogent theoretical explanation for the findings provided?
38. Are the results interpreted fully and cor-

rectly, or is the interpretation selective and/or extravagant?
39. Are any flaws in the study's design highlighted, together with recommendations for improvement?
40. Are the results interpreted with these limitations in mind?
41. Are any practical ramifications of the results discussed?
42. Do any ideas for future projects emerge?

'No' to any of the questions must raise reservations about the overall quality of the project.

REFERENCES

Every piece of work or research quoted in the report must be fully acknowledged and recorded in the reference section. These references should give the full name of the author, the date of the work, its title and where it was published (see page 110 on references).

Omissions in the references are suggestive of sloppiness which may then reflect adversely on the rest of the study.

Therefore:

43. Is every article, study, research report and book quoted in the reference section?
44. Do these references give all the required information?

OVERALL CONSIDERATIONS

And finally there are some general questions which need to be asked:

45. Was the project a worthwhile one, contributing to the knowledge base of midwifery?
46. Was it clearly written, so that the content was easily accessible to the reader?
47. Is the report scientific and objective both in the way in which it was conducted as well as the way in which it was analysed and written up?
48. Is the article devoid of jargon?
49. Has the research project advanced midwifery in any way?

These questions may seem pedantic and tedious but a poorly reported project may suggest a poorly conducted project. Remember that no research project is perfect. What is important though, is that the researcher recognizes this, justifies why design and analysis decisions were taken and interprets the results in the light of these. Asking the above questions of an article means that client/patient well-being will be safeguarded to some degree, since the reader will be in a position to make sound assessments of a research project before deciding whether to implement the findings into practice.

Statistical tests

It has been emphasized throughout this book that it is essential that the data from any research project are properly analysed. Where the research has involved testing an hypothesis either through the use of an experimental design or a correlational design, it is critical that the correct statistical test is used to find out whether the results support the prediction made in the hypothesis. If the wrong test is used then the results and conclusions will be invalid and in an area like midwifery which involves patient well-being, this could be potentially very damaging. The ways in which a decision could be made regarding the choice of correct test were outlined in Chapter 9. This chapter and the next five are all concerned with how to calculate those tests.

13

Non-parametric tests for same and matched subject designs

INTRODUCTION

As was mentioned in Chapter 9, the results from most of the designs you are likely to use can be analysed either by a non-parametric or a parametric statistical test. Each test does essentially the same job, but the parametric test is rather more sensitive. However, in order to use a parametric test, certain prerequisite conditions have to be fulfilled (see Ch. 9). If you cannot fulfil these or if you have any doubts then you should use the equivalent non-parametric test. All the tests in this chapter are *non-parametric ones for same and matched subject designs*. In the next chapter, the equivalent parametric tests for the same designs will be covered.

So, the statistical tests covered in this chapter are appropriate for any experimental design which involves either one group of subjects which is used in two or more conditions (same subject design) or alternatively two or more groups of subjects each of which is used in *one* condition only, but who are matched on certain key variables (matched subject design). (Have a look back to the examples given on page 84 in Chapter 9.) Therefore, the sort of designs we are talking about are:

1. *One group of subjects used in two or more conditions*: (same subject design)

   a. Two conditions (Fig. 13.1)
   or
   b. Three or more conditions (Fig. 13.2).

2. *Two or more groups of matched subjects, each of*

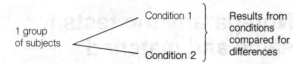

Figure 13.1 Same subject design: one group of subjects and two conditions.

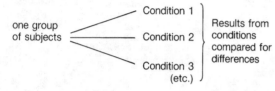

Figure 13.2 Same subject design: one group of subjects and three or more conditions.

| Subject group 1 | takes part in | Condition 1 | Results from conditions compared for differences |
| Subject group 2 | takes part in | Condition 2 | |

Figure 13.3 Matched subject design: two groups of matched subjects each taking part in one condition.

Subject group 1	takes part in	Condition 1	
Subject group 2	takes part in	Condition 2	Results from conditions compared for differences
Subject group 3 (and so on)	takes part in	Condition 3	

Figure 13.4 Matched subject design: three or more groups of matched subjects each taking part in one condition only.

which is used in one condition only: (matched subject designs)
a. Two matched groups only (Fig. 13.3)
or
b. Three or more matched groups (Fig. 13.4).

The designs which involve one group doing two conditions (Design 1a) or two matched groups doing one condition each (Design 2a) are analysed using the *McNemar* test if the data are only nominal, or the *Wilcoxon* test if the data are ordinal or interval/ratio. The designs which involve one group doing three or more conditions (Design 1b) or 3 (or more) matched groups doing one condition each (Design 2b) are ana-

Table 13.1 Non-parametric tests for related and matched subject designs

Design	Non-parametric text
1. One group of Ss taking part in two conditions. Results from conditions compared for differences.	McNemar test if the data are nominal or Wilcoxon test if the data are ordinal or interval/ratio
2. Two groups of matched Ss each taking part in one condition only. Results from conditions compared for differences.	McNemar test if the data are nominal or Wilcoxon test if the data are ordinal or interval/ratio
3. One group of Ss taking part in three or more conditions. Results from conditions compared for differences.	Friedman test or Page's *L* trend test (see pp 130–137 for which one to use). Both these can be used with ordinal or interval/ratio data
4. Three or more groups of matched Ss, each taking part in one condition only. Results from conditions compared for differences	Friedman test or Page's *L* trend test (see pp 130–137 for which one to use). Both these can be used with ordinal or interval/ratio data

lysed using either the *Friedman* test or the *Page's L* trend test (Table 13.1). Page 134 will explain which of those two you should select, since each one requires slightly different conditions.

NON-PARAMETRIC STATISTICAL TEST FOR USE WITH SAME OR MATCHED SUBJECT DESIGNS, TWO CONDITIONS AND NOMINAL DATA

McNemar test for the significance of changes

Just to remind you, this test is used when either you have one group of subjects who are measured or tested on two conditions (a same subject design) and the two sets of results are then compared for any differences between them; or when you compare two groups of subjects who are matched on all the critical variables which might influence the results (i.e. a matched group design). Each group is tested in *one* condition and the results are compared for differences between them. In other words you would use this test if you had either experimental Design 1a or 2a on pages 121–122.

The McNemar test is particularly suitable for 'before and after' type situations. However, there is one very important feature of this test; it is used with *nominal data*, that is, a level of measurement which simply allows you to allocate people or responses to named categories. Essentially what the McNemar test does is to record the changes from one category to the other, across the two conditions, to see if these changes are significant. When you calculate the McNemar test, you find a numerical value for χ^2, which you then look up in Table A2.1 to see if this figure represents significant differences between the two conditions or the two matched groups.

Example

Let us imagine you have noticed over the years the degree of fear most women experience prior to having an amniocentesis. It occurs to you that a pre-screening talk to explain what will happen, and to allow them to express any doubts or anxieties, may go a long way towards reducing their tension. You decide to try this and see whether your hunch is correct.

Your experimental hypothesis is:

H$_1$ A pre-screening talk will reduce fear levels in women about to undergo amniocentesis.

What would your null hypothesis be?
Is this a one-tailed or two-tailed hypothesis?

You select 20 pre-amniocentesis women and note whether they are frightened about the procedure.

You classify them as either:

1. little or no anxiety
or
2. high anxiety.

These are nominal data because you are simply allocating the women's responses to a named category. You then spend some time explaining to the women what will happen, discussing any

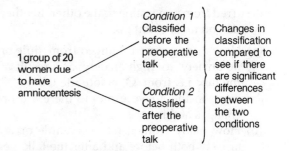

Figure 13.5 Design for experiment to assess effectiveness of preoperative talk for women due to have an amniocentesis.

Table 13.2 Patient anxiety about amniocentesis; Ø = little or no anxiety, X = high anxiety

Woman	Before talk	After talk
1	Ø	Ø
2	X	Ø
3	X	Ø
4	Ø	Ø
5	X	X
6	X	Ø
7	X	X
8	Ø	Ø
9	X	Ø
10	X	Ø
11	X	X
12	X	Ø
13	Ø	Ø
14	Ø	Ø
15	Ø	Ø
16	X	X
17	X	Ø
18	X	Ø
19	X	Ø
20	X	Ø

issues and problems they have etc. Following this session, the women are asked whether their anxiety levels have reduced. According to their response, you again allocate them to one of the categories, as before

You therefore have the design shown in Figure 13.5.

You have all the conditions required by the McNemar test, that is, a same subject design and nominal data.

You obtain the results shown in Table 13.2.

Calculating the McNemar test

1. You must first of all record the changes that

occurred from one testing to the other. In other words you must count up:

(a) How many women changed from 'little or no anxiety' to 'high anxiety' as a result of the talk, i.e. from 'Ø' before the talk to 'X' after. In the above example there are no changes of this kind.

(b) How many women had very little or no anxiety both before and after the talk, i.e. were 'Ø' before the talk and 'Ø' afterwards. In this example, there are six such women.

(c) How many women had high anxiety both before and after the talk, i.e. were 'X' before and 'X' after. Here there were four such women.

(d) How many women changed from feeling high anxiety before the talk to feeling little or no anxiety after, i.e. changed from 'X' before the talk to 'Ø' afterwards. Here there are ten.

2. These figures now have to be put in a table like the following (Fig. 13.6):

Cell A represents those women who changed from Ø to X (little anxiety to high anxiety, i.e. 0). This is calculation (a) above.

Cell B represents those women who had little or no anxiety before and after the talk (stayed at Ø, i.e. 6). This is calculation (b) above.

Cell C represents those women who had high

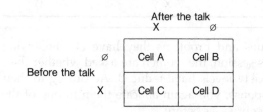

Figure 13.6 Table used in calculating the McNemar test.

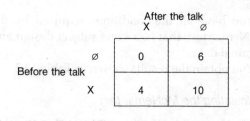

Figure 13.7 Table of Figure 13.6 with data entered.

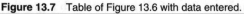

anxiety before and after the talk (stayed at X, i.e. 4). This is calculation (c) above.

Cell D represents those women who changed from high anxiety to low anxiety (changed from X to Ø, i.e. 10). This is calculation (d) above. So, if we enter these figures into the cells, the table looks like Figure 13.7.

Remember! You must organize your cells in the way indicated above, otherwise your calculations will be incorrect. In other words, whichever category is on the left-hand cell for the 'After' condition, the other category should be at the top for the 'Before' condition. The numbers in the cells should add up to the same as the number of patients tested. In this case, the number is 20.

3. Find the value of χ^2 from the formula:

$$\chi^2 = \frac{([A - D] - 1)^2}{A + D}$$

where A = the value in cell A (i.e. 0)
D = the value in cell D (i.e. 10)

If we substitute our figures we get:

$$\chi^2 = \frac{([0 - 10^*] - 1)^2}{10}$$
$$= \frac{(9)^2}{10}$$
$$= \frac{81}{10}$$

Therefore $\chi^2 = 8.1$

(*If you get a minus figure in the square brackets, ignore the minus and treat the figure as a plus; i.e. −10 becomes 10).

4. Before looking up the results to see if they represent a significant change in fear, you need a further value: the d.f. value. In the McNemar test, it is always 1.

Looking up the value of c^2 for significance

To see whether this value of 8.1 represents a significant difference in fear levels, turn to Table A2.1, which is the probability table associated with the McNemar test (and the Chi-squared or χ^2 test: see later). Down the left-hand column you will see d.f. values from 1 to 30. To their right are five numbers, called *critical values* of χ^2. To find out whether our χ^2 value is significant, look down the d.f. column until you find our d.f. value of 1. To the right you will see five critical values:

$$2.71 \quad 3.84 \quad 5.41 \quad 6.64 \quad 10.83$$

Each of these figures is associated with the probability value at the top of its column. For example, the critical value of 2.71 is associated with a probability value of 0.10, for a two-tailed test. You will notice that this table only refers to two-tailed hypotheses. Where you have a one-tailed hypothesis, look up the results in the way outlined, and simply halve the p value (see pp. 87–89).

For our χ^2 value to be significant, it has to be *equal to* or *larger than* one of the critical values to the right of d.f. = 1. Our χ^2 value of 8.1 is larger than 2.71, 3.84, 5.41 and 6.64 but smaller than 10.83. Therefore our value of χ^2 comes somewhere between 6.64 and 10.83. If you trace these figures up to the top of the table, you will see that 6.64 has an associated probability of 0.01 and that 10.83 has an associated probability of 0.001. Therefore, as our χ^2 value comes between 6.64 and 10.83, its associated probability must similarly be between 0.01 and 0.001. In other words the probability associated with $\chi^2 = 8.1$ is *less than* 0.01 (or 1%) and *larger than* 0.001 (or 0.1%). Convention dictates that we must always conclude that p is less than a given level and so here we would say that for $\chi^2 = 8.1$, p is *less than* 0.01 (or 1%) for a two-tailed hypothesis, therefore *0.005 for a one-tailed* hypothesis (i.e. *half* 0.01). If you look back to our hypothesis, you will see that we are predicting a specific direction to our results, i.e. a pre-screening talk will reduce fear levels; therefore, our hypothesis is one-tailed. Therefore, as our χ^2 value is larger than 6.64, that means that the probability of our results being due to random error is even less than 0.005. This is expressed as:

$$p < 0.005 \ (< \text{means 'less than'})$$

Had our χ^2 value been exactly 6.64 we would have expressed this as:

$$p = 0.005.$$

Interpreting the results

Our results are associated with a probability of less than 0.005 or 0.5%. This means there is less than 0.5% chance of the results being due to random error. If you remember, a p value of 5% or less was a standard cut-off point for claiming results to be significant. As 0.5% is less than 5% our results are significant. However, before going on to explain what this means, you must check that the changes in fear are in the direction you predicted, that is

high fear		low fear
before the	changed to	after the
talk		talk

It is possible to get significant results which are in the opposite direction to those predicted. In this case it would mean

low fear		high fear
before the	changed to	after the
talk		talk

These results, while significant, would not support your hypothesis. Therefore when you have a one-tailed hypothesis you must always check that your actual data are in the predicted direction.

If you look at the data in the table, you will see that the changes are in the predicted direction, and we can;

reject the null (no relationship) hypothesis
and
accept the experimental hypothesis.

We can state this in the following way:

Using a McNemar test on the data ($\chi^2 = 8.1$, d.f. = 1), the results were found to be significant at $p < 0.005$ for a one-tailed test. This suggests that a pre-screening talk significantly reduces the fear of women due to undergo amniocentesis.

It is very important to note, though, that there should be significant numbers involved to compute the McNemar test. If Cell A + Cell D $\div$ 2 comes to less than 5, you cannot use the McNemar. In such a case, it would be worth your while to collect sufficient data to satisfy the above requirement.

Activity 13.1 (Answers on page 238)

1. To practise looking up χ^2 values for the McNemar test, look up the following and say whether you would classify them as significant.
   - (i) $\chi^2 = 3.98$ d.f. = 1   one-tailed p
   - (ii) $\chi^2 = 6.71$ d.f. = 1   one-tailed p
   - (iii) $\chi^2 = 5.41$ d.f. = 1   two-tailed p
   - (iv) $\chi^2 = 2.59$ d.f. = 1   one-tailed p
   - (v) $\chi^2 = 10.96$ d.f. = 1   two-tailed p
   - (vi) $\chi^2 = 4.82$ d.f. = 1   two-tailed p

2. Calculate a McNemar test on the following data:
   As a Director of Midwifery Services, you wish to alter the shift system in order to accommodate changes accruing from the 'named-midwife' initiative, but have so far met with opposition from the midwives in the Unit. In fact on the last poll, only five out of 30 were prepared to alter their duties. You decide to send round an explanatory fact sheet, in the hope that presenting the reasons for your change might alter their views. At the end of the fact sheet you simply ask the midwives to indicate whether or not they would accommodate the altered duties.
   Your hypothesis is:

   H₁ Providing extra information about the reasons for changing the shifts system will modify the opinions of the midwives involved.

   Is this a one- or two-tailed hypothesis?
   You obtain the results shown in Table 13.3.

Table 13.3 Effect of extra information on opinions of midwives; √ for the change; X against the change

Midwife	Opinions prior to receipt of fact sheet	Opinions after the receipt of fact sheet
1	X	√
2	X	√
3	X	X
4	X	√
5	√	√
6	X	X
7	X	√
8	X	X
9	X	√
10	X	X
11	X	√
12	X	√
13	X	X
14	X	X
15	X	√
16	√	√
17	X	√
18	√	√
19	X	X
20	X	√
21	X	X
22	X	√
23	X	X
24	√	√
25	X	X
26	X	X
27	√	X
28	X	√
29	X	√
30	X	√

State what your χ^2 value is and what your p value is. Write this out in a similar format to that given on page 125.

NON-PARAMETRIC STATISTICAL TEST FOR USE WITH SAME AND MATCHED SUBJECT DESIGNS, TWO CONDITIONS AND ORDINAL OR INTERVAL/RATIO DATA

Wilcoxon signed-ranks test

To recap, this test is used when you have two conditions (either one control condition and one experimental condition or two experimental conditions) and you have either one group of subjects doing both conditions, or two groups of matched subjects, one group doing one condition and the other group the other condition (see Designs 1a and 2a on pages 121–122). The data for this test must be ordinal or interval/ratio.

Essentially what the Wilcoxon test does is to compare the performance of each S (or pair of matched Ss) in each condition to see if there is a significant difference between them. When you calculate this test, you end up with a numerical value for 'T' which you then look up in the probability tables for the Wilcoxon test to see if this value represents a significant difference between the conditions.

Example

Since pre-registration midwives were made supernumerary, it has become necessary that in order for students to obtain sufficient clinical experience, they have to be present in a passive observational capacity rather than an active one. It has been suggested to you that many women feel disconcerted about being observed during their care procedures, particularly when some intimate activity is being performed. Consequently, a rise in anxiety and tension levels may be experienced by women in such situations. You decide you will test the reported anxiety levels of a group of women undergoing ante-natal care both when there is a student midwife present and when there is no student midwife present. Therefore, you decide to test the following hypothesis:

H_1 Women receiving ante-natal care experience higher levels of anxiety when there is a student midwife present than when there is not.

What would your null hypothesis be?
Is this a one or two tailed hypothesis?

You devise a questionnaire which simply asks the women to indicate on a 5-point scale (ordinal data) how anxious they feel when being treated (a) when a student midwife is present and (b) when a student midwife is not present. On your scale, a score of 1 means 'not at all anxious' while 5 means 'very anxious'. You give this questionnaire to 15 women at an ante-natal clinic. Thus, you have the design shown in Figure 13.8:

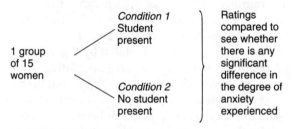

Figure 13.8 Design to test effect of presence of student midwife on patient anxiety.

You have all the conditions required by the Wilcoxon i.e. a same-subject design and ordinal data.

You administer your questionnaire to the 15 Ss (having, of course, included all the essential prerequisites for such a design, see Chapters 7 and 8) and you end up with the results shown in Table 13.4.

Calculating the Wilcoxon test

In order to find out whether these ratings differ significantly for each condition, you must take the following steps:

1. Add up the total (Σ) for condition A (Student present):

$$\Sigma A = 60$$

2. Add up the total (Σ) for condition B (No student present):

$$\Sigma B = 38$$

3. Find the mean ($\bar{x}$) for each condition

$$\bar{x} A = 4 \qquad \bar{x} B = 2.533$$

4. Calculate the difference (d) for each pair of

Table 13.4 Results of questionnaire and calculation of Wilcoxon test

Subject	Results		Calculations			
	1 Condition A Student present	2 Condition B* No student present	3 $d =$ A − B	4 Rank order of d	5 Rank of + differences	6 Rank of − differences
1	5	3	+2	(+) 5.5	+ 5.5	
2	4	3	+1	(+) 1.5	+ 1.5	
3	5	2	+3	(+) 9.5	+ 9.5	
4	2	5	−3	(−) 9.5		− 9.5
5	4	4	0	exclude		
6	3	3	0	exclude		
7	5	4	+1	(+) 1.5	+ 1.5	
8	5	3	+2	(+) 5.5	+ 5.5	
9	4	2	+2	(+) 5.5	+ 5.5	
10	4	2	+2	(+) 5.5	+ 5.5	
11	2	2	0	exclude		
12	3	1	+2	(+) 5.5	+ 5.5	
13	5	1	+4	(+) 11.5	+ 11.5	
14	4	2	+2	(+) 5.5	+ 5.5	
15	5	1	+4	(+) 11.5	+ 11.5	
Σ	60	38			+ 68.5	− 9.5
$\bar{x}$	4	2.533				

*It does not matter which condition is called A and which B.

scores by taking A – B, remembering to put in the + and – signs.

Therefore for S1 you would have 5 – 3 = +2 and so on. Put the results in column 3 (d = A – B).

5. You must then rank order these differences by giving a rank of 1 to the smallest difference, 2 to the next smallest and so on. When you do this, you must ignore the plus and minus signs. However, where the difference between a pair of scores is 0, you omit this pair altogether from any further analysis. Therefore, in this example, subjects 5, 6 and 11 are now excluded from any further analysis and we are reduced to 12 subjects.

You will also note that there are a number of d values which are identical, e.g. Ss 2 and 7 both have a d of + 1, Ss 1, 8, 9, 10, 12 and 14 all have a d value of + 2. Where this happens a special procedure is used – the 'tied rank' procedure.

Tied rank procedure To carry out the tied rank procedure, rank the scores as usual, giving a rank of 1 to the smallest, 2 to the next smallest (remember: we omit the 0s and ignore the + and – values). Continue this procedure until you come to the tied scores. Here, Ss 2 and 7 both have d values of 1. These two scores are the lowest and should therefore occupy the two lowest ranks i.e. ranks 1 and 2. So we add up these two ranks (1 + 2) and divide this by the number of d values that have the same score (i.e. 2 d values of 1).

$$\frac{1 + 2}{2} = 1.5$$

Therefore, the d values of 1 are both given the ranks of 1.5 (see column entitled Rank of d). We now find there are 6 d values of 2. These values occupy the next lowest ranks i.e. 3, 4, 5, 6, 7 and 8 (because ranks 1 and 2 have already been used up).

Therefore we add these ranks together:

$$3 + 4 + 5 + 6 + 7 + 8 = 33$$

and divide this by the number of d values having the value of 2 (i.e. 6 d values of 2) = 33 ÷ 6 = 5.5.

Thus, all the d-values of 2 are assigned the rank 5.5.

We now find there are 2 d values of 3 (Ss 3 and 4). These are the next two lowest scores and they would occupy the next two lowest ranks i.e. 9 and 10 (because ranks 1–8 have now been used up).

Therefore, we add these ranks together 9 + 10 = 19 and divide this by the number of d values which have the same value of 3 (i.e. 2 d values of 3) which is 19 ÷ 2 = 9.5.

Therefore, both the d values of 3 are given the rank of 9.5.

Now there are only two remaining d values, each of which is 4. These d values occupy the next two ranks i.e. 11 and 12 (because ranks 1–10 have now been used up). Therefore we add these ranks together (11 + 12 = 23) and divide this by the number of d values which have the same value of 4 (i.e. 2 d values of 4) = 11.5. Thus, the d values of 4 are each given the rank of 11.5.

Many people get very irritated by this ranking procedure, especially when calculating tied ranks, because a slip of just one figure can throw everything out. To avoid this, you may wish to write out all the ranks you will be using (which will be the same as the number of differences to be ranked) and cross them off as you use them. Here, then, we would write out the following ranks 1, 2, 3, 4, 5, 6, 7, 8, 9, 10, 11, 12 and strike them off as we go along.

Remember, the highest rank should be the same as the number of differences between scores you are ranking. Here we are ranking 12 d values, so the highest rank will be 12.

6. Now write in by each rank the plus or minus sign of the corresponding d value. Therefore, the first rank of 5.5 is given a plus sign because it has a corresponding d value of +2.

7. Put all the ranks with a + sign into column 5 'Rank of + differences'. Put all the ranks with a – sign into the column 6 'Rank of minus differences'.

8. Add up the ranks for the column 5 'Rank of + differences' to give the total (Σ) for the + ranks, i.e. +68.5.

Add up the ranks for the column 6 'Rank of – differences' to give the total (Σ) for the – ranks, i.e. –9.5.

9. Take the smaller of the two rank totals,

ignoring the plus or minus sign, as your value of T (i.e. $T = 9.5$).

10. Find N by counting up the number of subjects (or in the case of matched groups, pairs of Ss) omitting those who had d values of 0, i.e. $15 - 3 = 12$.

Looking up the value of T for significance

To see whether this T value of 9.5 represents a significant difference in the anxiety levels experienced by women when either a student midwife is present or not present, it must be looked up in the probability tables for the Wilcoxon test (Table A2.2).

Down the left-hand column you will see values of N, while across the top you will see 'Levels of significance' for one-and two-tailed tests. Under each of these are columns of figures which are called *critical values of T*.

To find out whether our T value is significant at one of the levels indicated, we must first locate our N value of 12 down the left-hand column. To the right of this you will see four numbers which represent the critical values of T for this number of Ss. These values are: 17 14 10 7. Each of these figures is associated with the corresponding p value indicated at the top of the column. For example, a critical value of 14 is associated with a probability of

0.05 for a two-tailed test
and 0.025 for a one-tailed test

In order for your T value to be significant at a given level, it has to be *equal to* or *smaller than* one of these four figures. So, taking our T value of 9.5, look at the first figure to the right of $N = 12$, i.e. 17. Our T value is smaller than 17, so look at the next figure: 14. Our T value is smaller than 14, so look at the next figure: 10. Our T value is smaller than 10, so look at the next figure: 7. Our T value is larger than 7. Therefore our T value comes somewhere between the critical values of 7 and 10 in the table. If you look at the top of the table, you will see that these values are associated with the probabilities of 0.01 and 0.005 for a one-tailed test and 0.02 and 0.01 for a two-tailed test.

Because we have a one-tailed hypothesis (more anxiety when a student midwife is present) this means our results are significant between the 0.01 and 0.005 (or 1%–2%) levels. Now, to be significant at a given level, the T value must be equal to or smaller than the critical value of T. Because it is smaller than 10 but larger than 7, we must comply with convention and select the value of 10, which is associated with a significance level of 1%. Had our T value equalled this figure exactly, we would say that our results are significant at p equals 0.01. However, our T value is smaller than 10, which means that its significance is actually less than 0.01. Therefore we express this as:

$$p < 0.01 \text{ (< means 'less than')}$$

This means that the probability of our results being due to random error is less than 1%.

Interpreting the results

Our T value is associated with a p value of < 0.01 level (i.e. $< 1\%$ level) which means that there is less than a 1% chance that our results are due to random error. If you remember, we said a good rule of thumb for claiming support for your hypothesis is a probability of 5% (or 0.05) or less. Because our T has a smaller p value than 5%, we can say that our results are significant. But, it is very important to note that you must check the averages for each set of data (A = 4, B = 2.533) to see whether the results are in the direction you predicted (i.e. larger with the student midwife present), since occasionally, you may get significant results which are actually the reverse of what you predicted and therefore would not support your hypothesis.

Here, the results are in the direction you predicted and therefore, we can say that your hypothesis has been supported (i.e. we can reject the null hypothesis).

We can state this in the following way:

Using a Wilcoxon test on the data ($T = 9.5$, $N = 12$), the results were found to be significant at $p < 0.01$ level for a one-tailed test. This suggests that women undergoing ante-natal care experience greater anxiety when a student midwife is present than when no student midwife is present.

(At what level would the results have been significant had the hypothesis been two-tailed?)

Activity 13.2 (Answers on page 238)

1. To practise ranking, rank order the following results using the guidelines above. Remember to rank from smallest to biggest, omitting any zero scores, ignoring the plus and minus signs of the d values, and giving the average rank for tied d values.

Table 13.5

Subject	Condition A	Condition B	d	Rank
1	10	9	+ 1	
2	8	9	− 1	
3	9	7	+ 2	
4	6	7	− 1	
5	5	4	+ 1	
6	8	3	+ 5	
7	7	6	+ 1	
8	9	9	0	
9	9	6	+ 3	
10	5	6	− 1	
11	7	3	+ 4	
12	8	4	+ 4	

2. To practise looking up T values, look up the following and say whether you would classify them as significant
   (i) $T = 7$ $N = 9$ one-tailed
   (ii) $T = 7$ $N = 15$ two-tailed
   (iii) $T = 15$ $N = 13$ one-tailed
   (iv) $T = 20$ $N = 16$ one-tailed
   (v) $T = 16$ $N = 12$ two-tailed
   (vi) $T = 32$ $N = 16$ one-tailed
   (vii) $T = 7$ $N = 12$ two-tailed
   (viii) $T = 12$ $N = 13$ one-tailed

3. Calculate a Wilcoxon on the following data:
   H_1 Reported satisfaction with care is greater when the mother has taken an active role in managing her labour than when she has taken a peripheral or passive role.
   (Is this a one- or a two-tailed hypothesis?)
   Brief method: Select two groups each of 12 women in the early stages of labour. The women are matched in pairs on all critical factors, such as parity, maternal and fetal well-being, social class, age etc. One group is encouraged to take an active part in the decision making during labour, while the other group takes very little or no part. One hour after delivery, both groups are asked to rate their satisfaction with care on a 7-point scale (1 = no satisfaction, 7 = very great satisfaction).

Table 13.6

Subject pair	Condition A Active role	Condition B Passive role
1	3	3
2	4	3
3	5	4
4	4	3
5	7	3
6	4	4
7	4	4
8	6	5
9	5	3
10	3	2
11	6	3
12	4	3

Write down the T value
           N value
           p value
and state whether or not your results are significant, using the format of the paragraph on page 129.

NON-PARAMETRIC STATISTICAL TESTS FOR USE WITH SAME AND MATCHED SUBJECT DESIGNS, THREE OR MORE CONDITIONS AND ORDINAL OR INTERVAL/RATIO DATA

Friedman test

This test is similar to the Wilcoxon in that it is used for related and matched subject designs. However, the Friedman is used when either

a. one group of subjects is tested under three or more conditions; the results from the conditions are compared for differences.
   or
b. three or more groups of matched subjects are each tested in one condition; the results from the groups are compared for differences.

You would use this test if you had either Design 1b or 2b on pages 121–122 and ordinal or interval/ratio data.

However, the Friedman test only tells you whether the results from each condition differ and not whether the results from one condition are better.

For this reason, any hypothesis which relates to the Friedman must predict general differences and not a specific direction to the results. In other words, it must be two-tailed. When calculating this test, you end up with a numerical value for χr^2 which you then look up in the probability tables associated with the Friedman test to see whether this represents a significant difference between your conditions.

Example

To illustrate this, let us suppose that you are a midwife tutor in a small school of health sciences. You have noticed that over the last 2 or 3 years students seem to do consistently worse on the physiology and biochemistry modules than they do on psychology and midwifery care modules. This may be to do with individual student preferences, but it may also reflect the calibre of the tutors responsible, the quality of their teaching support or of clinical supervision. However, before moving on to find the cause, you must first establish whether or not your observation is correct. Your hypothesis is:

H$_1$ Third-year direct entry midwifery students perform differently on four key curriculum topics.

This is a two-tailed hypothesis, as it predicts no direction to the differences.

To test this hypothesis, you randomly select 17 students in the final year of their training and compare their marks (on a 10-point scale; 1 = disastrous, 10 = excellent) in the four key curriculum topics: physiology, biochemistry, psychology and midwifery care.

You design, then, looks like Figure 13.9. Your data are shown in Table 13.7.

Calculating the Friedman test

In order to calculate the Friedman you must take the following steps:

1. Firstly, add up the scores for each condition:

$\Sigma A = 85$ $\Sigma B = 110$ $\Sigma C = 138$ $\Sigma D = 116$

2. Find out the means for each condition:

$\bar{x}A = 5$ $\bar{x}B = 6.471$ $\bar{x}C = 8.118$ $\bar{x}D = 6.824$

3. Rank the scores for each subject (i.e. across the row) giving the rank of 1 to the smallest score,

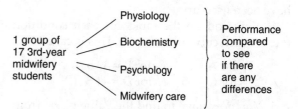

Figure 13.9 Design to test whether third-year direct entry midwifery students perform differently on four key curriculum topics.

Table 13.7

Subject	Condition A Physiology		Condition B Biochemistry		Condition C Psychology		Condition D Midwifery care	
	Score	Rank	Score	Rank	Score	Rank	Score	Rank
1	5	1	6	2	8	4	7	3
2	6	2.5	6	2.5	7	4	5	1
3	3	1	7	3.5	7	3.5	6	2
4	8	2	9	3	10	4	7	1
5	7	1.5	9	3.5	9	3.5	7	1.5
6	6	1.5	8	3	9	4	6	1.5
7	5	1	8	3	9	4	7	2
8	5	1	8	2.5	10	4	8	2.5
9	4	1	6	2	8	3	9	4
10	3	1	5	2	8	4	7	3
11	6	2	5	1	8	4	7	3
12	6	2.5	4	1	7	4	6	2.5
13	7	2	5	1	9	4	8	3
14	3	1	7	3	8	4	6	2
15	2	1	5	2	7	3.5	7	3.5
16	5	1	6	2.5	7	4	6	2.5
17	4	1	6	2	7	3.5	7	3.5
	$\Sigma = 85$ $\bar{x} = 5$	$T_C = 24$	$\Sigma = 110$ $\bar{x} = 6.471$	$T_C = 39.5$	$\Sigma = 138$ $\bar{x} = 8.118$	$T_C = 65$	$\Sigma = 116$ $\bar{x} = 6.824$	$T_C = 41.5$

a rank of 2 to the next smallest and so on. You will only need ranks 1–4 as there are only four scores for each subject. Where you have tied scores, use the tied rank procedure (see p. 128) i.e. add up the ranks these scores would have had if they had been different, and divide by the number of scores which are the same. Therefore, if we look at subject 2, she scored 5 in physiology, 6 in biochemistry, 6 in psychology and 7 in midwifery care. Thus 5 gets a rank of 1; the two 6s, had they been different would have had ranks of 2 and 3 (because rank 1 has now been used up); so we add 2 + 3 = 5, and divide this by the total number of scores which are the same (i.e. 2, because there are 2 scores of 6) = 2.5. This, then is the rank we give the 6s. The score of 7 in midwifery care gets a rank of 4 because ranks 1–3 have been used up.

4. Now add up the ranks for each condition (i.e. for each curriculum topic). This is called T_C.

T_C for A = 24 T_C for B = 39.5
T_C for C = 65 T_C for D = 41.5

5. You now have to find the value of χr^2 from the following formula:

$$\chi r^2 = \left[\left(\frac{12}{NC(C + 1)}\right)(\Sigma T_C^2)\right] - 3N(C + 1)$$

where N = number of Ss in the group (or in the case of matched designs, the number of sets of subjects) i.e. 17

C = number of conditions i.e. 4

T_C = total of the ranks for each condition
T_C for condition A = 24
T_C for condition B = 39.5
T_C for condition C = 65
T_C for condition D = 41.5

T_C^2 = each rank total squared i.e. 24^2; 39.5^2; 65^2; 41.5^2
= 576; 1560.25; 4225; 1722.25

Σ = sum or total of all the calculations following it

ΣT_C^2 = the sum of the squared ranks for each condition i.e.

576 + 1560.25 + 4225 + 1722.25
= 8083.5

Remember! Do all the calculations in brackets first, starting with divisions and multiplications and finally additions and subtractions.

Thus, if we substitute some values in the formula:

$$\chi r^2 = \left[\left(\frac{12}{17 \times 4(4 + 1)}\right) \times 8083.5\right] - 3 \times 17(4 + 1)$$

$$= \left[\left(\frac{12}{68 \times 5}\right) \times 8083.5\right] - 255$$

$$= [0.035 \times 8083.5] - 255$$

$$= 282.923 - 255$$

$$\chi r^2 = 27.923$$

Looking up the value of χr^2

To look up χr^2 in the tables, you also need the degrees of freedom value. This is the number of conditions minus 1, i.e. 4 – 1 = 3. As you will see, there are three main tables for the Friedman test: Tables A2.3a, A2.3b and A2.1. Table A2.3a is used where there are three conditions and only 2–9 subjects in each condition; Table A2.3b is for four conditions, with 2–4 Ss in each, and Table A2.1 is for anything larger, i.e. more conditions or more subjects.

Because we have four conditions and 17 subjects, we must use Table A2.1. (This table is also for use with the χ^2 test.) You will see that in the left-hand column, entitled d.f., there are various degrees of freedom values. Look down this column until you have found the d.f. for this example, i.e. 3. You will see five numbers called critical values to the right: 6.25, 7.82, 9.84, 11.34 and 16.27. Each of these values is associated with the level of probability shown at the top of its column, e.g. 11.34 is associated with a p value of 0.01. To be significant at a given level, our χr^2 value must be equal to or larger than the values here. So, if we take the first value 6.25, our χr^2 value is larger; it is also larger than 7.82, 9.84, 11.34 and 16.27. Therefore we take the value 16.27 and look up the column to see what the associated level of significance is, i.e. 0.001 or the 0.1% level. Because our χr^2 value of 27.923 is larger than the critical value 16.27, this means that our results are significant at less than (<) the 0.001 level. (Had our χr^2 value been 16.27 exactly, we would say our p value equals 0.001.)

This means that there is less than a 0.1% chance that our results are due to random error.

Note that because the Friedman only allows you to predict differences and not specific directions to the results, your hypothesis must be two-tailed and so this level of significance represents the level for a two-tailed hypothesis. Because our usual cut-off point is 5% and our p value is less than that, i.e. 0.1%, we can say that our results are significant at < 0.1% level.

Interpreting the results

The results are associated with a p value of less than 0.1%. This means that there is less than a 0.1% probability of our results being due to random error. As the standard cut-off point is 5%, we can reject our null hypothesis and say that our results are significant. In other words, students do perform differently in four key curriculum modules. We can express this in the following way:

> Using a Friedman test on the data ($\chi r^2 = 27.923$, $N = 17$), the results were found to be significant at $p < 0.001$, for a two-tailed test. This suggests that 3rd-year direct entry midwifery students perform significantly differently in four curriculum modules, and so supports the experimental hypothesis. The null hypothesis can therefore be rejected.

Do note, however, that the Friedman only allows us to identify differences and not to say on which topic students performed better. If, however, you do expect a trend in the results of a related or matched subject design (e.g. that students do worst in physiology, followed by biochemistry, followed by psychology and best in midwifery care, you would need the Page's L trend test (see next section).

If you had only three conditions and fewer subjects then you would use Table A2.3a. For example, supposing you had three conditions and seven subjects, and a χr^2 value of 7.5 you

would look to find your value of N across the top of the table, (remember N = the number of Ss or subject pairs). Under this you will see a column for the χr^2 value, and to the right the corresponding p value or significance level. So taking the column for $N = 7$, look down the χr^2 value to find 7.5. Since our χr^2 value must be equal to or larger than those given to be significant at a given level, we find that our value of 7.5 is larger than 7.143, but smaller than 7.714. We must take the critical value of 7.143 (because our χr^2 value must be equal to or larger than the critical value given) which gives us a corresponding p value of 0.027 or 2.7%.

However, because our χr^2 value of 7.5 is larger than 7.143, this means our p value is even less than (<) 0.027. Had our χr^2 value *equalled* the critical value of 7.143, we would say that our p value equals 0.027. So, our results have a p value of < 0.027. Using the standard cut-off of 0.05, we can say our results are significant. We can therefore reject the null hypothesis, and accept the experimental hypothesis.

Supposing, however, we had four conditions, and four subjects or pairs of subjects and a χr^2 value of 2.6, we would need to use Table A2.3b which is for use with four conditions and 2–4 Ss. Here we would find the column corresponding to our N value, and look down the χr^2 values to find our own of 2.6. Because our value has to be equal to or larger than the values shown to be significant at a given level, we can see that our χr^2 value of 2.6 is larger than 2.4 but smaller than 2.7. Therefore we have to take the value next smallest to our own, i.e. 2.4, which gives us a p value of 0.524 or 52.4%. Because of our standard 5% cut-off point, this p value cannot be classified as significant because it is larger. Therefore we would have to conclude that our results were not significant, our hypothesis was not supported and we would have to accept the null (no relationship) hypothesis.

Activity 13.3 (Answers on page 238)

1. To practise looking up χr^2 values, look up the following and say whether they are significant
   (i) $C = 4$ $N = 3$ $\chi r^2 = 7.4$ p
   (ii) $C = 4$ $N = 10$ $\chi r^2 = 9.92$ p
   (iii) $C = 3$ $N = 6$ $\chi r^2 = 5.72$ p

(iv) $C = 3$ $N = 12$ $\chi r^2 = 35.7$ p
(v) $C = 3$ $N = 8$ $\chi r^2 = 9.3$ p

2. Calculate a Friedman on the following data:

H1 The pain experienced in labour differs according to whether the mother was allowed to be mobile during the first stage, use a birthing chair or to be supine.

Brief method: Select seven women from each category of activity during the first stage of labour, ensuring that they are matched on certain key variables, such as parity, age, maternal condition, additional analgesia etc. Following delivery ask them to rate on a 5-point scale their degree of pain experienced. (1 = no pain, 5 = very severe pain). You might obtain the results shown in Table 13.8.

Table 13.8

Subject	Condition A Ambulant	Condition B Birthing chair	Condition C Supine
1	3	4	5
2	2	2	5
3	2	3	4
4	1	2	3
5	3	2	2
6	1	2	1
7	3	3	3

Write down the χr^2 value and the p value. State whether or not your results are significant, and what they mean, using the example given on page 133.

Page's L trend test

This test is an extension of the Friedman test, in that it is used when

a. the design is a related or matched subject one
b. the data is ordinal or interval / ratio
c. there are three or more conditions (i.e. one group of Ss doing three or more conditions, or three or more matched groups of Ss each doing one condition).

However, there is one salient difference: whereas the Friedman test can only be used to discover whether there are differences between the conditions without saying which condition is significantly better or worse than the others, the Page's L trend test is used when the experimenter has predicted a trend in the results; for example when comparing the quality of three colleges of midwifery, the experimenter, in the hypothesis, predicts that College A is better than College B, which in turn is better than College C. This contrasts with the sort of hypothesis which must

be used with the Friedman test, which would simply predict differences in quality between the three schools. Thus the sort of design we might have with the Page's L trend test is:

1. In a comparison of a group of students' attitudes to three types of teaching method, it is predicted that the seminar method will be most popular, followed by the lecture method with tutorials least popular. The design in Figure 13.10 could be used.

Alternatively, the following design is appropriate for use with the Page's L trend test:

2. In a comparison of three types of exercise techniques for post-partum stress incontinence, it is predicted that Exercise A will be more effective than Exercise B which will be more effective than Exercise C. Three groups of women, matched for age, duration of labour, perineal trauma, parity etc, are given one of the exercise regimes and compared for continence after 1 month (Fig. 13.11).

The Page's L trend test then essentially assesses whether there is a significant trend in the results. When calculating it you derive the value of L, which is then looked up in the probability tables associated with the Page's test to see whether this value represents a significant trend in your results.

Because you are predicting a *specific direction* to the results when you use a Page's L trend test, the hypothesis must be *one-tailed*.

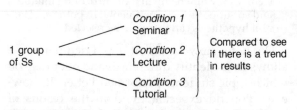

Figure 13.10 Design for assessing popularity of teaching methods.

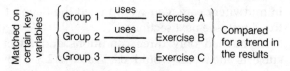

Figure 13.11 Design for assessing effectiveness of exercise techniques.

Example

Let us take the first hypothesis that in order to evaluate midwifery students' preferences for three types of teaching approach, you predict that the seminar method will be more popular than the lecture method, with the tutorial being least popular; a trend is predicted, i.e. seminar > lecture > tutorial (> means 'greater than').

You select a group of ten final year midwifery students and ask them to rate the three methods on a 5-point scale (5 = most preferred, 1 = least preferred). In order to analyse the results you must set out your data such that the scores you predict will be the smallest (i.e. tutorial) are placed on the left, and the scores you predict to be the largest are placed on the right as in Table 13.9.

Calculating the Page's L *trend test*

1. In order to calculate the value of L you must take the following steps: First find the total scores for each condition

$$\Sigma_1 = 20 \quad \Sigma_2 = 32 \quad \Sigma_3 = 38$$

Then find the mean score for each condition

$$\bar{x}_1 = 2 \quad \bar{x}_2 = 3.2 \quad \bar{x}_3 = 3.8$$

2. Rank the scores for each subject (or sets of matched Ss) across the row, as for the Friedman, giving the rank of 1 to the lowest score, the rank

of 2 to the next lowest etc. If you have two or more scores which are the same, you must give these the average rank (see page 128 on how to deal with tied scores), i.e you add up the value of the ranks they would have obtained had they been different and divide by the number of scores that are the same. Therefore, S1 has two scores of 3. Had these scores been the two lowest but different scores they would have had the ranks 1 and 2. These values are added together (3) and divided by 2 (because there are two scores of 3) to give the average rank, 1.5, which is entered alongside the scores of 3.

3. Add up the ranks for each condition, i.e.

$$T_C1 = 12 \quad T_C2 = 22.5 \quad T_C3 = 25.5$$

4. Find the value of L from the formula

$$L = \Sigma(T_C1 \times C) + \Sigma(T_C2 \times C) + \Sigma(T_C3 \times C)$$

Where: Σ means the total or sum of any symbols that follow it
T_C = total of ranks for each condition
    i.e. $T_C1 = 12$; $T_C2 = 22.5$; $T_C3 = 25.5$
C = numbers allotted to the conditions from left to right
    i.e. 1, 2 and 3
$(T_C \times C)$ = total of the ranks for each condition multiplied by the number assigned to the condition
    i.e. $T_C1 \times 1 = 12 \times 1$
    $T_C2 \times 2 = 22.5 \times 2$
    $T_C3 \times 3 = 25.5 \times 3$

Table 13.9

Subject	Condition 1 Tutorial		Condition 2 Lecture		Condition 3 Seminar	
	Score	Rank	Score	Rank	Score	Rank
1	3	1.5	4	3	3	1.5
2	2	1.5	2	1.5	4	3
3	3	1.5	3	1.5	5	3
4	1	1	3	3	2	2
5	2	1.5	3	3	2	1.5
6	2	1	4	2	5	3
7	1	1	2	2	4	3
8	3	1	4	2.5	4	2.5
9	2	1	4	2	5	3
10	1	1	3	2	4	3
	$\Sigma_1 = 20$	$T_C1 = 12$	$\Sigma_2 = 32$	$T_C2 = 22.5$	$\Sigma_3 = 38$	$T_C3 = 25.5$

$L = (12 \times 1) + (22.5 \times 2) + (25.5 \times 3)$
$= 12 + 45 + 76.5$
$= 133.5$

5. To look up your value of L, you also need two further values: C (the number of conditions, i.e. 3) and N (the number of Ss in the group or the number of sets of matched Ss, i.e. 10).

Looking up the value of L for significance

Turn to Table A2.4. Across the top you will see values of C (i.e. number of conditions) from 3 to 6, and down the left-hand column, values of N (i.e. number of Ss or sets of matched Ss) from 2 to 12. Look across the C values to find our value of $C = 3$ and down the N values to find our $N = 10$ value.

At their intersection point you will see three numbers: 134, 131, and 128. These are called critical values of L. If you look across these rows to the right-hand column, you will see that 134 represents a p value of 0.001; 131 represents a p value of 0.01 and 128 represents a p value of 0.05. To be significant at one of these levels, your L value must be equal to or larger than one of the numbers 134, 131 and 128. The obtained value of L in our example is 133.5. This is larger than 131, but smaller than 134. Therefore we must take the value of 131, which represents a significance level of 0.01 or 1%. But because our L value is larger than the critical value of 131, this means that the corresponding p value is less than (<) 0.01. This is expressed as $p < 0.01$. This means that there is less than a 1% chance of the results being caused by random error. Because you must be predicting a specific direction to your results in order to be using a trend test, your hypothesis, by definition, must be one-tailed. Therefore, all the values in this table are values for a one-tailed hypothesis.

Using our usual cut-off point of 5%, because the p value in our study is smaller, we can conclude that our results are significant at < 0.01 level. Thus we can reject the null hypothesis and conclude that there is a significant trend in the results as predicted in our hypothesis.

Interpreting the results

Our results have a probability value of < 0.01 which means that there is less than a 1% chance of their being due to random error. Because this p value is smaller than the usual cut-off point of 0.05, we can say that our results are significant. This means we can reject the null hypothesis and accept the experimental hypothesis.

This can be expressed in the following way:

Using a Page's L trend test on the data ($L = 133.5$, $N = 10$, $C = 3$), the results were found to be significant at $p < 0.01$ for a one-tailed hypothesis. This suggests that the experimental hypothesis has been supported, and that final year midwifery students prefer seminar teaching methods to lectures, with tutorials being the least preferred approach. The null hypothesis can therefore be rejected.

Activity 13.4   (Answers on pages 238–239)

1. To practise looking up L values, look up the following and decide at what level (if any) they are significant:
   (i) $N = 5$ $C = 4$ $L = 142.5$ p
   (ii) $N = 8$ $C = 5$ $L = 384$ p
   (iii) $N = 7$ $C = 3$ $L = 92$ p
   (iv) $N = 12$ $C = 6$ $L = 971$ p
   (v) $N = 10$ $C = 5$ $L = 455.5$ p
2. Calculate a Page's L trend test on the following data:
   H_1 It is hypothesized that sheepskins are more effective than terry towelling which in turn is more effective than cotton sheeting in reducing crying amongst premature babies.
   Method: Take three groups, each of eight premature babies, matched for weeks' gestation, age, sex, medication, birth weight etc., and nurse each group on one of the three surfaces. After I week compare the average number of minutes per day spent crying. The results are shown in Table 13.10:

Table 13.10

Subject trio	Condition 1 Sheepskins		Condition 2 Cotton sheeting		Condition 3 Terry towelling	
	Score	Rank	Score	Rank	Score	Rank
1	40		25		30	
2	55		30		40	
3	35		35		45	
4	20		30		40	
5	30		20		30	
6	50		45		50	
7	55		45		50	
8	60		50		60	

State your L and p values, using the sample format given on page 136.

Remember! Put the scores which are predicted to be lowest in the left-hand column and those predicted to be highest in the right-hand column. In other words, you will need to rearrange the table.

Remember, too, that the data in this example are of an interval/ratio type, which can be used with both non-parametric and parametric tests.

14

Parametric tests for same and matched subject designs

INTRODUCTION

All the statistical tests described in this chapter, like those in the previous one, are used to analyse the results from same subject or matched subject designs; in other words, those designs which either use one group of subjects for all the conditions, or alternatively, two or more groups of matched subjects who do one condition each (see pp. 65–68 for the designs).

There is one major difference, however; all the tests in this chapter are *parametric*, which means that they require certain conditions to be fulfilled before they can be used, in particular that the data must be of an interval/ratio level. This requirement concerning the level of data can never, ever be violated. Parametric tests are also rather more difficult to calculate than non-parametric tests. You should always remember that for any given design, the relevant parametric and non-parametric tests do the same job: they assess whether there are significant differences (or in the case of correlations, similarities) between the conditions, but the parametric tests are more sensitive to these differences.

The designs we are interested in then are as follows:

1. *One group of subjects used in all the conditions:* (same subject design)

a. Two conditions only (Fig. 14.1)
or
b. Three or more conditions (Fig. 14.2)

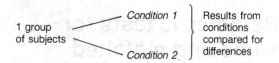

Figure 14.1 One group of subjects tested under two conditions.

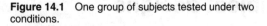

Figure 14.2 One group of subjects tested under three or more conditions.

2. *Two or more groups of matched subjects, each of which is used in one condition only:* (matched subject designs)

a. Two matched groups only (Fig. 14.3)
b. Three of more matched groups (Fig. 14.4)

Results from designs which use one group of subjects in both of two conditions (Design 1a) or two groups of matched subjects, each doing one condition (Design 2a) are analysed using the related *t*-test (Table 14.1). Results from designs using one group of subjects who take part in all three (or more) conditions (Design 1b) or three or more groups of matched subjects each doing one condition (Design 2b) are analysed using the one-

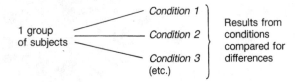

Figure 14.3 Two groups of matched subjects each tested under one condition.

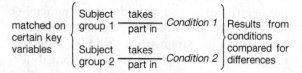

Figure 14.4 Three or more groups of matched subjects, each tested under one condition.

Table 14.1 Parametric tests for related and matched subject designs

Design	Parametric test
1a. One group of Ss tested in two conditions	Related *t*-test
2a. Two groups of matched Ss, each tested in one condition only	Related *t*-test
1b. One group of Ss tested under three or more conditions	One-way anova for related designs, to be used with the Scheffé multiple range test
2b. Three or more groups of matched Ss, each tested in one condition only	One-way anova for related designs, to be used with the Scheffé multiple range test

way analysis of variance (or anova as it is usually known) for related designs. In addition we shall look at the Scheffé multiple range test which is used in conjunction with the anova (see the relevant section).

It should be noted that the *t*-test is sometimes referred to as the 'Student-*t*' in some texts.

PARAMETRIC STATISTICAL TEST FOR USE WITH ONE GROUP OF SUBJECTS AND TWO CONDITIONS OR TWO GROUPS OF MATCHED SUBJECTS, DOING ONE CONDITION EACH

Related *t*-test

Just to recap, this test is used for exactly the same designs as the Wilcoxon, in other words, one group of subjects who take part in both of two conditions (a same subjects design) and the results from the two conditions are then compared for differences. Alternatively, the related *t*-test is used where you have two groups of matched subjects, who do one condition each (a matched subject design) and again the results from the two conditions are compared to see if there are differences between them.

The related *t*-test is especially suitable for 'before and after' type designs, for instance, when you wish to compare the effects of a treatment on one group of subjects.

When calculating the *t*-test, you find the value of *t*, which you then look up in the probability tables for the *t*-test to see whether this value represents significant differences between the results from each condition. Remember that parametric tests are more difficult to calculate than non-parametric tests, so do not panic when you look at the formula. As long as you work through the stages systematically, you will have no difficulty.

Example

Let us imagine you are a community midwife and a recurring problem that new mothers report to you is the incidence of early evening crying in their new babies. While these babies appear to be too young to be suffering from infantile colic, you decide to recommend a proprietary colic treatment anyway, to see if it has any impact. Your experimental hypothesis then is

H$_1$ Excessive early evening crying in neonates can be significantly reduced by a standard infant colic preparation.

This is a one-tailed hypothesis as it predicts a specific direction to the results.

Brief method: To test your hypothesis, you select eight babies who have been reported to cry excessively during the early evening. You ask the mothers to make a note over a 3-day period of the length of time (in minutes) their baby spends crying. You then calculate the average time per baby. The mothers are then given a standard colic treatment and after 1 week are again asked to record the crying time over three evenings. You again compute the average for each baby.

Therefore you have the design shown in Figure 14.5.

Your results are shown in Table 14.2.

Calculating the related t test

To calculate the related *t* test, you must:

1. Add up the scores for each condition to give the total (Σ), i.e.:

$$\Sigma A = 461 \qquad \Sigma B = 401$$

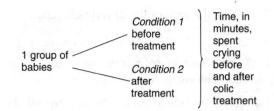

Figure 14.5   Design of experiment to assess whether babies spend less time crying following administration of colic treatment.

Table 14.2   Incidence in early evening crying in newborn babies

Subject	Condition 1 Mean time crying in minutes before colic preparation	Condition 2 Mean time crying in minutes after colic preparation	Calculations from statistical test	
			d (A–B)	*d*^{2}
1	49	42	+ 7	49
2	57	45	+ 12	144
3	72	65	+ 7	49
4	64	65	– 1	1
5	50	60	– 10	100
6	45	35	+ 10	100
7	59	40	+ 19	361
8	65	49	+ 16	256
Σ	461	401	Σ*d* = 60	Σ*d*^{2} = 1060
$\bar{x}$	57.625	50.125		

2. Calculate the mean score ($\bar{x}$) for each condition, i.e.:

$$\bar{x} A = 57.625 \qquad xB = 50.125$$

3. Calculate the difference (*d*) between each subject's pair of scores and enter this in column 4; i.e. for each subject take the score of Condition B away from the score of Condition A (e.g. for S1, 49 – 42 = 7). Remember to put in the plus and minus signs for each *d* value.

4. Add these differences up to give Σ*d*, remembering to take account of the plus and minus values, i.e.:

$$\Sigma d = 60$$

5. Square each difference to give *d*^{2}, e.g. 7^2 = 49, and enter these in column 5 (*d*^{2}).

6. Add up the *d*^{2} values to give Σ*d*^{2}, i.e:

$$\Sigma d^2 = 1060$$

7. Square the total of the differences, i.e.:

$$60^2 = 3600 = (\Sigma d)^2.$$

It is important to recognise the difference in meaning between

Σd^2 (Stage 6) which means to add up all the squared differences
and $(\Sigma d)^2$ (Stage 7) which means to add up all the differences and square the total.

8. Find the t from the following formula:

$$t = \frac{\Sigma d}{\sqrt{\dfrac{N\Sigma d^2 - (\Sigma d)^2}{N-1}}}$$

where Σd = the total of the differences (i.e. 60)
$(\Sigma d)^2$ = the total of the differences, squared (i.e. 3600)
Σd^2 = the total of the squared differences (i.e. 1060)
N = number of subjects, or pairs of matched subjects (i.e. 8)
$\sqrt{}$ = the square root of the final calculation of everything under the square root sign.

If we substitute some values, then:

$$t = \frac{60}{\sqrt{\dfrac{8 \times 1060 - 3600}{8-1}}}$$

$$= \frac{60}{\sqrt{\dfrac{8480 - 3600}{7}}}$$

$$= \frac{60}{\sqrt{697.143}}$$

$$= \frac{60}{26.404}$$

$$t = 2.272$$

Looking up the value of t

To see whether this t value is significant you need one further value, the degrees of freedom, which here is the number of subjects minus 1, i.e. $8 - 1 = 7$. Turn to Table A2.5. You will see down the left-hand margin a number of d.f. values.

Look down the column until you find the d.f. value of 7.

To the right of that you will see 6 critical values of t in the main body of the table:

1.415   1.895   2.365   2.998   3.499   5.405

If your value of t is equal to or larger than any of the given values, it is significant at the level indicated at the top of the column. For example, 3.499 has an associated p value of 0.005 for a one-tailed test and 0.01 for a two-tailed test. So, if we look at the numbers, we can see that our t value of 2.272 is larger than 1.895 but smaller than 2.365. This means that the probability associated with our t value of 2.272 is somewhere between 0.05 and 0.025 for a one-tailed hypothesis. In other words the p value for $t = 2.272$ must be smaller than 0.05 (or 5%) and larger than 0.025 (or $2\frac{1}{2}$%). We would therefore say that for our study and our one-tailed hypothesis, that the results are significant at less than 0.05 (or 5%). (Because of convention, we would never say that p is greater than 0.025 and so we must focus on the value of 1.895 in the table.)

We express this as: $p < 0.05$ (< means 'less than') (Had our t value been exactly the same as the critical value of 1.895 in the table, we would have said that $p = 0.05$.)

Interpreting the results

Our results have an associated probability of less than 0.05, which means that the chances of random error accounting for the outcome of our experiment are less than 5 in 100. Because the usual cut-off point for claiming that the results are significant is 5%, we can conclude that our results are significant, at less than the 5% level. However, because we have a one-tailed hypothesis we can only say that our hypothesis has been supported if the results are in the direction predicted. This means that providing the average amount of time spent crying is greater before the colic preparation given than it is afterwards, we can reject the null hypothesis and accept that our experimental hypothesis has been supported. Since the averages are 57.625 and 50.125 minutes respectively, the results are in the predicted direction and we can conclude that the proprietary colic treatment significantly reduces crying time in young babies. We can state this as follows:

> Using a related t-test on the data ($t = 2.272$, $N = 8$), the results are significant at $p < 0.05$, for a one-tailed test. The experimental hypothesis has been supported, suggesting that crying time in new babies is significantly reduced following administration of a standard colic remedy. The null hypothesis can therefore be rejected.

Remember, had the average time been reversed (i.e. more time following the colic preparation) we could not claim that the hypothesis had been supported.

Activity 14.1   (Answers on page 239)

1. To practise looking up t values, look up the following and say whether or not they are significant and at what level.
   (i)   d.f. = 11 $t = 2.406$ one-tailed p
   (ii) d.f. = 14 $t = 1.895$ two-tailed p
   (iii) d.f. = 19 $t = 2.739$ one-tailed p
   (iv) d.f. = 7 $t = 3.204$ one-tailed p
   (v)   d.f. = 9 $t = 2.973$ two-tailed p
2. Calculate a related t-test on the following data:
   H_1 Direct entry student midwives with 'A'-level biology do better on their 1st year theory exam than students without 'A'-level biology.
   Is this hypothesis one- or two-tailed?
   Method: Select two groups, each of 12 students, matched on certain key features such as overall 'A'-level points, attendance levels, quality of teaching etc. Of these, one group has 'A'-level biology and the other does not. Compare the performance of the two groups on their 1st year theory exam. The marks are as in Table 14.3.

Table 14.3   Marks of student midwives for the 1st year theory exam

Subject pair	Condition 1 'A'-level biology	Condition 2 No 'A' level biology	Calculations from statistical test	
			d	d^2
1	64	68		
2	59	60		
3	72	62		
4	68	58		
5	58	49		
6	70	62		
7	65	61		
8	62	50		
9	73	71		
10	45	49		
11	56	54		
12	67	68		

State the t-value, the d.f. value, and the p value expressed in a similar format to that on this page.

PARAMETRIC STATISTICAL TESTS FOR USE WITH ONE GROUP OF SUBJECTS AND THREE OR MORE CONDITIONS OR THREE OR MORE GROUPS OF MATCHED SUBJECTS

One-way analysis of variance (anova) for related and matched subject designs

The one-way anova for related and matched subject designs is the parametric equivalent of the Friedman test. In other words it is used for designs which either use one subject group in three or more conditions and the results from these conditions are compared for differences between them. Or alternatively, it is used where the experimenter has got three or more groups of *matched* subjects who do one condition each. The results from each condition are compared for differences (see Designs 1b and 2b pp. 139–140).

It is called a 'one-way' anova because it only deals with experiments which manipulate one independent variable. If you ever hypothesized a relationship between two independent variables and a DV (see Ch. 6) you would require a two-way anova, or in extremis a relationship between three independent variables and a DV, then you would require a three-way anova. However, these are outside the scope of this book and the reader is referred to Greene & D'Oliveira (1982) and Ferguson (1976).

Like all parametric tests, the data must be of an interval/ratio level, and the remaining three conditions should be more or less fulfilled.

When calculating an anova you find the value of 'F' which is then looked up in the probability tables for anovas to find out whether this value represents a significant difference between conditions. Like the Friedman test, the anova only tells us whether there are overall differences between conditions, and not the direction of the differences and so the hypothesis must be two-tailed.

Example

Because the anova is quite complicated to calculate, it may be helpful to explain the purpose of it beforehand. Let us imagine that you have noticed that your delivery suite midwives seem to show a high degree of clinical skill but they seem less competent in their supervision of students and in their interpersonal skills. Obviously, if your observations are correct, you will need to do some staff development on the weaker areas. You therefore decide to make an evaluation of a group of ten delivery suite midwives in the three different aspects of their job — clinical skills, interpersonal skills and supervision skills.

Your hypothesis then is:

H₁ Delivery suite midwives show different levels of professional competence in three aspects of their job: clinical, supervisory and interpersonal skills. To see if there is any difference in the competence shown in these areas you decide to compare the performance of the group on each aspect, giving marks out of 20. As this is an interval/ratio scale of measurement, we can fulfil this requirement of a parametric test.

Therefore we have the design shown in Figure 14.6.

Further suppose that you have collected and set out the results which look as shown in Table 14.4.

You are hypothesizing that the performance of the group varies according to the aspect of the job, and therefore you would expect there to be significant differences or variations between the condition totals (126, 105 and 101). This, obviously, is one potential source of variation in the results and is called a between-conditions comparison. However, because each subject is assessed on all three conditions, we can also compare the overall performances of the subjects, to see if there is any variation in competence between the midwives, i.e. a comparison of all the T_s totals. This comparison allows us to look at another potential source of variation in the scores: a between-the-subjects comparison. This is illustrated in Figure 14.7 for the example given above using the data from the first five subjects.

The solid vertical lines in Figure 14.7 indicate the comparisons which can be made between

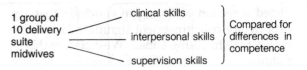

Figure 14.6 Design for the comparison of differences in levels of various skills in midwives: experimental design.

Table 14.4

Subject	Condition 1 Clinical	Condition 2 Interpersonal	Condition 3 Supervisory	Total for Ss: T_S
1	15	12	11	38
2	12	9	8	29
3	13	10	11	34
4	10	10	12	32
5	17	14	10	41
6	8	12	11	31
7	11	12	9	32
8	14	9	9	32
9	16	8	12	36
10	10	9	8	27
Total	T_C $T_C1 = 126$	$T_C2 = 105$	$T_C3 = 101$	Grand total = 332

conditions, to see if there is any difference in performance on each aspect of the job, as was hypothesized. This comparison concentrates on one source of potential variation in the results: the between-conditions variation. The dotted horizontal lines indicate the comparisons which can be made between subjects, to see if there is any difference in the overall performances among the subjects. This comparison concentrates on a second potential source of variation in the results: the between-subject variation. There is, of course, a third source of potential variation in scores: that due to random error.

If we consider these sources of variation for a moment, it can be seen that ideally what we would hope to find from our anova is:

a. significant differences between the performance of the job tasks, i.e. a significant between conditions comparison, since this was what was hypothesized, and

b. no significant differences between the subjects, since this would suggest that they were a fairly representative and similar sample.

The purpose of the one-way related anova is

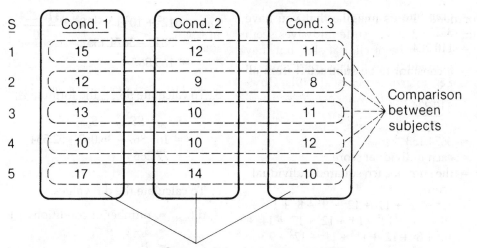

Figure 14.7   There is variation between the subjects and variation between conditions.

to find out whether any of these sources of varia-tion are responsible for significant differences in results.

In order to do this, we need a number of values:

the sums of squares	(SS)
the degrees of freedom	(d.f.)
the mean squares	(MS)
the F ratios	(F)

for each source of variation. When these have been calculated they are entered into a table the format of which is shown in Table 14.5.

Table 14.5

Source of variation scores	Sums of of squares (SS)	Degrees of freedom (d.f.)	Mean squares (MS)	F ratios (F)
Variation between conditions, i.e. aspects of job	SS_{bet}	d.f.$_{bet}$	MS_{bet}	F_{bet}
Variation between subjects' overall performance	SS_{subj}	d.f.$_{subj}$	MS_{subj}	F_{subj}
Variation due to random error	SS_{error}	d.f.$_{error}$	MS_{error}	
Total	SS_{tot}	d.f.$_{tot}$		

Firstly, do not panic—the calculations are surprisingly easy, if rather laborious! Follow the steps described below (the data are on page 144).

Calculating the one-way anova

1. We must first calculate the SS values for each source of variation. To do this, you will need several values:

ΣT_C^2 = sum of the squared totals for each condition
i.e. $126^2 + 105^2 + 101^2$
= 15 876 + 11 025 + 10 201
= 37 102

ΣT_S^2 = sum of each subject's performance squared
i.e. $38^2 + 29^2 + 34^2 + 32^2 + 41^2 + 31^2 + 32^2 + 32^2 + 36^2 + 27^2$
= 1444 + 841 + 1156 + 1024 + 1681 + 961 + 1024 + 1024 + 1296 + 729
= 11 180

n = number of Ss or sets of matched Ss
= 10

C = number of conditions
= 3

N = total number or scores, i.e. $n \times C$
= 30

Σx = grand total
= 332

$(\Sigma x)^2$ = grand total squared
  = 332^2
  = 110 224

$\dfrac{(\Sigma x)^2}{N}$ = a constant to be subtracted from all SS

  = $\dfrac{110\,224}{30}$

  = 3674.133

x = each individual score

Σx^2 = the sum of each squared individual score

  = $15^2 + 12^2 + 11^2 + 12^2 + 9^2 + 8^2 + 13^2 +$
   $10^2 + 11^2 + 10^2 + 10^2 + 12^2 + 17^2 + 14^2 +$
   $10^2 + 8^2 + 12^2 + 11^2 + 11^2 + 12^2 + 9^2 +$
   $14^2 + 9^2 + 9^2 + 16^2 + 8^2 + 12^2 + 10^2 +$
   $9^2 + 8^2$

  = 3840

2. To calculate the SS_{bet} the formula is:

$$\frac{\Sigma T_C^{\,2}}{n} - \frac{(\Sigma x)^2}{N}$$

$= \dfrac{126^2 + 105^2 + 101^2}{10} - \dfrac{110\,224}{30}$

  = 3710.2 − 3674.133

  = 36.067

3. To calculate the SS_{subj} the formula is:

$$\frac{\Sigma T_S^{\,2}}{C} - \frac{(\Sigma x)^2}{N}$$

$= \dfrac{38^2 + 29^2 + 34^2 + 32^2 + 41^2 + 31^2 + 32^2 + 32^2 + 36^2 + 27^2}{31}$

  $- \dfrac{110\,224}{30}$

  = 3726.667 − 3674.133

  = 52.534

4. To calculate the SS_{tot} the formula is:

$$\Sigma x^2 - \frac{(\Sigma x)^2}{N}$$

  = $15^2 + 12^2 + 11^2 + 12^2 + 9^2 + 8^2 + 13^2 +$
   $10^2 + 11^2 + 10^2 + 10^2 + 12^2 + 17^2 +$
   $14^2 + 10^2 + 8^2 + 12^2 + 11^2 + 11^2 +$
   $12^2 + 9^2 + 14^2 + 9^2 + 9^2 + 16^2 + 8^2 +$

$12^2 + 10^2 + 9^2 + 8^2 - \dfrac{110\,224}{30}$

  = 3840 − 3674.133

  = 165.867

5. To calculate SS_{error} the formula is:

$$SS_{tot} - SS_{bet} - SS_{subj}$$

  = 165.867 − 36.067 − 52.534

  = 77.266

6. To calculate the d.f. values:

d.f.$_{bet}$ = number of conditions − 1
  = 3 − 1
  = 2

d.f.$_{subj}$ = number of Ss − 1 (or sets of matched Ss − 1)
  = 10 − 1
  = 9

d.f.$_{tot}$ = $N - 1$
  = 30 − 1
  = 29

d.f.$_{error}$ = d.f.$_{tot}$ − d.f.$_{bet}$ − d.f.$_{subj}$
  = 29 − 2 − 9
  = 18

7. To calculate the MS values:

MS_{bet} = $\dfrac{SS_{bet}}{\text{d.f.}_{bet}}$

  = $\dfrac{36.067}{2}$

  = 18.034

MS_{subj} = $\dfrac{SS_{subj}}{\text{d.f.}_{subj}}$

  = $\dfrac{52.534}{9}$

  = 5.837

MS_{error} = $\dfrac{SS_{error}}{\text{d.f.}_{error}}$

  = $\dfrac{77.266}{18}$

  = 4.293

8. To calculate the F ratios:

F ratio for the between conditions variation

$$= \frac{MS_{bet}}{MS_{error}}$$

$$= \frac{18.034}{4.293}$$

$$= 4.201$$

F ratio for the between subjects variation

$$= \frac{MS_{subj}}{MS_{error}}$$

$$= \frac{5.837}{4.293}$$

$$= 1.36$$

We can now fill in our table using these values (Table 14.6).

Looking up the values of the F ratios

We need to look up these F ratios to find out whether they represent significant differences between the conditions and/or between the subjects. Turn to Tables A2.6a–d which are the probability tables for the anova.

Table a shows the critical values of F at $p < 0.05$.

Table b shows the critical values of F at $p < 0.025$.

Table c shows the critical values of F at $p < 0.01$.

Table 14.6

Source of variation in scores	Sums of squares *SS*	Degrees of freedom d.f.	Mean squares *MS*	*F* ratios
Variation in scores between conditions i.e. aspects of job	36.067	2	18.034	4.201
Variation in scores between subjects	52.534	9	5.837	1.36
Variation in scores due to random error	77.266	18	4.293	
Total	165.867	29		

Table d shows the critical values of F at $p < 0.001$.

Note again, that as the anova can only tell us whether there are general differences and *not* whether these differences are in specific direction, these values are for a two-tailed hypothesis.

On each of these Tables you will see that there are values called v_1 across the top and v_2 down the left-hand column. These are d.f. values. To look up the F ratio for the between conditions comparison, we need the d.f.$_{bet}$ value and the d.f.$_{error}$ value. Taking Table A2.6a first, locate the d.f.$_{bet}$ (i.e. 2) across the top row, and the d.f.$_{error}$ (i.e. 18) down the left-hand column. Where they intersect is the critical value of F for these d.f. values. If our F ratio of 4.21 is equal to or larger than the critical value, it is significant at the p value stated at the top of the table. As 4.201 is larger than 3.55, we can conclude that our results have an associated probability of less than 5%. But can we do any better? Turn to Table A2.6b and repeat the process. Because our value of 4.201 is smaller than the intersection value of 4.56 our results are not significant at the 0.025 level. Therefore, the probability that our results are due to random error is less than 0.05.

This is expressed, then, as $p < 0.05$.

To find out whether there are differences between the subjects' overall performances (i.e. whether the F ratio of 1.36 is significant), we need the d.f.$_{subj}$ value (in this case 9) and the d.f.$_{error}$ value (in this case 18). Look across the v_1 values in Table A2.6a for 9, and down the left-hand column for 18. You will see that there is no v_1 value of 9, so you must take the next smallest. At the intersection point the critical value is 2.51. As our F ratio is smaller than this, the results can be said to be not significant. In other words, there is no significant difference between subjects in their overall performance.

Interpreting the results

Our results have an associated probability level of less than 5%, which means that the chances of random error accounting for the results are less than 5 in 100. Since the usual cut-off point is 5%, we can say that our results are significant, which means that the delivery suite midwives perform some parts of their job better than others. However, the between-subjects F ratio is not significant, which suggests that the midwives concerned did not differ from each other in terms of their overall job performance.

If we take these two results together we can conclude that the delivery suite midwives do indeed perform differently on each aspect of their job, and since there is no significant difference in the overall quality of the midwives concerned we may assume that the differences are due to some factor associated with their department, training, attitudes etc. We can express this in the following way:

> Using a one-way anova for related subject samples on the data ($F = 4.201$, $N = 10$) it was found that the results were significant at $p < 0.05$. This suggests that there are significant differences in performance levels on the three aspects of the midwife's job investigated. These differences cannot be attributed to variations in the subjects since the F ratio for the between-subjects calculations was not significant ($F = 1.36$, $p = NS$). Therefore, the null hypothesis can be rejected.

It must be remembered that the anova only tells you that there are significant differences between the conditions and not which condition has better/worse scores. For instance in this example, we know that midwives perform differently on three aspects of their job but we do not know whether the difference lies between:

> clinical and interpersonal
> or
> clinical and supervisory
> or
> interpersonal and supervisory
> or
> all three.

In order to find out you need to use the Scheffé multiple range test in the next section. However, the Scheffé can only be used if the results from the anova are significant.

Activity 14.2 (Answers on page 239)

1. To practise looking up F ratios, look up the following and state whether or not they are significant and at what level:
   (i) F ratio$_{bet}$ = 4.96   d.f.$_{bet}$ = 2   d.f.$_{error}$ = 10 p
   (ii) F ratio$_{subj}$ = 4.22   d.f.$_{subj}$ = 7   d.f.$_{error}$ = 15 p
   (iii) F ratio$_{subj}$ = 2.21   d.f.$_{subj}$ = 11   d.f.$_{error}$ = 20 p
   (iv) F ratio$_{bet}$ = 5.15   d.f.$_{bet}$ = 14   d.f.$_{error}$ = 8 p
   (v) F ratio$_{subj}$ = 3.14   d.f.$_{subj}$ = 9   d.f.$_{error}$ = 14 p
   (vi) F ratio$_{bet}$ = 3.98   d.f.$_{bet}$ = 10   d.f.$_{error}$ = 12 p

   Remember! Use all the Tables to find the smallest p value possible.

2. Calculate a one-way anova for related designs on the following data:
   H$_1$ There is a relationship between the type of analgesia used during labour and the length of the second stage.

   Brief method: Select three groups each of six women, matched on age, parity, health etc. Each group is given one of three different types of analgesia during the first stage of labour. The length of the second stage is then calculated in minutes for each subject.

Table 14.7

S	Condition A Inhalation analgesia	Condition B Narcotics	Condition C Epidural
1	15	16	11
2	12	14	14
3	10	14	12
4	14	15	12
5	22	19	13
6	17	18	15

State your F ratios, d.f. values and p values in the manner suggested on page 147.

Scheffé multiple range test

The analysis of variance only tells you whether there are overall differences between the conditions and not where these differences lie. As a result, it is not possible from this test alone to conclude whether the scores from one condition are significantly better or worse than those from another. If you look back to the example given, the anova only allows us to conclude that delivery suite midwives perform differently in aspects of their job; it does not permit us to say that their performance on one task is better than their performance on another. However, if you look at the results for each condition (p. 144) it appears that the clinical scores are better than the interpersonal scores, with the supervisory scores being worst. We can find out whether the differences between these sets of results are significant by comparing each pair of mean scores using the Scheffé multiple range test. In other words, we can compare:

1. the mean clinical score with the mean interpersonal score
2. the mean clinical score with the mean supervisory score
3. the mean interpersonal score with the mean supervisory score

to find out if the differences in performance in each area are significant. The Scheffé test should be carried out after you have calculated the anova because it uses some of the values from the anova table. Remember, too, that it should be carried out only if the results from the anova are significant.

There are a number of other multiple range tests which perform the same function, but the Scheffé has been selected because it is considered to be the best (McNemar, 1963) and also because it can be used if there are unequal numbers of subjects in each condition. Obviously this latter point does not apply in same subject and matched subject designs (since you will, by definition, have the same number of scores in each condition) but since the Scheffé can also be used with a one-way anova for unrelated designs and unequal subject numbers this feature is a useful one.

When calculating the Scheffé, you find two values. Firstly, F is calculated for each comparison of means you wish to make, and secondly F^1 is calculated. Each F is compared with the F^1 value. If it is equal to or larger than the F^1 value, then the result is significant.

Calculating the Scheffé

There are three possible comparisons we can make using the Scheffé on our sample data:

1. Clinical vs. interpersonal scores
2. Clinical vs. supervisory scores
3. Interpersonal vs. supervisory scores.

To make these comparisons, take the following steps:

1. Calculate the mean score for each condition

$$\bar{x}_1 = 12.6; \quad \bar{x}_2 = 10.5; \quad \bar{x}_3 = 10.1$$

2. Find the value of F for the first comparison (i.e. Clinical vs Interpersonal) using the following formula:

$$F = \frac{(\bar{x}_1 - \bar{x}_2)^2}{\dfrac{MS_{error}}{n_1} + \dfrac{MS_{error}}{n_2}}$$

where $\bar{x}_1$ = mean for Condition 1
  = 12.6
$\bar{x}_2$ = mean for Condition 2
  = 10.5
MS_{error} = mean square value for the random error variation (from the anova calculations)
  = 4.293
n_1 = number of subjects in Condition 1
  = 10
n_2 = number of subjects in Condition 2
  = 10

If these values are substituted, then

$$F = \frac{(12.6 - 10.5)^2}{\dfrac{4.293}{10} + \dfrac{4.293}{10}}$$

$$= \frac{4.41}{0.858}$$

$$= 5.14$$

3. Repeat the calculations for the other two comparisons, using the appropriate means and n values.

Thus for the comparison of the clinical and supervisory scores, the formula is:

$$F = \frac{(\bar{x}_1 - \bar{x}_3)^2}{\dfrac{MS_{error}}{n_1} + \dfrac{MS_{error}}{n_3}}$$

$$= \frac{(12.6 - 10.1)^2}{\dfrac{4.293}{10} + \dfrac{4.293}{10}}$$

$$= 7.284$$

and for the comparison of the interpersonal and supervisory scores, the formula is:

$$F = \frac{(\bar{x}_2 - \bar{x}_3)^2}{\dfrac{MS_{error}}{n_2} + \dfrac{MS_{error}}{n_3}}$$

$$= \frac{(10.5 - 10.1)^2}{\dfrac{4.293}{10} + \dfrac{4.293}{10}}$$

$$= 0.187$$

4. Using the d.f.$_{bet}$ and d.f.$_{error}$ values derived from the anova (i.e. 2 and 18 respectively), turn to Table A2.6a and locate the d.f.$_{bet}$ value across the v_1 row, and the d.f.$_{error}$ down the v_2 column. At the intersection point, you will find the value of 3.55. This is the critical value for F at the $< 5\%$ or < 0.05 level of significance. The $< 5\%$ level is selected because of the extreme stringency of the Scheffé test. If a smaller p value were to be selected, you would be far less likely to obtain significant results on the Scheffé. However, should you ever get any results that look as though they are considerably more significant than the 5% level, you can repeat steps 4–6 with Tables A2.6b (1%), A2.6c (2½%) and A2.6d (0.1%).

5. Calculate F^1 using the formula:

$$F^1 = (C - 1) F°$$

where C = the number of conditions
    = 3
$F°$ = the figure at the intersection point of the appropriate d.f. values in the Table
    = 3.55
F^1 = (3 – 1) 3.55
    = 7.1

6. Compare the F values derived from the calculations in steps 2 and 3 with the F^1 value above. If the F value is equal to or larger than the F^1 value it is significant.

Therefore, taking our F values of

5.14
7.284
0.187

we can see that only one is larger than the F^1 value, i.e. the comparison between the clinical and supervisory scores.

Interpreting the results

The results from the Scheffé test indicate that there is only one significant difference between pairs of performance scores, that is between the clinical and supervisory scores (at $p < 0.05$). This suggests that the main reason for the significant results of the anova is the difference between delivery suite midwives in clinical and supervisory skills.

Activity 14.3 (Answers on page 239)

Carry out a Scheffé test on the following results:
H$_1$ There is a difference in the efficacy of four teaching approaches used with new parents in parentcraft classes.

   Method: A group of six parents attending parentcraft classes are given comparable information in four different ways about what to do at the onset of labour: role-play, film, lecture, and individual reading. They are then asked to evaluate the effectiveness of each technique by awarding it marks out of 20. A one-way anova for related designs was computed on the scores and the following relevant results obtained:

d.f.$_{bet}$ = 3
d.f.$_{error}$ = 15
MS_{error} = 3.87

The mean scores for each condition were:

Condition 1 Role-Play 11.2
Condition 2 Film 13.1
Condition 3 Lecture 10.7
Condition 4 Reading 8.4

15

Non-parametric tests for different (unrelated) subject designs

INTRODUCTION

The statistical tests described in this chapter are used when the experimental design involves two or more than two different unmatched groups of subjects who are compared on a certain task, activity etc. All the tests covered in this chapter are non-parametric ones, which means that they:

- are less sensitive
- are easier to calculate
- can be used on nominal, ordinal or interval/ratio data.

Therefore, if you cannot fulfil the conditions required for parametric tests, you should use its non-parametric equivalent. The designs involved in this chapter, then, are:

1. *Two different, unmatched subject groups compared on a certain task, activity etc.*

| Subject group 1 | takes part in | Condition 1 | Results from |
| Subject group 2 | takes part in | Condition 2 | conditions are compared for differences |

or

2. *Three or more different, unmatched subject groups compared on a certain task, activity etc.*

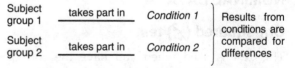

Subject group 1	takes part in	Condition 1	
Subject group 2	takes part in	Condition 2	Results from conditions are compared for differences
Subject group 3	takes part in	Condition 3	

Table 15.1 Tests for different subjects designs

Design	Non-parametric test
1. Two different groups of subjects, compared on a task.	Chi-squared test if data are nominal Mann-Whitney U test (if data are other than nominal, i.e. ordinal or interval/ratio).
2. Three or more different groups of subjects, compared on a task.	Extended chi-squared test if data are nominal Kruskal-Wallis (if just a difference in results is predicted and the data are other than nominal, i.e. ordinal or interval/ratio). Jonckheere trend test (if a trend in the results is predicted and the data are other than nominal, i.e. ordinal or interval/ratio).

Results from Design 1 are analysed using the Chi-squared (χ^2) test if the data are nominal or the Mann-Whitney U test if they are other than nominal (i.e. ordinal or interval/ratio).

Results from Design 2 are analysed using the extended chi-squared (χ^2) test if the data are nominal or the Kruskal-Wallis test if the data are other than nominal (i.e. ordinal or interval/ratio). If a trend in the results is predicted, such that subject group 1 is expected to perform better than subject group 2, with subject group 3 performing worst, the Jonckheere trend test is used as long as the data are other than nominal (Table 15.1).

NON-PARAMETRIC STATISTICAL TEST FOR USE WITH TWO DIFFERENT SUBJECT GROUPS AND NOMINAL DATA

Chi-squared (χ^2) test

This test is used when you have the sort of experimental design which uses two different unmatched groups of subjects who are compared on a task, activity etc. The data for the χ^2 test (pronounced Kie-squared) must be *nominal*.

To refresh your memory, the nominal level of measurement only allows you to allocate your subjects to named categories (e.g. Entonox/ Trilene; medio-lateral/J-shape; breech/cephalic); it does not allow you to measure your subjects' responses along a dimension, i.e. how much

Entonox administered, how extensive the medio-lateral incision etc. Check Chapter 4 to make sure you are happy with this concept. As you can see, a subject may only be allocated to one category, since it is impossible to be both breech and cephalic, or to have a medio-lateral incision and a J-shape. Because of this the χ^2 can only be used when different subjects are allocated to different categories, i.e. an unrelated design.

With the χ^2 test you may only use two nominal categories and two subject groups. For example you may wish to find out whether there is a difference between male and female fetuses in terms of likelihood of threatened miscarriage. You have two groups:

'male fetus' and 'female fetus'

and two nominal categories:

'threatened miscarriage' and 'no threatened miscarriage.'

Should you ever wish to allocate two groups to more than two nominal categories you must use the *extended* χ^2 (See p. 164).

It should also be noted that when you use the χ^2 test, you should ensure that at least 20 subjects will be in each group. While this may sound off-putting, it rarely takes too much time to collect this amount of data. You do not need to use equal numbers of subjects in each group. When you calculate the χ^2 test, you find a numerical value for χ^2 which you then look up in the probability tables associated with the χ^2 test to see if this value represents a significant difference between the result you observed and those that could be expected by chance.

Example

Let us suppose you were interested in finding out whether there is a relationship between fertility problems and gender of the baby. Your hypothesis is:

H_1 Women who have a history of fertility problems are more likely to deliver a male baby than are women who have no history of fertility problems.

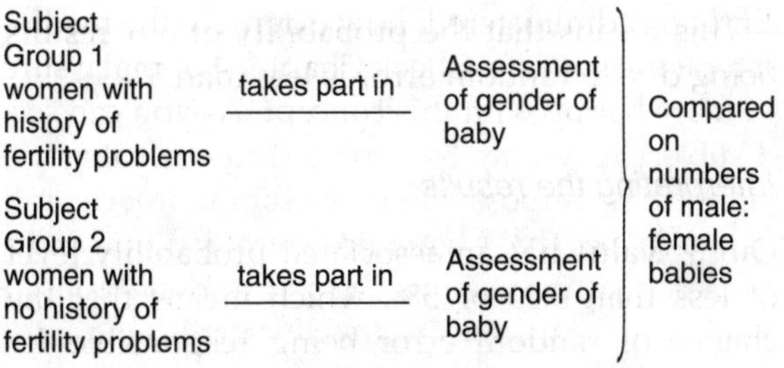

Subject
Group 1
women with ――――takes part in――――Assessment
history of   of gender of
fertility problems   baby   } Compared
                                                                     on
                                                                     numbers
Subject   of male:
Group 2   female
women with ――――takes part in――――Assessment   babies
no history of   of gender of
fertility problems   baby

Figure 15.1   Effect of fertility problems on gender of baby.

Brief method: You select 30 pregnant women who have a history of fertility problems and 32 pregnant women who have no history of fertility problems. Upon delivery, you note the number of male and female babies born to each group.

This is a nominal level of measurement because you are using two categories: male and female, and are simply allocating the babies to one of these groups.

You have a design which looks like Figure 15.1.

In other words you have two groups of subjects who can be allocated to *two* nominal categories (male or female).

You end up with the results shown in Table 15.2.

Calculating the χ^2 test

1. The first step you must always take is to set your data out in a 2 × 2 table as shown in Table 15.2. The subject groups should go down the side and the nominal categories across the top, although it does not matter which category is on the left, nor which subject group is at the top. Label your Cells A, B, C, and D in the same way as in the table (i.e. from left to right).

Table 15.2   Format of data when calculating the χ^2 test

	Male babies	Female babies	Marginal totals
Subject group 1 Fertility problems	A 21	B 9	A + B 30
Subject group 2 No fertility problems	C 14	D 18	C + D 32
Marginal totals	A + C 35	B + D 27	Grand total N 62

2. You must now add up the marginal totals for each row and each column, i.e.:

$$A + B = 21 + 9$$
$$= 30$$
$$C + D = 14 + 18$$
$$= 32$$
$$A + C = 21 + 14$$
$$= 35$$
$$B + D = 9 + 18$$
$$= 27$$

3. Calculate the grand total N either by adding up the vertical marginal totals, i.e.

$$30 + 32 = 62$$

or by adding up the horizontal marginal totals, i.e.

$$35 + 27 = 62$$

(The answer will be the same.)

4. Find χ^2 from the formula:

$$\chi^2 = \frac{N\left[(AD - BC) - \frac{N}{2}\right]^2}{(A + B)(C + D)(A + C)(B + D)}$$

where N = the grand total, i.e. 62
$$AD = \text{Cell A} \times \text{Cell D} = 21 \times 18$$
$$= 378$$
$$BC = \text{Cell B} \times \text{Cell C} = 9 \times 14$$
$$= 126$$

The values under the division line are all the marginal totals:

$$A + B = 30$$
$$C + D = 32$$
$$A + C = 35$$
$$B + D = 27$$

Therefore, if we substitute these values in the formula:

$$\chi^2 = \frac{62\left[(378 - 126^*) - \frac{62}{2}\right]^2}{30 \times 32 \times 35 \times 27}$$
$$= \frac{3028142}{907200}$$
$$\chi^2 = 3.338$$

(*If you get a minus number from the calculations in the inner brackets, ignore the minus sign)

5. Before this χ^2 value can be looked up in the probability tables to see if it represents a significant difference, the d.f. value is required. Use the d.f. formula of:

$$(r-1)(c-1)$$

where r = the number of rows
c = the number of columns
$= (2-1) \times (2-1)$
$= 1$

Obviously, in a 2×2 table like this, the d.f. will always equal 1.

Looking up the value of χ^2 for significance

To find out whether the χ^2 value of 3.338 represents a significant difference in gender of babies delivered to women who have a history of fertility problems and those who have not, it must be looked up in the probability tables associated with the χ^2 test (Table A2.1). Down the left-hand column you will see d.f. values from 1–30. Look down this column until you find the d.f. value of 1. To the right of this are five numbers, called critical values of χ^2:

2.71   3.84   5.41   6.64   10.83.

Each of these critical values is associated with the probability level at the top of its column, e.g. the critical value of 5.41 is associated with 0.02 for a two-tailed test. You will see that the p values in the table are only associated with two-tailed hypotheses. If you have a one-tailed hypothesis, as we have here, simply look up your χ^2 value as described, find the two-tailed p value and halve it (see pp. 87–89).

In order for our χ^2 value of 3.338 to be significant at one of these levels, it has to be equal to or larger than one of these numbers. Our value is larger than 2.71 but smaller than 3.84. Therefore, the probability associated with our obtained χ^2 value must be less than 0.05 (or 5%) but larger than 0.025 (or 22%) for a one-tailed hypothesis. (Remember we have had to halve the p values in the table which are for two-tailed hypotheses). The convention is that we say that p is less than 0.05 (or 5%) rather than greater than 0.025 (or 22%). This is expressed as $p < 0.05$.

This means that the probability of our results being due to random error is less than 5%.

Interpreting the results

Our χ^2 value has an associated probability level of less than 0.05 or 5%, which means that the chance of random error being responsible for the results is less than 5%. Because a 5% cut-off point is usually used to claim that the results support the experimental hypothesis, we can say that our results are significant.

However, before we can finally conclude that the hypothesis has been supported, just go back to the 2×2 table and check the results are in the predicted direction, because it is quite possible sometimes to obtain significant results which are opposite to those predicted in the hypothesis and so would *not* support the hypothesis.

Here we find that more of the fertility problem group have delivered male babies (21 vs. 14) and more of the non-fertility problem group have delivered female babies (18 vs. 9). Therefore the results are as predicted. We can reject the null (no difference) hypothesis on this basis. This can be expressed in the following way:

Using a χ^2 test on the data (χ^2 = 3.338, d.f. = 1) the results were found to be significant at $p < 0.05$, for a one-tailed test. This suggests that the null hypothesis can be rejected and that women who have a history of fertility problems are more likely to deliver male babies.

Activity 15.1   (Answers on page 239)

1. In order to practise looking up χ^2 values, look up the following and say what the associated p value is and whether or not it is significant.
   (i) χ^2 = 4.02   one-tailed   d.f. = 1 p
   (ii) χ^2 = 5.91   two-tailed   d.f. = 1 p
   (iii) χ^2 = 3.84   two-tailed   d.f. = 1 p
   (iv) χ^2 = 2.62   two-tailed   d.f. = 1 p
   (v) χ^2 = 6.95   one-tailed   d.f. = 1 p

2. Calculate a χ^2 test on the following:
   H$_1$ Midwife-tutors are more likely to undertake research than are clinical midwives of comparable years of experience since qualifying. (Is this a one- or two-tailed hypothesis?)
   Method: You randomly select 35 midwife-tutors and 42 clinical midwives and ask them whether or not they have ever undertaken any research.
   The results are as in Table 15.3.

Table 15.3

	Research	No research
Midwife-tutors	25	10
Clinical midwives	15	27

State your χ^2 value, p value, using the sample format given on page 154.

NON-PARAMETRIC STATISTICAL TEST FOR USE WITH TWO DIFFERENT, UNMATCHED SUBJECT GROUPS AND ORDINAL OR INTERVAL/RATIO DATA

Mann-Whitney *U* test

This test is used to analyse results from experiments which have compared *two different, unmatched* groups of subjects on a task (see Design 1, page 151). The Mann-Whitney U test simply compares the results from each group to see if they differ significantly. This test can only be used with ordinal or interval/ratio data. It cannot be used with nominal data.

When calculating this test, you end up with a numerical value for U which you look up in the probability tables associated with the Mann-Whitney test, to see if the U value does, in fact, represent a significant difference between the groups.

Example

Suppose you were interested in testing the hypothesis that there is a relationship between the loss of colostrum in the third trimester and the production of breast milk following delivery.

Your hypothesis would be:

H_1 Women who secrete colostrum during the last trimester produce different amounts of breast milk post-delivery compared with women who do not experience colostrum secretion.

Brief method: In order to test this hypothesis you select 15 women who reported no loss of colostrum during the third trimester of pregnancy and 13 women who experienced regular

Group 1
15 women with no loss of colostrum — assessed on — Supply of breast milk

Group 2
13 women with colostrum secretions — assessed on — Supply of breast milk

} compared for differences in amount

Figure 15.2 Design of experiment to test whether colostrum secretions in late pregnancy are related to breast milk production post-partum.

secretions. Four weeks after delivery you record on a 9-point scale whether the women have an adequate supply of breast milk (1 = none, 9 = excessive).

Therefore, we have the design shown in Figure 15.2.

(Note that because we don't have to match the subjects, you can use different numbers in each group.) You might end up with the results shown in Table 15.4.

Calculating the Mann-Whitney U *test*

To calculate the Mann-Whitney, take the following steps:

1. First calculate the totals (Σ) and means for each condition:

Table 15.4

Subject	*Condition 1* No colostrum secretions	Rank	Subject	*Condition 2* Colostrum secretions	Rank
1	6	18	1	7	22.5
2	5	12.5	2	9	27.5
3	7	22.5	3	6	18
4	3	2.5	4	5	12.5
5	5	12.5	5	6	18
6	4	7	6	7	22.5
7	4	7	7	7	22.5
8	3	2.5	8	8	25.5
9	8	25.5	9	9	27.5
10	6	18	10	6	18
11	5	12.5	11	5	12.5
12	4	7	12	4	7
13	3	2.5	13	5	12.5
14	3	2.5			
15	4	7			
Total	70	159.5		84	246.5
Mean	4.667			6.462	

i.e.   Condition 1   Total: 70
                       Mean :   4.667
       Condition 2   Total :   84
                       Mean :   6.462

2. Taking the whole set of scores together (i.e. all 28 scores) rank them giving the rank of 1 to the lowest, 2 to the next lowest and so on. Where there are 2 or more scores the same, use the tied rank procedure (see p. 128), i.e. add up the ranks the scores would have obtained had they been different and divide this number by the number of scores that are the same. Thus 3 is the lowest score, but there are four scores of 3. Therefore add up the ranks 1, 2, 3 and 4 (the ranks they would have obtained had they been different) and divide by 4 because there are 4 scores of 3, i.e.

$$\frac{1 + 2 + 3 + 4}{4} = 2.5$$

Assign the rank of 2.5 to all the scores of 3. (See columns labelled rank.) Remember! Put the scores from both conditions together, as though they were just one set of scores, when you do the ranking. Many students forget to do this.

3. Add the rank totals for each condition separately. i.e. Rank total 1 = 159.5, Rank total 2 = 246.5

4. Select the larger rank total, i.e. 246.5 to use in the formula below.

5. Find U from the formula:

$$U = n_1 n_2 + \frac{n_x(n_x + 1)}{2} - T_x$$

Where n_1 = the number of subjects in Condition 1 (i.e. 15)

n_2 = the number of subjects in Condition 2 (i.e. 13)

T_x = the larger rank total (i.e. 246.5)

n_x = the number of Ss in the condition with the larger rank total (i.e. Condition 2 = 13)

Therefore if we substitute these values

$$U = 15 \times 13 + \frac{13(13 + 1)}{2} - 246.5$$

$$= 195 + 91 - 246.5$$

$$= 39.5$$

6. Because there are unequal numbers in each condition, it is necessary to repeat the calculations for the smaller rank total (i.e. 159.5) as well.

Here T_x becomes the smaller rank total (159.5) and n_x becomes the number of subjects in the condition with the smaller rank total (i.e. Condition 1 = 15 subjects).

$$U_2 = 15 \times 13 + \frac{15(15 + 1)}{2} - 159.5$$

$$= 195 + 120 - 159.5$$

$$= 155.5$$

We now have two values of U:

$$U = 39.5$$
$$U_2 = 155.5$$

We need to look up the smaller of these two U values in the appropriate table (A2.7a–d).

Note: If you use equal numbers of subjects in each condition, you only need to carry out the first calculation of U, using the larger rank total and the appropriate n value. If you use unequal numbers you will have to find both U values and select the smaller one.

Looking up the value of U for significance

In order to find out whether our U value of 39.5 represents a significant difference in amount of breast milk produced four weeks post-partum, you have to look up this value in Tables A2.7a–d. There are *four* probability tables for the Mann-Whitney, each one representing different p values (see headings). Table A2.7a represents the smallest (most significant) p values, while Table A2.7d represents the largest (least significant) p value. To look up your U value you also need:

$$n_1 \text{ value (15)}$$
$$n_2 \text{ value (13)}$$

Starting with Table A2.7a, look across the top row until you find your n value of 15, and down the left-hand column for your n_2 value of 13. Where these two points intersect is the number 42. In order to be significant at a given level, your U value must be equal to or smaller than the value at the intersection point. As 39.5 is smaller than 42, our results are significant at either 0.005 for a one-tailed test or 0.01 for a two-tailed test. As we only predicted a general difference in amount of breast milk produced without specifying which group would produce more, we have a two-tailed hypothesis. Therefore, our results are significant at the 0.01 or 1% probability level. But, if you notice, our U value of 39.5 is actually smaller than the value of 42 at the intersection point. This means our results are even more significant than the 1% level. This is expressed as:

$$p < 0.01 \text{ or } < 1\%$$

Had our U value been the same as the value at the intersection point, the results would have been significant at exactly the 0.01 or 1% level. This would have been expressed as:

$$p = 0.01 \text{ (or } 1\%)$$

However, our results have a probability of less than 1% which means that the chance of random error accounting for our results is less than 1%.

Supposing, however, our U value had been 52.5, with our n values the same. Using Table A2.7a, we would find that the intersection value is 42. Because our U of 52.5 is larger than this value, it would not be significant at the probability levels of 0.005 and 0.01 given in the heading. Therefore, we would move on to Table A2.7b. At this intersection point for $n_1 = 15$, $n_2 = 13$, the value is 47. Our U value is larger than this and so cannot be classified as significant at this level either. Turn on to Table A2.7c. The intersection value here is 54. Our U value is smaller and so would be significant at the < 0.05 level for a two-tailed test.

If you ever find your U value is larger than the relevant intersection values in Table A2.7d, your results would not be significant.

Interpreting the results

Our U value has an associated probability level of less than 1% which means that there is less than a 1% chance of random error causing the results. If you remember, it was said that a good cut-off point for claiming that your results were significant and supported your hypothesis was the 5% level or less. Since our p value is less than 5% we can claim our results are significant; our null (no relationship) hypothesis can therefore be rejected and the experimental hypothesis supported.

Although the hypothesis did not predict which of the two groups of women would produce more milk, it is useful to compare the means from each condition to see which group was, in fact, more productive. Here the mean scores are 4.667 and 6.462 for no colostrum and colostrum respectively, which means that the colostrum group was more productive. This can be stated in the following way:

> Using a Mann-Whitney U test to analyse the data ($U = 39.5$, $n_1 = 15$, $n_2 = 13$), the results were found to be significant at $p < 0.01$ for a two-tailed hypothesis. This means that the production of colostrum during the third trimester is related to the amount of milk produced 4 weeks postpartum. Further inspection of the results suggest that women who secreted colostrum in late pregnancy had a greater amount of breast milk following delivery.

Activity 15.2   (Answers on page 240)

1. To practise looking up U values, look up the following and state whether or not they are significant and at what level.

   (i) $n_1 = 12$ $n_2 = 12$ $U = 33.5$ two tailed p
   (ii) $n_1 = 10$ $n_2 = 10$ $U = 27$ one tailed p
   (iii) $n_1 = 14$ $n_2 = 12$ $U = 37.5$ one-tailed p
   (iv) $n_1 = 20$ $n_2 = 18$ $U = 87.5$ one tailed p
   (v) $n_1 = 15$ $n_2 = 15$ $U = 70.5$ one-tailed p
   (vi) $n_1 = 18$ $n_2 = 15$ $U = 92.5$ two-tailed p

2. Calculate a Mann-Whitney U test on the following:
   H_1 Women who eat a diet high in animal fats during pregnancy are more likely to experience severe carpal tunnel syndrome during the last trimester than are women who have a vegetarian diet.
   Brief method: Randomly select 14 women in the last trimester who eat a diet high in animal fats and another group of 14 women at the same stage of pregnancy who eat a vegetarian diet and compare the degree of carpal tunnel syndrome using a 7-point scale (1 = no problem, 7 = extreme pain and tingling). The results might be as shown in Table 15.5.

Table 15.5

Subject	*Condition 1* Diet high in animal fat	Rank	Subject	*Condition 2* Vegetarian diet	Rank
1	5		1	3	
2	4		2	3	
3	5		3	5	
4	6		4	4	
5	3		5	2	
6	3		6	1	
7	4		7	3	
8	5		8	4	
9	6		9	5	
10	5		10	5	
11	6		11	3	
12	6		12	3	
13	4		13	4	
14	3		14	2	

State the *U* value and the *p* value in a format similar to that suggested earlier.

NON-PARAMETRIC STATISTICAL TESTS FOR USE WITH THREE OR MORE DIFFERENT, UNMATCHED SUBJECT GROUPS AND ORDINAL OR INTERVAL/RATIO DATA

Kruskal-Wallis test

This test is simply an extension of the Mann-Whitney test, in that it is used:

- when different subject groups are involved
- when the data are ordinal, or interval/ratio
- when the conditions for its parametric equivalent cannot be fulfilled.

However, while the Mann-Whitney can only be used to analyse the results from designs with two different groups of subjects, the Kruskal-Wallis is used with designs employing three or more different groups of subjects (Figure 15.3).

The Kruskal-Wallis, however, only tells you whether there are differences between these groups and not which results are better or worse than the others. Therefore, the associated hypothesis must be two-tailed (i.e. just predicting differences in the results with no specific direction to them). Should you ever predict a trend in your results, e.g. that Group 1 will perform better than Group 2, which in turn will perform better than

Subject group 1 — takes part in — *Condition 1*
Subject group 2 — takes part in — *Condition 2*
Subject group 3 (etc.) — takes part in — *Condition 3*
} Compare results from the groups to see if there are differences between them

Figure 15.3 A different-subject design with three or more groups of subjects. The Kruskal-Wallis test is used to analyse the results.

Group 3 etc with this sort of unrelated design, you would use a Jonckheere trend test to analyse your results. However, with the Kruskal-Wallis, you calculate the value of *H*, which you then look up in the probability tables associated with the Kruskal-Wallis test, to find out whether the *H* value represents significant differences between the groups.

Example

Imagine you are interested in the severity of incontinence in the last month of pregnancy depending on the position of the fetus.

Your hypothesis is:

H_1 There is a relationship between the severity of stress incontinence during the last month of pregnancy, according to whether the fetus is in an anterior, posterior or breech presentation.

Brief method: To test your hypothesis, you select ten women whose babies are lying in an anterior position, ten whose babies are lying in a posterior position and ten whose babies are in a breech position. You then ask them to rate on a 5-point scale, the severity of the stress incontinence experienced (1 = none, 5 = very severe).

Your design looks like Figure 15.4.

Your results look like Table 15.6.

Calculating the Kruskal-Wallis test

1. Calculate the totals and mean scores for each condition:

Condition 1 Total = 24 $\bar{x} = 2.4$
Condition 2 Total = 39 $\bar{x} = 3.9$
Condition 3 Total = 25 $\bar{x} = 2.5$

Table 15.6

Subject*	Condition 1 Anterior	Rank	Subject	Condition 2 Posterior	Rank	Subject	Condition 3 Breech	Rank
1	3	16	1	4	24	1	2	8
2	4	24	2	5	29	2	3	16
3	2	8	3	5	29	3	3	16
4	·2	8	4	4	24	4	4	24
5	1	2.5	5	4	24	5	1	2.5
6	3	16	6	3	16	6	3	16
7	4	24	7	2	8	7	2	8
8	1	2.5	8	3	16	8	1	2.5
9	2	8	9	5	29	9	3	16
10	2	8	10	4	24	10	3	16
Total	24	117.0		39	223		25	125.0
Mean	2.4			3.9			2.5	

*Because this is a different, unmatched subject design, you do not have to have equal numbers of subjects in each group, although it is easier if you do.

Subject Group 1 (10 pregnant women)	takes part in	Condition 1 Anterior
Subject Group 2 (10 pregnant women)	takes part in	Condition 2 Posterior
Subject Group 3 (10 pregnant women)	takes part in	Condition 3 Breech

Compared for differences

Figure 15.4 Design to test whether there is a relationship between the severity of stress incontinence and the position of the fetus.

2. Taking *all* the scores together, as though they were a single set of 30 scores, rank the scores, giving a rank of 1 to the lowest score, a rank of 2 to the next lowest etc. Where 2 or more scores are the same, apply the average ranks procedure (see p. 128), i.e. add up the ranks the scores would have obtained had they been different and divide this number by the total number of scores that are the same. Thus, in the example, 1 is the lowest score, but there are four scores of 1. Had these been different, they would have been ranked 1, 2, 3 and 4. So add these ranks up (10) and divide by 4 because there were four scores of 1 (i.e. 2.5). Give the rank of 2.5 to all the scores of 1. Remember that you have now used up ranks 1–4, so you must start with 5 next.

Remember! Rank all the scores together, as though they were just one set of 30 scores.

3. Add the rank total for each condition separately to give T:

$$T_C1 = 117.0$$
$$T_C2 = 223$$
$$T_C3 = 125.0.$$

4. Find the value of H from the following formula:

$$H = \left[\frac{12}{N(N+1)} \left(\sum \frac{T_C^2}{n_C} \right) \right] - 3(N+1)$$

where N = total number of subjects (i.e. 30)
n_C = number of subjects in each group (i.e. $n_1 = 10$; $n_2 = 10$; $n_3 = 10$)
T_C = rank totals for each condition (i.e. $T_C1 = 117$; $T_C2 = 223$; $T_C3 = 125$)
T_C^2 = rank total for each condition *squared* (i.e. 117^2; 223^2; 125^2)
$\sum$ = total of any calculations following
$\sum \frac{T_C^2}{n_C}$ = each rank total squared and divided by the number of subjects in that condition

i.e. $\dfrac{117^2}{10} + \dfrac{223^2}{10} + \dfrac{125^2}{10}$

Substituting these values:

$$H = \left[\frac{12}{30(30+1)} \times \left(\frac{117^2}{10} + \frac{223^2}{10} + \frac{125^2}{10} \right) \right] - 3 \times 31$$

$$= \left[\frac{12}{930} \times (1368.9 + 4972.9 + 1562.5)\right] - 93$$

$$= (0.013 \times 7904.3) - 93$$

$$= 102.756 - 93$$

$$= 9.756$$

Looking up the H value for significance

To find out whether $H = 9.756$ represents significant differences between the results from each group, you will also need the d.f. value. This is the number of conditions minus 1, i.e. $3 - 1 = 2$. Turn to Tables A2.1 and A2.8. Table A2.8 covers the probability levels for experiments using three groups of subjects, with 1–5 subjects in each group, while Table A2.1 covers the probability levels for experiments with more subjects and more conditions. (This is also the Chi-squared table.)

Because we have ten subjects in each condition we use Table A2.1. Down the left-hand column you will see various d.f. values. Look down the column until you find our d.f. of 2. To the right of this are five numbers:

$$4.60 \quad 5.99 \quad 7.82 \quad 9.21 \quad 13.82$$

These are called *critical values* and each one is associated with the probability level indicated at the top of the column, e.g. 7.82 has a p value of 0.02. To be significant at a given level, our H value has to be equal to or larger than one of these numbers. So, with our H of 9.756, we can see that it is larger than 9.21, but smaller than 13.82. This means that for our two-tailed hypothesis, the probability associated with the obtained H value of 9.756 must be somewhat less than 0.01 (or 1%) but somewhat greater than 0.001 (or 1%). To comply with convention, we would say that p is less than 0.01 (or 1%). (Remember with the Kruskal-Wallis, we can only predict general differences in our results, therefore any hypothesis must be two-tailed). This is expressed as $p < 0.01$ or $< 1\%$. This means that there is less than a 1% chance that our results are due to random error. (Had our H value been equal to the critical value, p would have been 0.01 exactly. This would have been expressed as $p = 0.01$ or 1%.)

Interpreting the results

Our H value of 9.756 has a probability of < 0.01 (or $< 1\%$) which means that the probability of random error accounting for the results is less than 1%. As you will remember, it was noted earlier that the usual cut-off point for assuming support for the experimental hypothesis is the 5% level or less. As our p value is less than 1%, it is smaller than the cut-off point of 5% and therefore we can say that our results are significant. This means we can reject the null hypothesis and accept the experimental hypothesis. This can be expressed in the following way:

> Using a Kruskal-Wallis test on the data ($H = 9.756$, $N = 30$) the results were found to be significant at $p < 0.01$. This suggests that there is a significant difference in the degree of stress incontinence during the last month of pregnancy according to the fetal position. This means that the experimental hypothesis has been supported.

Remember that the Kruskal-Wallis will only tell you that there are differences between your conditions and not which position causes most stress incontinence. If you had hypothesized a trend in the results, e.g.

> Anterior presentations produce more incontinence than posterior presentations which in turn produce worse incontinence than breech presentations

and had used the same unmatched design, you would use a Jonckheere trend test to analyse your results (see p. 161).

Because we used more than five Ss in our experiment, we had to use Table A2.1 to look up our H value. Suppose, however, that we had used instead, five Ss in Condition 1, four in Condition 2 and three in Condition 3, and had obtained an H value of 5.438. We would now need to use Table A2.8. You will see that there is a heading 'Size of groups', under which there is every permutation of n values. Your n values are $n_1 = 5$, $n_2 = 4$ and $n_3 = 3$. Therefore you need to find these n values (in any order) in the columns and to the right of these you will see six values of H:

7.4449

7.3949

5.6564

5.6308
4.5487
4.5231

and to their right, the relevant p values. (You do not need the d.f. value here.)

To be significant at a given level, our H value must be equal to or larger than the critical values here. Our hypothesized H value of 5.438 is larger than 4.5487 but smaller than 5.6308. These values are associated with probabilities of 0.050 and 0.099, and so our obtained H value must have a probability of less than 0.099 but greater than 0.050. Because of convention, we would say that our H of 5.438 has a probability of less than 0.099. Because our cut-off point is 0.05, we must accept the null (no relationship) hypothesis, i.e. our results would not be significant.

Activity 15.3   (Answers on page 240)

1. To practise looking up H values, look up the following and state whether or not they are significant and at what level.
   (i) $n_1 = 3$ $n_2 = 4$ $n_3 = 3$ $H = 5.801$ p
   (ii) $n_1 = 5$ $n_2 = 5$ $n_3 = 4$ $H = 5.893$ p
   (iii) $n_1 = 12$ $n_2 = 10$ $n_3 = 10$ $n_4 = 10$ d.f. = 3 $H = 8.5$ p
   (iv) $n_1 = 3$ $n_2 = 3$ $n_3 = 5$ $H = 7.0234$ p
   (v) $n_1 = 10$ $n_2 = 12$ $n_3 = 14$ $n_4 = 14$ $n_5 = 14$ d.f. = 4
      $H = 15.23$ p
   (vi) $n_1 = 10$ $n_2 = 10$ $n_3 = 8$ $n_4 = 10$ d.f. = 3 $H = 6.86$ p
2. Calculate a Kruskal-Wallis on the following data:
   H$_1$ Compliance with postnatal exercise instructions varies according to whether the instructions are (a) oral, (b) written by the midwife or (c) written by the woman herself.
   Method: Select 15 women within 1 week of parturition and randomly allocate five to oral instructions, five to midwife-written instructions and five to self-written instructions. After 1 week compare their self-reported compliance (on a 5-point scale where 5 = did every exercise daily, 1 = did no exercises at all). The results are as in Table 15.7.

Table 15.7

Sub-ject	Condi-tion 1 Oral	Rank	Sub-ject	Condi-tion 2 Midwife	Rank	Sub-ject	Condi-tion 3 Self	Rank
1	3		1	3		1	4	
2	2		2	3		2	3	
3	2		3	3		3	4	
4	3		4	2		4	3	
5	1		5	3		5	5	

State the H and p values in the format recommended earlier.

Jonckheere trend test

This test is used with the same experimental designs as the Kruskal-Wallis, i.e.

- three or more different (unmatched) subject groups are being compared
- the data is ordinal or interval/ratio
- the conditions required for a parametric test cannot be fulfilled (see p. 151 for the design).

However, the one major difference which determines whether you use a Kruskal-Wallis or Jonckheere trend test relates to your hypothesis. If you simply predict that there will be differences between the groups, without specifying which group will perform best or worst then you use the Kruskal-Wallis. However, if you predict a trend in your results, e.g. Group A will do better than Group B who in turn will do better than Group C then you are predicting a definite direction to your results and you should use the Jonckheere to analyse them. Therefore any hypothesis associated with the Jonckheere must be one-tailed.

When calculating the Jonckheere, you end up with a numerical value for S, which you look up in the probability tables associated with the Jonckheere test, to see whether this value represents a significant trend in the results.

It should be stressed here that you must have the same numbers of subjects in each group for the Jonckheere. This is not necessary for the Kruskal-Wallis, but it is essential here.

Example

Therefore if we look back to the example which predicts a relationship between fetal position and severity of stress incontinence, all that was predicted was a difference in the severity of the incontinence without specifying which position would lead to the worst incontinence. Consequently, a Kruskal-Wallis test was used. If, however, we re-stated the hypothesis to predict a specific direction to the results i.e.

H$_1$ Anterior fetal positions lead to worse stress incontinence than do posterior fetal conditions which in turn lead to worse stress incontinence than breech presentations.

Subject Group 1 (10 pregnant women) — takes part in — Condition 1 Breech

Subject Group 2 (10 pregnant women) — takes part in — Condition 2 Posterior

Subject Group 3 (10 pregnant women) — takes part in — Condition 3 Anterior

} Groups are compared on stress incontinence predicting that Group 3 will be worse than Group 2 who, in turn, will be worse than Group 1.

Figure 15.5 Anterior positions are predicted to lead to worse stress incontinence than posterior positions, with breech presentations leading to least incontinence.

Table 15.8

Subject	Breech	Subject	Anterior	Subject	Posterior
1	3	1	4	1	2
2	4	2	5	2	3
3	2	3	5	3	3
4	2	4	4	4	4
5	1	5	4	5	1
6	3	6	3	6	3
7	4	7	2	7	2
8	1	8	3	8	1
9	2	9	5	9	3
10	2	10	4	10	3

we would need a different statistical test to analyse the results i.e. the Jonckheere trend test. We would therefore have the design in Figure 15.5.

If we use the previous data, we can see whether or not there was a definite trend in results. These results are as in Table 15.8.

Calculating the Jonckheere trend test

So, taking the data from the previous example, we first have to set out the conditions such that the condition expected to obtain the lowest scores is on the left, and the condition expected to obtain the highest scores is on the right, the remaining condition in the middle. In other words, the conditions must be ordered from lowest on the left, to highest on the right, with any intermediary conditions ordered accordingly.

So, because we have predicted that the breech position will produce the least stress inconti-

nence followed by the posterior fetal position with the anterior fetal presentation producing the worst, we must re-order the above data to put the breech group on the left, the posterior group in the middle and the anterior group on the right (Table 15.9).

To calculate the Jonckheere:

1. First calculate the mean score for each condition (Condition 1 = 2.4, Condition 2 = 2.5 and Condition 3 = 3.9)

2. Starting with the extreme left-hand condition and the first score (i.e. 3) count up all the scores to the right of Condition 1 (i.e. in Conditions 2 and 3) which are larger than this score. Do not count any scores which are the same.

Therefore, in Condition 2, only Subject 4 with a score of 4 achieved a higher score, while in Condition 3, Subjects 1, 2, 3, 4, 5, 9 and 10 all obtained higher scores. This means that in total, 8 scores in Conditions 2 and 3 are higher than the score of 3. This number is put in brackets by Subject 1, Condition 1's score. Do exactly the same for the second score (4) in Condition 1. There are no scores in Condition 2 which are larger and 3 scores in Condition 3 which are larger. Thus the total of 3 is put in brackets by Subject 2, Condition 1. Continue in this way for the rest of the scores in Condition 1.

Do the same for each score in Condition 2, although, of course, you will only be comparing these with Condition 3 since it is only these scores which are to the right of Condition 2.

Table 15.9

Subject	Condition 1 Breech	Subject	Condition 2 Posterior	Subject	Condition 3 Anterior
1	3 (8)	1	2 (9)	1	4
2	4 (3)	2	3 (7)	2	5
3	2 (15)	3	3 (7)	3	5
4	2 (15)	4	4 (3)	4	4
5	1 (18)	5	1 (10)	5	4
6	3 (8)	6	3 (7)	6	3
7	4 (3)	7	2 (9)	7	2
8	1 (18)	8	1 (10)	8	3
9	2 (15)	9	3 (7)	9	5
10	2 (15)	10	3 (7)	10	4
$\bar{x}$	2.4		2.5		3.9

Because Condition 3 has no scores to the right the procedure terminates with the last subject in Condition 2.

3. Before we can calculate S, we need two more values: A and B. To find A: Add up all scores in brackets to give the value A, i.e.

$$A = 8 + 3 + 15 + 15 + 18 + 8 + 3 + 18 + 15 + 15 + 9 + 7 + 7 + 3 + 10 + 7 + 9 + 10 + 7 + 7$$
$$\therefore A = 194$$

4. In order to find out the maximum value A could have been, had all the scores in Conditions 2 and 3 been bigger than those in Condition 1 and all the scores in Condition 3 been bigger than those in Condition 2, find the value B from the formula:

$$B = \frac{C(C - 1)}{2} \times n^2$$

where n = number of Ss in each condition
C = number of conditions
i.e. $n = 10$
$C = 3$

$$B = \frac{3(3 - 1)}{2} \times 10^2$$

$$= 300$$

4. Calculate S using the following formula:

$$S = (2 \times A) - B$$
$$= (2 \times 194) - 300$$
$$S = 88$$

Looking up the value of S for significance

To look up $S = 88$, turn to Table A2.9 where you will see two tables — the top one for significance levels of $< 5\%$ and the lower one for levels of $< 1\%$. Both are for one-tailed hypotheses because a specific direction to the results must be predicted in order to use the Jonckheere test. Start with the top table first. In order to look up your S value, you need the number of conditions and the number of subjects in each condition (i.e. 3 and 10 respectively). Look across the top row for the appropriate value of n and down the left-hand column for the appropriate value of C. At the intersection point you will find the figure 88. If our S value is equal to or larger than this

figure, then the results are significant at the level stated in the heading of the table. As our S value is exactly 88, our results are significant at the < 0.05 or $< 5\%$ level. This means that there is less than a 5% probability that our results are due to random error.

Had our S value been larger than the intersection figure of 88 (say 131), we would move down to the second table which is associated with a probability level of < 0.01 and repeat the process. The intersection figure is 124, which means the result is larger than this value and the probability of our results being due to random error is less than 0.01 or 1%.

Interpreting the results

Because our usual cut-off point is 5%, and our results have a probability level of $< 5\%$ the results can be classified as significant and we can reject the null (no relationship) hypothesis. There is less than a 5% chance that random error is responsible for our results. This means that there is a significant trend in our results with breech presentations producing least incontinence followed by posterior fetal presentations and then anterior fetal presentations. This can be expressed thus:

> Using a Jonckheere trend test on the data ($S = 88$, $n = 10$), the results were found to be significant at $< 5\%$ level. This means that there is a significant trend in the degree of stress incontinence according to fetal position, with breech presentations producing least incontinence followed by posterior presentations and then anterior presentations which produce the worst stress incontinence. The null hypothesis can be rejected.

Activity 15.4   (Answers on page 240)

1. To practise looking up S values, look up the following and state whether or not they are significant and at what level.

   (i) $C = 3$ $n = 6$ $S = 61$ p
   (ii) $C = 5$ $n = 5$ $S = 68$ p
   (iii) $C = 5$ $n = 8$ $S = 151$ p
   (iv) $C = 3$ $n = 10$ $S = 124$ p
   (v) $C = 3$ $n = 7$ $S = 55$ p
   (vi) $C = 4$ $n = 5$ $S = 48$ p

2. Calculate a Jonckheere trend test on the following data:

   H_1 There is a difference in the number of ante-natal appointments kept, according to the social class to which the mother belongs, with women from social class 3 being better than social class 2, who in turn are better than social class 4.

Method: Randomly select eight women belonging to each of the social classes and calculate the percentage of kept appointments. The data are as shown in Table 15.10.

Table 15.10

Sub-ject	Condition 1 Social class 3	Sub-ject	Condition 1 Social class 2	Sub-ject	Condition 3 Social class 4
1	100	1	100	1	75
2	90	2	100	2	70
3	100	3	80	3	50
4	75	4	75	4	30
5	75	5	60	5	60
6	80	6	80	6	80
7	90	7	50	7	70
8	70	8	50	8	75

Remember! You must arrange your data such that the condition expected to have the lowest results is on the left, while the condition expected to have the highest results is on the right. State the values of A, B, S, and p; express the results in the format given earlier in the section.

NON-PARAMETRIC STATISTICAL TEST FOR USE WITH THREE OR MORE DIFFERENT SUBJECT GROUPS AND NOMINAL DATA

Extended chi-squared (χ^2) test

As the name implies this test is an extension of the χ^2 test described earlier in the chapter. Like the earlier test it is used:

- with different subject groups
- with nominal data (re-read Ch. 4 if you need to refresh your memory on levels of measurement)
- when the remaining conditions required for a parametric test cannot be fulfilled (see p. 151 for the designs).

However, there is an important point which relates to the extended χ^2 test. The ordinary χ^2 test only allows you to use two groups of subjects which you can allocate to *two* nominal categories.

This means you arrange your data in a 2 × 2 table as in Figure 15.6.

However, the extended χ^2 allows you to use:

a. two groups of subject and three (or more) nominal categories.

This means you arrange your data in a 2 × 3 table as in Figure 15.7.

b. three (or more) groups of subjects and two nominal categories.

This means you arrange your data in a 3 × 2 table, as in Figure 15.8.

c. three (or more) groups of subjects and three (or more) nominal categories, etc.

This means you arrange your data in a 3 × 3 table as in Figure 15.9.

So you may want to ask two groups of women, one from Social Class II and the other from Social Class IV whether they intend to breast feed. Their

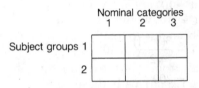

Figure 15.6 A 2 × 2 table for calculating the χ^2 test.

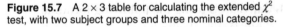

Figure 15.7 A 2 × 3 table for calculating the extended χ^2 test, with two subject groups and three nominal categories.

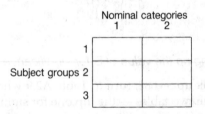

Figure 15.8 A 3 × 2 table for calculating the extended χ^2 test, with three subject groups and two nominal categories.

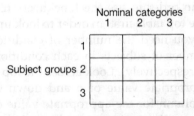

Figure 15.9 A 3 × 3 table for calculating the extended χ^2 test, with three subject groups and three nominal categories.

choice of answers are 'Yes', 'No' and 'Don't know'. Because you have two groups of Ss and three nominal categories you would have a 2×3 table and would need to analyse the data using an extended χ^2 test.

(By the way, I recognize that the heading of this sub-section may be confusing, in that it implies the extended χ^2 can only be used with three or more subject groups, whereas it can be used with two groups as long as they are being allocated to more than two nominal categories. I apologize for this, but as you can see, a clear, succinct title was difficult to achieve.)

The extended χ^2 test only tells you whether there are overall differences between the groups and not where these differences lie. As a result any hypothesis associated with the extended χ^2 must be two-tailed, in that it cannot predict a specific direction to the results.

The data you obtained in your experiment are called the observed data. The main point of the χ^2 test is to compare your observed data with the data you would have expected had your results been due to totally random distributions. In other words you are comparing the results obtained from your experimental hypothesis (observed data) with those predicted by your null (no relationship) hypothesis (expected data). Obviously, the greater the discrepancies between the observed and the expected data, the more likely your results are to be significant. Always ensure that you have tested sufficient subjects to obtain expected frequencies of more than 5. The easiest way to do this is by using at least 20 subjects in each group. You do not need to use equal numbers of subjects in each group.

When calculating the extended χ^2, the value of χ^2 is found and this is then looked up in the probability tables associated with the test to find out whether this value represents significant differences between the observed and expected frequencies.

Example

Suppose in the course of your work you noted that ante-natal care seemed to be rather less useful for ethnic minority groups than for the majority white caucasian group, perhaps because of language barriers or cultural mores.

Your hypothesis is:

H$_1$ Ante-natal provision is differentially useful for Asian, African Caribbean and Caucasian mothers.

Brief method: You randomly select 30 Asian women, 35 African Caribbean women and 53 Caucasian women at comparable stages of pregnancy from an ante-natal clinic. You simply ask them whether or not they are satisfied with the quality of care they have received (two nominal categories). Thus you have:

Group 1
Asian
}
Compared for differences in satisfaction with ante-natal care

Group 2
African Caribbean

Group 3
Caucasian

There are, then, three unrelated groups of subjects. Each subject's response is allocated to one of two categories (satisfied/not satisfied) and the relative numbers in each category are compared using the extended χ^2.

Imagine that you have carried out some research to test the hypothesis just quoted and you have obtained the following data:

Asian women	satisfied	9
	not satisfied	21
African Caribbean women	satisfied	22
	not satisfied	13
Caucasian women	satisfied	25
	not satisfied	28

These data are then set out in the table shown in Figure 15.10. (Ensure that the cells are numbered in this way, i.e. from left to right.)

Make sure your subject groups are down the left-hand side, and the nominal categories across the top, although the order in each case is irrelevant.

Calculating the extended χ^2 test

So, to calculate the χ^2 test, take the following steps:

	Satisfied	Not satisfied	Marginal totals of subjects
Group 1 Asian	Cell 1 9 E = 14.237	Cell 2 21 E = 15.763	30
Group 2 African Caribbean	Cell 3 22 E = 16.61	Cell 4 13 E = 18.39	35
Group 3 Caucasian	Cell 5 25 E = 25.153	Cell 6 28 E = 27.848	53
Marginal totals	56	62	Grand total (N) 118

Figure 15.10 An example of data for the extended χ^2 test, with three subject groups and two nominal categories.

1. Add up the numbers in each row to give the marginal total for:

a. Asian women, i.e. $9 + 21 = 30$
b. African Caribbean women, i.e. $22 + 13 = 35$
c. Caucasian women, i.e. $25 + 28 = 53$

2. Add up the numbers in each column to give the marginal totals for:

a. satisfied, i.e. $9 + 22 + 25 = 56$
b. not satisfied, i.e. $21 + 13 + 28 = 62$

3. Add up either the marginal totals for patients, i.e.

$$30 + 35 + 53 = 118$$

or the marginal totals for levels of satisfaction, i.e.

$$56 + 62 = 118$$

to give the grand total (N)
therefore $N = 118$

4. Calculate the expected frequency (E) for each cell by multiplying the two relevant marginal totals together and dividing by N.

$$\text{Cell 1, } E = \frac{30 \times 56}{118}$$

$$= 14.237$$

$$\text{Cell 2, } E = \frac{30 \times 62}{118}$$

$$= 15.763$$

$$\text{Cell 3, } E = \frac{35 \times 56}{118}$$

$$= 16.61$$

$$\text{Cell 4, } E = \frac{35 \times 62}{118}$$

$$= 18.39$$

$$\text{Cell 5, } E = \frac{53 \times 56}{118}$$

$$= 125.153$$

$$\text{Cell 6, } E = \frac{53 \times 62}{118}$$

$$= 27.848$$

Enter each expected frequency in the lower right-hand corner of the appropriate cell.

5. Calculate the following formula for χ^2:

$$\chi^2 = \sum \frac{(O - E)^2}{E}$$

where
O = observed frequencies for each cell (i.e. your actual data)
E = expected frequencies for each cell
Σ = sum or total of all calculations to the right of the sign.

$$\text{Cell 1} = \frac{(9 - 14.237)^2}{14.237}$$

$$= 1.926$$

$$\text{Cell 2} = \frac{(21 - 15.763)^2}{15.763}$$

$$= 1.74$$

$$\text{Cell 3} = \frac{(22 - 16.61)^2}{16.61}$$

$$= 1.75$$

$$\text{Cell 4} = \frac{(13 - 18.39)^2}{18.39}$$

$$= 1.58$$

$$\text{Cell 5} = \frac{(25 - 25.153)^2}{25.153}$$

$$= 0$$

$$\text{Cell 6} = \frac{(28 - 27.848)^2}{27.848}$$

$$= 0$$

6. All these values are added together to give χ^2

$$\chi^2 = \sum \frac{(O - E)^2}{E}$$

i.e.: 1.926 + 1.74 + 1.75 + 1.58 + 0 + 0 = 6.996
Therefore χ^2 = 6.996

7. To look up the value χ^2 6.996, you will also need the degrees of freedom (d.f.) value, i.e.

$$(r - 1) \times (c - 1)$$

where r = number of rows (3)
c = number of columns (2)
Therefore, d.f. = $(3 - 1) \times (2 - 1) = 2$

Looking up the value of χ^2 for significance

Turn to Table A2.1. You will see down the left-hand column, different d.f. values. Find our d.f. = 2 value. To the right of this are five numbers, called *critical values* of χ^2:

4.60   5.99   7.82   9.21   13.82

Each critical value is associated with the p value at the top of its column, e.g. 9.21 has a p value of 0.01. To be significant at a particular level, our χ^2 value must be equal to or *larger* than one of these critical values. (Remember that the extended χ^2 can only determine whether there are overall differences in the results, so the associated hypothesis must be two-tailed.)

Our χ^2 value of 6.996 is larger than 5.99 but smaller than 7.82. This means that our results are not good enough to be significant at 0.02, but they are slightly better than the 0.05 level. Therefore, by convention we express this as $p < 0.05$ (less than 0.05). Had our χ^2 value been 5.99 exactly we would have expressed this as $p = 0.05$. This means that our χ^2 value is significant at the < 0.05 level or < 5% level. In other words, the chances of our results being due to random error are less than 5%.

Interpreting the results

Our χ^2 value has an associated probability value of < 0.05. This means that there is less than a 5% chance that our results could be accounted for by random error. As the usual cut-off point of 5% or less is used to claim support for the experimental hypothesis and our results have a probability of less than 5%, we can say they are significant. The null hypothesis can be rejected and the experimental hypothesis accepted. This means that there is a significant relationship between ethnic origin and level of satisfaction with ante-natal care.

This can be expressed in the following way:

Using the extended χ^2 on the data (χ^2 = 6.996, d.f. = 2) the results were found to be significant at $p < 0.05$ for a two-tailed test. This suggests that ethnic origin (Asian, African Caribbean and Caucasian) are significantly associated with satisfaction with ante-natal care.

Activity 15.5   (Answers on page 240)

1. To practise looking up χ^2 values, look up the following and state whether or not they are significant.
   (i) χ^2 = 3.45   d.f. = 2 p
   (ii) χ^2 = 8.91   d.f. = 3 p
   (iii) χ^2 = 6.77   d.f. = 2 p
   (iv) χ^2 = 9.42   d.f. = 4 p
   (v) χ^2 = 7.95   d.f. = 2 p

2. Calculate an extended χ^2 on the following data.
   You are concerned about the missed appointments at the ante-natal clinic and think it may be to do with the difficulty of getting to the clinic by public transport.
   Your hypothesis, then, is:
   H_1 Keeping an ante-natal appointment is related to the ease of access to the hospital, when using public transport.
   So you select 25 patients who have a single bus journey with no changes, 30 who have to make one change of bus and 29 who have to make more than one change of bus. You simply note whether or not they missed their next appointment.
   You obtain the data in Figure 15.11.
   Calculate an extended χ^2 on this data and state what the χ^2 value is and the p value. Present your results in the format suggested earlier.

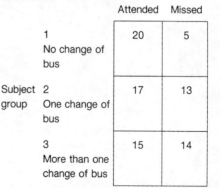

		Attended	Missed
	1 No change of bus	20	5
Subject group	2 One change of bus	17	13
	3 More than one change of bus	15	14

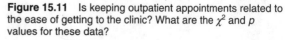

Figure 15.11   Is keeping outpatient appointments related to the ease of getting to the clinic? What are the χ^2 and p values for these data?

CHAPTER CONTENTS

16

Parametric tests for different (unrelated) subject designs

INTRODUCTION

The statistical tests described in the last chapter are used to analyse results from unrelated designs, i.e. any design which uses two or more than two groups of different, unmatched subjects. They are also used when the conditions necessary for a parametric test (see Ch. 9) cannot be fulfilled. The tests covered in this chapter are the parametric equivalent to those in the previous chapter, in other words they are used when:

- two or more than two different (unmatched) groups of subjects are used in the research and the results from each are compared for differences.
- when the conditions essential for a parametric test can be fulfilled (especially the interval/ratio level of measurement).

Therefore, the sorts of designs involved are:

1. *Two different, unmatched subject groups, compared on a task* (Fig. 16.1).

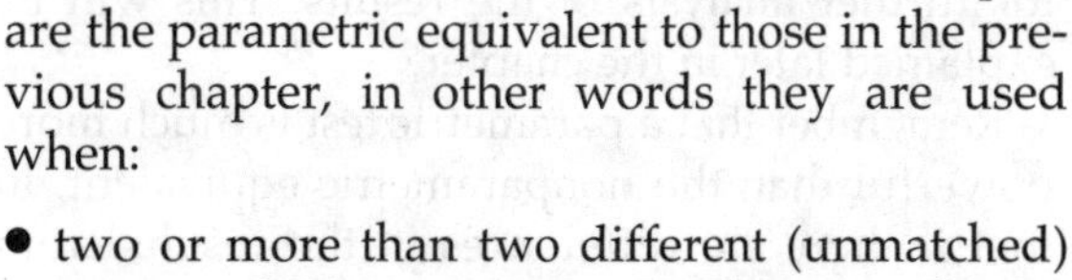

Figure 16.1 Different subject design: two groups of different, unmatched subjects each taking part in one condition.

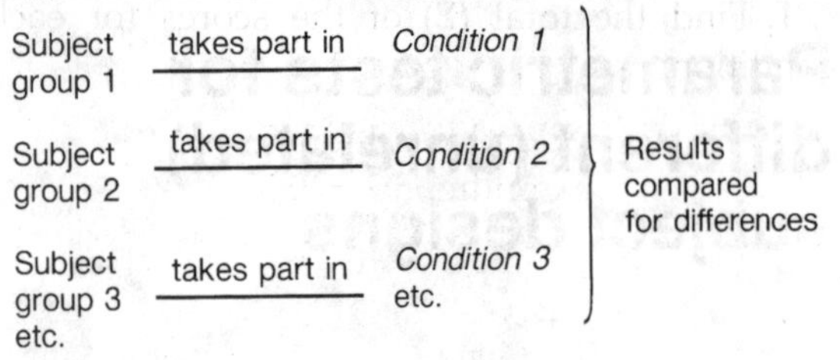

Figure 16.2 Different subject design: three, or more, groups of different, unmatched subjects each taking part in one condition.

2. *Three or more different, unmatched subject groups, compared on a task* (Fig. 16.2).

Results from experiments using Design 1 (two unmatched groups) are analysed by the unrelated *t*-test, while results derived from experiments using Design 2 (three or more unmatched groups) are analysed by the one way analysis of variance (anova) for unrelated designs (Table 16.1). In addition, the Scheffé multiple range test can be used in conjunction with the anova for further analysis of the results. This will be explained later in the chapter.

Remember that a parametric test is much more powerful than the nonparametric equivalent, in that if there are differences in the results from the different subject groups, the parametric test is more likely to pick them up. This said, there are, however, a number of points you should remember:

1. The parametric test and its non-parametric equivalent do essentially the same job in that

Table 16.1 Parametric tests for different (unrelated) subject designs

Design	Parametric test
1. Two groups of different, unmatched subjects, each taking part in one condition. Results from conditions compared for differences.	Unrelated *t*-test
2. Three or more groups of different, unmatched subjects, each taking part in one condition. Results from conditions compared for differences.	One-way analysis of variance (anova) for unrelated designs and Scheffé multiple range test

they compare results from the subject groups to find out whether any differences between them are significant.
2. In order to use a parametric test you must ensure that you fulfil the necessary conditions. (see p. 81).
3. If you are in any doubt as to whether a parametric test should be used, always use the non-parametric equivalent.
4. Parametric tests, although more sensitive, are more difficult to calculate.

PARAMETRIC STATISTICAL TEST FOR USE WITH TWO GROUPS OF DIFFERENT SUBJECTS

Unrelated *t*-test

This test is used when the experimental design compares two separate or different unmatched groups of subjects participating in different conditions (see Design 1, previous page). It is the parametric equivalent of the Mann-Whitney *U* test. The fact that it is parametric means, principally, that you must have interval/ratio data. Do note that you do not need to have equal numbers in each group. When calculating the unrelated *t*-test, you find the value of *t* which you then look up in the probability tables associated with the *t*-test to find out whether the *t*-value represents a significant difference between the results from your two groups.

Example

Imagine that satellite ante-natal clinics have just been introduced into your health authority in an attempt to increase the take up of ante-natal care. You are interested in comparing the percentage of kept appointments under this new system with those at conventional hospital units. Your hypothesis is:

H_1 The percentage of missed ante-natal appointments is lower at satellite clinics than at hospital clinics.

(This is a one-tailed hypothesis because it predicts that the percentage of missed appointments will be lower at the satellite clinics.)

Group 1
Satellite
ante-natal ——— *Condition 1*
clinics   average percentage
                appointments missed

Group 2
Hospital
ante-natal ——— *Condition 2*
clinics   average percentage
                appointments missed

⎫
⎬ Compared
⎭ for
   differences

Figure 16.3 Is the percentage of missed appointments lower at satellite than at hospital ante-natal clinics?

Brief method: You select ten satellite clinics and ten hospital ante-natal clinics and calculate the average percentage of missed appointments over the last 12 months for each clinic. You have the design shown in Fig. 16.3.

In other words you are comparing the results of two different groups of subjects — a design and type of measurement which require an unrelated *t*-test.

You obtain the results shown in Table 16.2.

Calculating the unrelated t-test

In order to calculate *t*, you should take the following steps (the unrelated *t*-test formula looks very formidable, but please do not panic! As long as you work through the following stages systematically, you should not have too much difficulty).

1. Find the total (Σ) of the scores for each condition:

$$\text{Condition } 1 = 345$$
$$\text{Condition } 2 = 285$$

2. Find the average score ($\bar{x}$) for each condition: i.e.

$$\bar{x} \text{ for Condition } 1 = 34.5$$
$$\bar{x} \text{ for Condition } 2 = 28.5.$$

3. Square every individual score and enter the results in the columns headed X_1^2 and X_2^2, i.e.

Subject 1, Group 1, scored 40, which when squared becomes 1600.

4. Add up the squared scores for each condition separately to give ΣX^2, i.e.

$$\Sigma X_1^2 = 12\ 325$$
$$\Sigma X_2^2 = 8725$$

5. Take the total for each condition separately, and square it, to give $(\Sigma X)^2$, i.e.

$$(\Sigma X_1)^2 = 345^2$$
$$= 119\ 025$$
$$(\Sigma X_2)^2 = 285^2$$
$$= 81\ 225$$

Do make a note of the difference between the symbol ΣX^2 which means: 'square each individual score and then add up all the squared scores', and $(\Sigma X)^2$ which means: 'add up all the

Table 16.2

	Group 1*, Hospital			Group 2, Satellite		
Subject	Scores (X_1)		X_1^2	Subject	Scores (X_2)	X_2^2
1	40		1600	1	20	400
2	30		900	2	25	625
3	35		1225	3	30	900
4	25		625	4	25	625
5	30		900	5	15	225
6	40		1600	6	40	1600
7	45		2025	7	35	1225
8	35		1225	8	40	1600
9	25		625	9	25	625
10	40		1600	10	30	900
$\Sigma X_1 =$	345	$\Sigma X_1^2 =$	12325	$\Sigma X_2 =$	285	$\Sigma X_2^2 =$ 8725
$\bar{x}_1 =$	34.5			$\bar{x}_2 =$	28.5	

*It does not matter whether the satellite ante-natal clinic is Condition 1 or 2.

individual scores for the condition and then square the result'.

6. Now (take a deep breath!) calculate t from the formula:

$$t = \frac{\bar{x}_1 - \bar{x}_2}{\sqrt{\dfrac{\left(\Sigma X_1{}^2 - \dfrac{(\Sigma X_1)^2}{n_1}\right) + \left(\Sigma X_2{}^2 - \dfrac{(\Sigma X_2)^2}{n_2}\right)}{(n_1 - 1) + (n_2 - 1)}} \times \sqrt{\left(\dfrac{1}{n_1} + \dfrac{1}{n_1}\right)}}$$

where
$\bar{x}_1$ = mean of scores from Condition 1
   = 34.5
$\bar{x}_2$ = mean of scores from Condition 2
   = 28.5
$\Sigma X_1{}^2$ = the square of each individual score from Condition 1 totalled
   = 12 325
$\Sigma X_2{}^2$ = the square of each individual score from Condition 2 totalled
   = 8725
$(\Sigma X_1)^2$ = the total of the individual scores from Condition 1 squared
   = 345^2
   = 119 025
$(\Sigma X_2)^2$ = the total of the individual scores from Condition 2 squared
   = 285^2
   = 81 225
n_1 = number of Ss in Condition 1
   = 10
n_2 = number of Ss in Condition 2
   = 10

If we substitute these values in the formula:

$$t = \frac{34.5 - 28.5}{\sqrt{\dfrac{\left(12\,325 - \dfrac{119\,025}{10}\right) + \left(8725 - \dfrac{81\,225}{10}\right)}{(10 - 1) + (10 - 1)}} \times \sqrt{\left(\dfrac{1}{10} + \dfrac{1}{10}\right)}}$$

$$= \frac{6}{\sqrt{\dfrac{422.5 - 602.5}{18} \times \dfrac{1}{5}}}$$

$$= \frac{6}{\sqrt{56.944 \times 0.2}}$$

$$= \frac{6}{3.375}$$

$$t = 1.778*$$

*(Note: it does not matter if your t value is + or –, because you ignore the sign anyway.)

7. Calculate the degrees of freedom from the formula:

$$\text{d.f.} = (n_1 - 1) + (n_2 - 1)$$
$$= (10 - 1) + (10 - 1)$$
$$= 18$$

Looking up the value of t for significance

To look up the value $t = 1.778$, with d.f. = 18, turn to Table A2.5. Down the left-hand column, you will find values of d.f. Look down the column until you find d.f. = 18. To the right of this, you will see six numbers, called critical values of t:

1.330   1.734   2.101   2.552   2.878   3.922

Each critical value represents a different level of probability as indicated by the bold type at the top of the table. Therefore, 2.552, for example, is associated with a probability of 0.01 for a one-tailed and 0.02 for a two-tailed test. To be significant at one of these levels, our t value must be equal to or larger than the associated critical t value in the table.

Our t value is larger than 1.734, but smaller than 2.101. This means that for our one-tailed hypothesis, the probability associated with our t value of 1.778 comes somewhere between 0.05 (5%) and 0.025 (22%). In other words the probability for $t = 1.778$ is less than 5%, but greater than 22%. According to convention, we always say that p is less than a given level, and so here the p value for $t = 1.778$ is less than 5% (or 0.05). This is expressed as:

$$p < 0.05 \text{ (or 5\%)}$$
(< means 'less than')

This means that the chances of random error accounting for our results are less than 5%. Has our t value been 1.734 exactly, the associated probability level would have equalled 0.05. This would be expressed as $p = 0.05$.

(n.b. it does not matter if your t value is + or − because you ignore the sign anyway.)

Interpreting the results

Our t value of 1.778 has an associated probability level of less than 5%, which means that the possibility of random error being responsible for the outcome of our experiment is less than 5 in 100. As the usual cut-off point for claiming support for the experimental hypothesis is 5% we can say that our results are significant. However, because we predicted a specific direction to the results (i.e. a one-tailed hypothesis), we must check that the results are in the predicted direction (i.e. that satellite ante-natal clinics have a higher percentage of kept appointments); sometimes significant results are obtained which are in the opposite direction to the hypothesis and therefore do not support it.

Here, if we look at the mean scores for each condition, we can see that the average percentage of missed appointments for the hospital condition is larger (34.5 as opposed to 28.5). Therefore, the experimental hypothesis has been supported. This can be stated in the following way:

> Using an unrelated t-test on the data ($t = 1.778$, d.f. = 18) the results were found to be significant ($p < 0.05$ for a one-tailed hypothesis). The null hypothesis can therefore be rejected. This means that satellite ante-natal clinics have fewer missed appointments than hospital ante-natal clinics.

Activity 16.1   (Answer on page 240)

1. To practise looking up t values, look up the following and state whether or not they are significant and at what level:
   (i) $t = 2.149$ d.f. = 10   one-tailed p
   (ii) $t = 2.596$ d.f. = 16   two-tailed p
   (iii) $t = 3.055$ d.f. = 12   two-tailed p
   (iv) $t = 1.499$ d.f. = 15   one-tailed p
   (v) $t = 3.204$ d.f. = 18   two-tailed p

2. Calculate an unrelated t-test on the following data
   H_1 Absenteeism is greater amongst midwives working under the traditional random allocation system than amongst those operating as 'named midwives'.
   Brief method: Randomly select 15 midwives operating on a random allocation-to-client basis and 12 'named' midwives and note the number of units of absence for each over the previous 12 months.
   The results are shown in Table 16.3.

Table 16.3

Condition 1 Random allocation		Condition 2 Named midwife	
Subject	Score	Subject	Score
1	18	1	17
2	22	2	12
3	10	3	15
4	14	4	10
5	25	5	19
6	19	6	8
7	17	7	5
8	28	8	14
9	18	9	18
10	14	10	21
11	15	11	20
12	22	12	16
13	23		
14	19		
15	24		

State the t, d.f. and p values, using the format outlined earlier.

PARAMETRIC STATISTICAL TEST FOR USE WITH THREE OR MORE GROUPS OF DIFFERENT SUBJECTS

One-way analysis of variance (anova) for unrelated (different subject) designs

The one-way anova for unrelated designs is the parametric equivalent of the Kruskal-Wallis test, i.e. it is used to compare results from three or more conditions, with different, unmatched subject groups in each condition (see Figure 16.2, page 170 for the design)

It is used when the prerequisite conditions for a parametric test can be fulfilled, the most important of which is that the data are of an interval/ratio level.

The one-way anova is so-called because it analyses results from experiments where only one independent variable is manipulated. (All the statistical tests and designs covered in this book relate solely to the manipulation of one IV.) More complex designs which manipulate two IVs simultaneously are analysed using a two-way anova; those which manipulate three IVs simultaneously require a three-way anova. (Refresh your memory by re-reading Chapter 6). All this is outside the domain of this book, but the reader is referred to Ferguson (1976) for more information on this topic.

The anova only tells you whether there are general, non-specified differences in the results from the different conditions — it does not tell you which group is better than the others. (To find this out, once you have calculated your anova, you will need to use the Scheffé test — but more of that later.) Because of this, any hypothesis associated with the anova must, of necessity, be two-tailed.

Essentially, what the one-way unrelated anova does is to tell you whether the differences in scores from each condition are sufficiently large to be classified as significant. But if you look back to the outline design on page 170 you will see that different subject groups are doing different conditions. Therefore, any variation between the scores from the conditions must also reflect the variations between the subject groups.

This source of variation is called *between conditions* variance. However, because different subjects are involved in each condition, it is conceivable that any outcome in the results is due not to differences between conditions, but to individual differences amongst the subjects, of inherent variations in personality, ability, reactions to the study etc., i.e. the result of random error. Thus, this is another source of potential variation in the results and is known as *error variance*.

Obviously, you would wish your results to be the outcome of the different conditions and not random error. Thus, the degree of between condition variance should be much larger than the error variance. What the one-way unrelated anova does is to tell you whether your results are due to real differences between the experimental conditions or alternatively to random error in the form of individual differences.

Example

An actual example might clarify all this. Induced labours are thought to be quicker than are those which start spontaneously.

Suppose you are interested in looking at the impact various forms of induction have on the

second stage of labour. You decide to compare the effects of prostaglandin pessaries, artificial rupture of the membranes (ARM) and oxytocin. Your hypothesis is:

H_1 Prostaglandin pessaries, ARM and oxytocin have different effects on the length of the second stage of labour.

(Note the inevitable change to a two-tailed hypothesis in the latter example). Obviously, what you are predicting here are differences in length of the second stage of labour between the groups of women as a result of different induction methods. Therefore, you are anticipating a significant degree of between-group variation. However, suppose you picked your subjects badly, such that all the fittest and most motivated women were in the ARM group. Almost inevitably, this type of induction would produce the fastest times, not because of the nature of the induction, but because of the idiosyncrasies of the subjects. In other words random error would account for your results. Obviously, the sort of situation which has all the most motivated and fittest subjects inadvertently allocated to one group is very unlikely to occur, particularly if you randomly allocate your subjects to conditions, but the point is this: your results could be due to genuine differences in terms of induction, or to some quirks of your subjects. Obviously, you want your results to be due to the former and what the one-way unrelated anova does is to tell you how probable it is that your results *are* due to the IV and not to random error.

Thus, when you calculate the one-way unrelated anova, you have to find out the degree of variation in the scores due to the differences between experimental conditions (between conditions variance) and that due to random error (error variance). This will give you an F ratio which you then look up in the probability tables associated with the anova to see if it represents a significant result. Please note, however, that the following formula is only appropriate for designs with equal numbers of subjects in each group.

Let us suppose, then, that you randomly selected ten women who had their labours induced by prostaglandin pessaries, ten by ARM

Group 1 10 women	receive	Condition 1 ARM
Group 2 10 women	receive	Condition 2 Prostaglandin pessaries
Group 3 10 women	receive	Condition 3 Oxytocin

Compared on the length of the second stage of labour

Figure 16.4   Comparison of three different methods of inducing labour.

and ten by oxytocin. You monitor the length of the second stage of labour of each woman. Thus we have the sort of design shown in Figure 16.4.

When we calculate the one-way unrelated anova we need to set out a table for the sources of variance in scores as in Table 16.4.

You obtain the scores shown in Table 16.5.

Table 16.4

Source of variance	Sums of squares (SS)	Degrees of freedom (d.f.)	Mean squares (MS)	F ratio
Variation in results due to treatment (between conditions)	SS_{bet}	$d.f._{bet}$	MS_{bet}	F_{bet}
Variation in results due to random error	SS_{error}	$d.f._{error}$	MS_{error}	
Total	SS_{tot}	$d.f._{tot}$		

Table 16.5

	Condition 1 ARM	Condition 2 Prostaglandin pessaries	Condition 3 Oxytocin
1	40	20	25
2	30	25	30
3	35	30	40
4	25	25	35
5	30	15	25
6	40	40	25
7	45	35	20
8	35	40	30
9	25	25	35
10	40	30	35
	$\Sigma T_1 = 345$	$\Sigma T_2 = 285$	$\Sigma T_3 = 300$

Calculating the one-way anova for unrelated designs

To calculate the sums of squares (SS) for each source of variation, take the following steps:

1. Calculate the value ΣT_C^2, which is the sum of the squared total for each condition, i.e.

$$T_1^2 = 345^2$$
$$= 119\,025$$
$$T_2^2 = 285^2$$
$$= 81\,225$$
$$T_3^2 = 300^2$$
$$= 90\,000$$
$$\therefore \Sigma T_C^2 = 119\,025 + 81\,225 + 90\,000$$
$$= 290\,250$$

2. Find the value of n, which is the number of subjects in each condition

$$n = 10$$

3. Calculate the value of N, which is the total number of scores, i.e.

$$N = 10 + 10 + 10$$
$$= 30$$

4. Calculate $(\Sigma x)^2$ which is the grand total of all the scores, squared, i.e.

$$(\Sigma x)^2 = (345 + 285 + 300)^2$$
$$= 930^2$$
$$= 864\,900$$

5. Calculate the value of $\dfrac{(\Sigma x)^2}{N}$ (this value is subtracted from all calculations), i.e.

$$\frac{(\Sigma x)^2}{N} = \frac{(930)^2}{30}$$
$$= \frac{864\,900}{30}$$
$$= 28\,830$$

6. Thus to calculate the SS_{bet}, use the formula:

$$\frac{\Sigma T_C^2}{n} - \frac{(\Sigma x)^2}{N} = \frac{345^2 + 285^2 + 300^2}{10} - \frac{864\,900}{30}$$
$$= \frac{119\,025 + 81\,225 + 90\,000}{10} - 28\,830$$
$$= 195$$

7. Calculate SS_{tot} from the following formula:

$$\Sigma x^2 - \frac{(\Sigma x)^2}{N}$$

where Σx^2 = the square of each individual score, all added together, i.e.

$$\begin{aligned}
\Sigma x^2 &= 40^2 + 30^2 + 35^2 + 25^2 + 30^2 + 40^2 + 45^2 + 35^2 + \\
&\quad 25^2 + 40^2 + 20^2 + 25^2 + 30^2 + 25^2 + 15^2 + 40^2 + \\
&\quad 35^2 + 40^2 + 25^2 + 30^2 + 25^2 + 30^2 + 40^2 + 35^2 + \\
&\quad 25^2 + 25^2 + 20^2 + 30^2 + 35^2 + 35^2 \\
&= 30\ 400
\end{aligned}$$

$$\therefore SS_{tot}\ 30\ 400 - 28\ 830$$
$$= 1570$$

8. Calculate SS_{error} from the formula $SS_{tot} - SS_{bet}$

$$= 1570 - 195$$
$$= 1375$$

9. Calculate the d.f. values

$$\begin{aligned}
d.f._{bet} &= \text{number of conditions} - 1 \\
&= 3 - 1 \\
&= 2 \\
d.f._{tot} &= N - 1 \\
&= 30 - 1 \\
&= 29 \\
d.f._{error} &= d.f._{tot} - d.f._{bet} \\
&= 29 - 2 \\
&= 27
\end{aligned}$$

10. Divide each SS value by its own d.f. value to obtain the MS value, i.e.

$$\begin{aligned}
MS_{bet} &= \frac{SS_{bet}}{d.f._{bet}} \\
&= \frac{195}{2} \\
&= 97.5 \\
MS_{error} &= \frac{SS_{error}}{d.f._{error}} \\
&= \frac{1375}{27} \\
&= 50.926
\end{aligned}$$

11. Calculate the F ratio by using

$$\frac{MS_{bet}}{MS_{error}}$$

Table 16.6

Source of variance	SS	d.f.	MS	F ratio
Variation due to treatment, i.e. between conditions	195	2	97.5	1.915
Variation due to random error	1375	27	50.926	
Total	1570	29		

$$= \frac{97.5}{50.926}$$
$$= 1.915$$

Insert all these values into the appropriate slots in your anova table (see p. 175) as in Table 16.6.

To look the F ratio up in Tables A2.6a–d, you need the d.f. values for each source of variation, i.e. 2 and 27. If you turn to Tables A2.6a–d you will see that they each deal with critical values of F for different significance levels:

Table A2.6a = $p < 0.05$
Table A2.6b = $p < 0.025$
Table A2.6c = $p < 0.01$
Table A2.6d = $p < 0.001$

Starting with Table A2.6a which represents the largest and therefore least significant probabilities ($p < 0.05$) you will see various numbers associated with v_1, which are the d.f._{bet} values across the top, and v_2 values down the left-hand side which are the d.f._{error} values. Therefore, locate your d.f._{bet} of 2 along the top and the d.f._{error} of 27 down the left-hand column. Where these two lines intersect you will see the number 3.35. To be significant at the $p < 0.05$ level, our F value has to be equal to or larger than the given value of 3.35. Since $F = 1.915$ is smaller, we must conclude our results are not significant.

Interpreting the results

Because our F value of 1.915 is smaller than the number observed at the appropriate intersection point on Table A2.6a, we have to conclude that our results are not significant at < 0.05, and that the probability of our results being due to random error is greater than 5%. Since the normal cut-off level for claiming support for the experimental hypothesis is 5% or less, we have to accept the null (no relationship) hypothesis. This means that there is no relationship between type of induction of labour (ARM, prostaglandin pessaries or oxytocin) and length of the second stage of labour. This can be expressed as:

Using a one-way anova for unrelated designs ($F = 1.915$, $d.f._{bet} = 2$, $d.f._{error} = 27$) the results were not significant (p is greater than 5% for a two-tailed hypothesis). Therefore the null hypothesis must be accepted. This indicates that there is no relationship between type of induction of labour (ARM, prostaglandin pessaries and oxytocin) and length of the second stage of labour.

Had our F value been larger, say 5.234, it would obviously have been significant on Table A2.6a's probabilities. But could we do any better? Turn to Table A2.6b ($p < 0.025$) and repeat the process. The value at the intersection point using d.f. values of 2 and 27 is 4.24. Our F value is larger than this and so is significant at the < 0.025 level. Repeat the process with Table A2.6c ($p < 0.01$). The value at the intersection point is 5.49. Our F ratio is smaller and so is not significant at this level. Therefore, in this case we would conclude that the F value of 5.234 is significant at the $p < 0.025$ level.

Remember that because an anova only tells us whether there are differences and not in which direction these difference lie, the p values are for a two-tailed hypothesis. Had you obtained significant results and you wanted to find out which group had significantly shorter second-stage labour than the others, you would need to use the Scheffé (see next section). However, it must be stressed that you should only use the Scheffé if you obtained significant results from your anova.

Activity 16.2   (Answers on page 240)

1. To practise looking up F ratios, look up the following and state whether or not they are significant and at what level:
   (i) d.f. = 3   d.f. = 12 $F = 6.103$ p
   (ii) d.f. = 2   d.f. = 10 $F = 15.76$ p
   (iii) d.f. = 3   d.f. = 15 $F = 4.01$ p
   (iv) d.f. = 3   d.f. = 12 $F = 5.95$ p

2. Calculate a one-way unrelated anova on the following data:

H_1 Weight gain during months 3–5 as a percentage of total weight gained during pregnancy differs according to whether the pregnancy is the first, second or third.
  Brief method: Select seven women with a first pregnancy, seven with a second pregnancy and seven with a third pregnancy. Monitor weight gain for each woman throughout the pregnancy and calculate that gained during months 3–5 as a percentage of the total. Compare the three groups. Results are shown in Table 16.7.

Table 16.7

	1st pregnancy	2nd pregnancy	3rd pregnancy
1	25	15	10
2	35	30	20
3	30	20	20
4	20	15	25
5	20	25	15
6	25	30	10
7	15	15	20

State your F ratio and p value in a format similar to that suggested. Also, present your values in an anova table.

Scheffé multiple range test for use with one-way anovas for unrelated designs

The analysis of variance only tells us whether there are significant differences between the results from each condition. It does not tell us which group(s) did better or worse than the others. For example, let us take the example given in Activity 16.2 that weight gained during months 3–5 is different for para 0, para 1 and para 2 women. Further, let's imagine that the results were significant. These results only tell us that weight gain is greater in some groups than others, but it doesn't tell us whether one group gains significantly more or less weight than the others. In other words, we cannot tell from the results of the anova alone whether there are significant differences between:

Para 0 and Para 1
  and/or
Para 0 and Para 2
  and/or
Para 1 and Para 2

If we want to find this out, we must use a Scheffé multiple range test.

There are three important points which relate to the use of the Scheffé:

- the Scheffé can only be used if the results from the anova are significant.
- the formula for the Scheffé has already been presented in conjunction with the one-way anova for related samples. The formula for the Scheffé for use with the anova for unrelated samples is the same but is presented again here for ease and clarity.
- the Scheffé can only be carried out after an anova has been performed. It cannot be used independently.

Essentially what the Scheffé does is to compare the mean scores from each condition to see if the difference between them is significant.

When calculating the Scheffé you have to find two values; F is computed first for each comparison of means you wish to make. This is then compared with a second value: F^1. If any F is equal to or larger than F^1 then the difference between the two relevant means is significant.

Example

Let us take the example given in Activity 16.2 i.e. that there is a relationship between the percentage weight gained during months 3–5 and parity. Suppose you repeated the experiment with six subjects in each group this time and you obtained the following data shown in Table 16.8.

You can perform a one-way anova for unrelated designs on the data. The outcome looks like Table 16.9.

This means that there are significant differences in weight gained during months 3–5 as a percentage of the total accordance to parity.

Table 16.8

Subject	Condition 1 Para 0	Condition 2 Para 1	Condition 3 Para 2
1	35	20	10
2	30	25	15
3	33	30	15
4	30	20	20
5	25	25	20
6	25	15	10
Σ	178	135	90
$\bar{x}$	29.667	22.5	15.0

Table 16.9

Source of variace	SS	d.f.	MS	F ratio
Variation due to treatment, i. e. between the conditions	645.445	2	322.723	15.088
Variation due to random error	320.833	15	21.389	
Total	966.27			

$F = 15.088$ is significant at $p < 0.001$.

However, in order to find out whether one group gains significantly more weight than another we need to compare:

1. Para 0 and Para 1
2. Para 0 and Para 2
3. Para 1 and Para 2

using the Scheffé multiple range test.

Calculating the Scheffé multiple range test

1. Calculate the mean score for each group:

i.e. Condition 1 Para 0 = 29.667 $(\bar{x}_1)$
Condition 2 Para 1 = 22.5 $(\bar{x}_2)$
Condition 3 Para 2 = 15.0 $(\bar{x}_3)$

2. Find the value of F for the first comparison you wish to make, i.e. Para 0 vs. Para 1, using the following formula:

$$F = \frac{(\bar{x}_1 - \bar{x}_2)^2}{\dfrac{MS_{error}}{n_1} + \dfrac{MS_{error}}{n_2}}$$

where $\bar{x}_1$ = mean for Condition 1
= 29.667
$\bar{x}_2$ = Mean for Condition 2
= 22.5
MS_{error} = the MS_{error} value from the anova table
= 21.389
n_1 = the number of subjects in Condition 1
= 6
n_2 = the number of subjects in Condition 2
= 6

Substituting these values:

$$F = \frac{(29.667 - 22.5)^2}{\dfrac{21.389}{6} + \dfrac{21.389}{6}}$$

$$= \frac{(7.167)^2}{3.565 + 3.565}$$

$$= \frac{51.366}{7.13}$$

$$= 7.204$$

3. Repeat the calculations for the second comparison, i.e. Para 0 vs. Para 2. Substitute the appropriate means and n values:

$$F = \frac{(\bar{x}_1 - \bar{x}_3)^2}{\dfrac{MS_{error}}{n_1} + \dfrac{MS_{error}}{n_3}}$$

$$= \frac{(29.667 - 15)^2}{\dfrac{21.389}{6} + \dfrac{21.389}{6}}$$

$$= 30.171$$

4. Repeat the calculations for the third comparison, i.e. Para 1 vs. Para 2. Substitute the appropriate means and n values.

$$F = \frac{(\bar{x}_2 - \bar{x}_3)^2}{\dfrac{MS_{error}}{n_2} + \dfrac{MS_{error}}{n_3}}$$

$$= \frac{(22.5 - 15)^2}{\dfrac{21.389}{6} + \dfrac{21.389}{6}}$$

$$= 7.889$$

5. To calculate F^1, use d.f.$_{bet}$ and the d.f.$_{error}$ values derived from the anova table (i.e. 2 and 15 respectively). Turn to Table A2.6a: critical values of F at $p < 0.05$. Locate d.f.$_{bet}$ (2) across the top row and d.f.$_{error}$ (15) down the left-hand column. At their intersection point, you will see the figure 3.68.

Find the F^1 from the formula:

$$F^1 = (C - 1) F°$$

where $F°$ is the figure at the intersection point

$$= 3.68$$

C is the number of conditions

$$= 3$$

$$F^1 = (3 - 1) 3.68$$

$$= 7.36$$

6. Compare each F value derived from the comparison of pairs of means with the F^1 value above. If the F value is equal to or larger than F^1, then the result is significant at $p < 0.05$ (because we used the $p < 0.05$ table to calculate F^1).

If we take our F values:

1. 7.204
2. 30.171
3. 7.889

we can see that only comparison (1) is not significant (Para 0 and Para 1).

This means that the differences between Para 0 and Para 2, and Para 1 and Para 2 are significant and that there is less than a 5% probability that the results are due to random error.

It is important to point out that to derive F^1 we used the $p < 0.05$ table. The reason for this relates to the extreme stringency of the Scheffé; if we were to derive F^1 from the smaller p value tables, we would rarely get significant results using this test.

However, should you ever obtain results from the Scheffé which look as though they might be significant at a lower p value, just re-calculate F^1 using Tables A2.6a–d. Here, the F value of 30.71 (comparison 2 above) seems to be significant at a smaller probability level. If we recalculate F^1 using Table A2.6d ($p < 0.001$) we get

$$(3 - 1) 11.34$$
$$F^1 = 22.68$$

The F value of 30.171 is larger than this and so this comparison (Para 0 vs. Para 2) is significant at $p < 0.001$.

Interpreting the results

We have obtained the following results:

1. The comparison between the Para 0 and Para 1 was not significant. This means that any differences between these two groups could be explained by random error. Therefore there is no significant difference in weight gained during months 3–5 as a percentage of total weight gain between these groups.

2. The comparison between the Para 0 and

Para 2 is significant at $p < 0.001$. This means that there is less than a 0.1% chance that the differences between these groups are attributable to random error. Therefore, we can conclude that the Para 0 group gains significantly more weight during months 3–5 as a percentage of total weight gain than the Para 2 group (mean scores 29.667 and 15.0 respectively).

3. The comparison between the Para 1 and Para 2 is significant at $p < 0.05$ with Para 1 women gaining more weight. Therefore, there is less than a 5% probability that random error could account for the differences between these groups.

These results might be expressed in the following way:

> Having calculated a one-way anova for unrelated designs on the data and obtained significant results ($F = 15.088$, $p < 0.001$), comparisons of means were performed using the Scheffé multiple range test. The results indicated that (a) there

was no significant difference between the Para 0 and Para 1 groups ($F = 7.204$); (b) the comparison between the Para 0 and Para 2 group was significant at $p < 0.001$ ($F = 30.171$); (c) the comparison between the Para 1 and Para 2 groups was significant at $p < 0.05$ ($F = 7.889$).

Activity 16.3   (Answers on pages 240–241)

Carry out a Scheffé on the following results:
H_1 There is a difference in length of labour depending upon the strength of contractions during early first stage.

Brief method: Randomly select ten women in the early first stage of labour experiencing light contractions, ten in the early first stage experiencing moderate contractions and ten in the early first stage experiencing strong contractions. Comparisons of the length of labour for the groups using a one-way anova for unrelated designs yielded the following results:

$F = 6.01$; $p < 0.01$
$\text{d.f.}_{bet} = 2$
$\text{d.f.}_{error} = 27$
$MS_{error} = 2.11$
$\bar{x}_1$ (strong contractions) $= 6.3$
$\bar{x}_2$ (moderate contractions) $= 7.75$
$\bar{x}_3$ (light contractions) $= 10.15$

17

Non-parametric and parametric statistical tests for correlational designs

INTRODUCTION

All the tests described in this chapter are for use with correlational designs rather than experimental designs. Let us recap on the characteristics of correlational designs.

Firstly, while the experimental design is concerned with finding differences between sets of scores, the correlational design looks for the degree of association between them. Furthermore, with a correlational design neither of the two variables in the hypothesis is manipulated. Therefore, there is no IV or DV. As a result, a correlational design cannot ascertain which variable is having an effect on the other and thus, no cause and effect can be determined. All that can be concluded is whether or not there is any association in the scores for each of the two variables. Although this failure to ascribe cause and effect in correlational designs means that the researcher ends up with less precise information than would be obtained from experimental designs, it should also be pointed out that correlational designs are more acceptable if any ethical considerations are involved, because the researcher is not manipulating anything. Therefore, correlational designs are frequently used in medical research.

The way in which this association between sets of scores is assessed involves using the appropriate statistical test, which calculates a correlation coefficient between the sets of scores. This will result in a figure somewhere between −1 and +1. The closer the figure is to −1, the stronger the negative correlation between the scores. This means that large scores on one variable are associated with small scores on the other. The closer the figure is to +1, the stronger the positive correlation between the scores. In other words, high scores on one variable are associated with high scores on the other (and by definition, low scores on one variable are associated with low scores on the other.) The closer the correlation coefficient is to 0, the weaker the relationship is between the scores.

To carry out a correlational design, you would usually select just one group of subjects. These subjects would represent a whole range of scores on one of the variables in the hypothesis. The implication of this is that in order to cover a range of numbers, the data must be ordinal or interval/ratio. (It is possible to carry out a correlational study with non-dimensional nominal data, but the analysis possible is not very powerful and so such correlations are not often carried out.) You would then measure each subject on the other variable to find out if there was a relationship between them. For instance, if we take the example that the greater the number of cigarettes smoked during pregnancy, the lower the neonatal birth weight, we could select a group of women who vary in terms of the number of cigarettes they smoked, i.e. represented a whole range of scores on the smoking variables, as in Table 17.1.

We would then collect information on the birth weight of their babies. We would expect that the woman who smoked fewest cigarettes would have the biggest baby, while the one who

Table 17.1

Subject	No. of cigarettes
1	0
2	15
3	10
4	20
5	30
6	0
7	5
8	25
9	40
10	20

Table 17.2

Subject	Cigarettes	Neonatal birth weight
1	0	3.8 kg
2	15	3.3 kg
3	10	3.5 kg
4	20	3.1 kg
5	30	2.7 kg
6	0	4.0 kg
7	5	3.0 kg
8	25	2.5 kg
9	40	2.8 kg
10	20	3.2 kg

smoked most would have the smallest, with the other women ranging in between accordingly (see Table 17.2).

By computing the appropriate statistical test, we could find out whether there is a correlation between these scores. Such a design differs from an experimental design in that although the experimental design would also predict a relationship between smoking and neonatal birth weight, it would have to manipulate the smoking variable in order to assess its effects on birth weight. This would be done by selecting two groups of women, smokers and non-smokers, measuring the birth weights of their babies, and comparing the results to see if there are differences between the groups.

Obviously, whether you use an experimental or a correlational design depends on what you are predicting and the sort of research area you are involved in. If you are still unsure about the differences in assumptions and approach between experimental and correlational designs, re-read Chapter 6. When you have done this, plan out a correlational and an experimental design for the hypothesis in Activity 17.1.

Activity 17.1 (Answers on page 241)

H_1 There is a relationship between a woman's age and the length of time taken to conceive.

Statistical tests for correlational designs

The tests that are covered in this chapter are appropriate for two sorts of correlational design:

Table 17.3

Design	Non-parametric test	Parametric test
One group of subjects; *two* sets of scores compared for the degree of association between them	Spearman rank order correlation coefficient If you wish to predict scores on one variable from your knowledge of scores on the other use a linear regression equation	Pearson product moment correlation coefficient If you wish to predict scores on one variable from your knowledge of scores on the other, use a linear regression equation
One group of subjects; *three or more* sets of scores compared for the degree of association between them	Kendall's coefficient of concordance	–

Table 17.4

Non-parametric test	Parametric test
Spearman rank order correlation coefficient if the data is at least ordinal, or interval/ratio	Pearson product movement correlation coefficient if the data is interval/ratio

1. Those that compare *two* sets of scores to see if there is a correlation between them. In addition, a further test will be provided in this section, which allows you to predict scores on one variable, if you know the scores on the other.

2. Those that compare *three or more* sets of scores to see if there is a correlation between them.

Both non-parametric and parametric tests (Table 17.3) are included in this chapter. Each will be outlined separately.

Statistical tests which compare two sets of scores

Within this section, we shall look at two statistical tests, each of which can be used to assess the correlation between two sets of scores. In other words, you would typically take a group of subjects who represented a whole range of scores on one variable, and you would compare these with just one set of scores on the other variable, to see if they were associated in some way. Like the statistical tests for experimental designs, you can use either a non-parametric test to analyse your results, or, as long as you can fulfil the necessary

conditions, (see p. 81) a parametric test. The most important of these conditions is the sort of data you have. In order to use a parametric test, you must have interval/ratio data. The tests are shown in Table 17.4.

NON-PARAMETRIC STATISTICAL TEST FOR CORRELATIONAL DESIGNS WHICH COMPARE TWO SETS OF SCORES

Spearman rank order correlation coefficient test

Example

Let's suppose you were interested in the hypothesis:

H_1 There is a negative correlation between duration of pregnancy (in weeks) and the severity of nausea experienced.
(This is a one-tailed hypothesis, as it predicts a negative correlation, i.e. a direction to the results).

Brief method: You select nine women at various stages of pregnancy and ask them to rate on a 7-point scale the severity of nausea experienced (1 = no nausea, 7 = extreme nausea). You are anticipating that as pregnancy progresses, so nausea diminishes (Table 17.5).

Because one set of scores (the nausea) is only ordinal, we cannot fulfil the conditions necessary for a parametric test and so the Spearman must be used. It should be remembered that it does not matter at all that one variable is of an interval/ratio type (number of weeks gestation) and that the other is of an ordinal type, since all this correlational test does is to tell you whether the highest scores on one variable are associated with the

Table 17.5

Subject	Results from the experiment		Calculations from the statistical test			
	Variable A* Weeks' gestation	Variable B Nausea felt on a 7-point scale	Rank A	Rank B	d $(A - B)$	d^2 $(A - B)^2$
1	4	5	2	7.5	−5.5	30.25
2	10	3	5	4.5	+0.5	0.25
3	15	1	8	2	+6	36
4	7	3	3	4.5	−1.5	2.25
5	2	6	1	9	−8	64
6	21	1	9	2	+7	49
7	14	1	7	2	+5	25
8	12	4	6	6	0	0
9	8	5	4	7.5	−3.5	12.25
						$\Sigma d^2 = 219$

*It does not matter which is Variable A and which is B

highest or lowest scores on the other, irrespective of the nature of the scores. Therefore, as long as your data are not nominal, you can compare anything using the Spearman: weight with height, centimetres dilated with pain etc.

When calculating the Spearman you will find a correlation coefficient called r_s or rho, which you then look up in the probability tables associated with the Spearman test to see whether this value represents a significant correlation between the two variables.

Calculating the Spearman test

To calculate the Spearman test, take the following steps:

1. Rank order the scores on Variable A, giving the rank of 1 to the smallest score, the rank of 2 to the next smallest and so on. Enter these ranks in the Column 'Rank A'. Repeat the procedure for the scores in variable B and enter the ranks in the column 'Rank B'.

If some scores are the same, follow the procedure for tied ranks (see p. 128). In other words add up the ranks these scores would have had if they had been different and divide this total by the number of scores that are the same. For example, in variable B, the lowest score is 1, but subjects 3, 6 and 7 all had this score. Thus, had these scores been different they would have had the ranks 1, 2 and 3. Therefore, add these ranks

up, and divide by 3, (because there are three scores of 1), i.e.

$$\frac{1 + 2 + 3}{3} = 2$$

Assign the average rank of 2 to each score of 1.

2. For each subject take the Rank B score from the Rank A score to give d.

Enter these differences in the column entitled 'd $(A - B)$', i.e.

$$\text{subject 1, Rank } A - \text{Rank } B = 2 - 7.5$$
$$= -5.5$$

3. Square each d to give d^2, and enter this in the appropriate column, entitled 'd^2'

$$-5.5^2 = 30.25$$

4. Add up all the d^2 figures to give Σd^2. (Σ means 'sum or total of')

$$\Sigma d^2 = 219$$

5. Find r_s from the following formula:

$$r_s = 1 - \frac{6 \Sigma d^2}{N(N^2 - 1)}$$

Where Σd^2 = the total of all the d^2 values
= 219
N = the number of subjects or pairs of scores
= 9

If we substitute these values then

$$r_s = 1 - \frac{6 \times 219}{9(81 - 1)}$$

$$= 1 - \frac{1314}{720}$$

$$= 1 - 1.825$$

$$r_s = -0.825$$

(Do *not* forget to put in the + or – sign in front of the r_s figure, since this indicates a positive or negative correlation respectively.)

Looking up the value of r_s

Turn to Table A2.10. Down the left-hand column you will find values of *N*, while across the top you will see levels of significance for a one-tailed test and for a two-tailed test. Firstly, find your value of *N* down the left-hand column. To the right you will see four numbers, called *critical values* of r_s:

0.600   0.683   0.783   0.833

Each of these values is associated with the level of significance indicated at the top of the column, e.g. 0.600 is associated with

0.05 for a one-tailed test.
0.10 for a two-tailed test.

If your r_s value is equal to or larger than one of these four critical values, then your results are associated with the probability level indicated at the top of the appropriate column.

Our r_s value of –0.825 (ignore the minus sign for the time being) is larger than 0.783, but smaller than 0.833. This means that for our one-tailed hypothesis, the probability associated with our r_s value of 0.825 must be less than 0.01 (or 1%) but greater than 0.005 (or 2%). Convention dictates that we say that our *p* value is *less than* 0.01 (rather than saying it is greater than 0.005). In other words the probability of our results being due to random error is even less than 0.01 or 1%. This is expressed as:

$p < 0.01$ (or < 1%) (< means 'less than')

Had our r_s value been equal to the critical value of 0.783 the associated probability level would be exactly 0.01. This would be expressed as:

$$p = 0.01 \text{ (or 1\%)}$$

Interpreting the results

Our r_s value of –0.825 is associated with a probability level of less than 1%. This means that the chance of random error accounting for our results is less than 1 in 100. Now, given that the usual cut-off point for claiming results as significant is 5% or less, we can say that the results obtained in this experiment are significant. As we had a one-tailed hypothesis we must check that the results are in the predicted direction before claiming that our hypothesis has been supported. We have an r_s value of minus 0.825. This means that the two variables are negatively correlated; in other words, the greater the gestational stage, the less the nausea. This is exactly what was predicted and so we can safely reject the null hypothesis and accept the experimental hypothesis. This can be expressed in the following way:

Using a Spearman test on the data ($r_s = -0.825$, $N = 9$) the results were found to be significant ($p < 0.01$ for a one-tailed test). This means that there is a negative correlation between the variables, such that the greater the gestational stage, the less the degree of nausea experienced. The null hypothesis can therefore be rejected.

Activity 17.2   (Answers on page 241)

1. To practise looking up r_s values, look up the following and state whether or not they are significant and at what level.
   (i) $r_s = 0.784$ $N = 10$ one-tailed   *p*
   (ii) $r_s = 0.812$ $N = 6$ two-tailed   *p*
   (iii) $r_s = 0.601$ $N = 16$ two-tailed   *p*
   (iv) $r_s = 0.506$ $N = 12$ two-tailed   *p*
   (v) $r_s = 0.631$ $N = 18$ one-tailed   *p*

2. Calculate a Spearman on the following data:
   H₁   There is a relationship between the length of waiting time in an ante-natal clinic (in minutes) and the degree of satisfaction with care (on a 7-point scale, 7 = very high, 1 = very low).
   Method: You select a group of ten pregnant women who have been waiting varying lengths of times in an ante-natal clinic and ask them to rate their satisfaction with their care.
   The data are shown in Table 17.6.

Table 17.6

S	Condition A Waiting time	Condition B Satisfaction
1	45	4
2	65	3
3	50	5
4	30	5
5	75	2
6	40	6
7	55	5
8	80	2
9	35	6
10	70	3

State your r_s and p values in a format similar to the one outlined earlier.

PARAMETRIC STATISTICAL TEST FOR CORRELATIONAL DESIGNS WHICH COMPARE TWO SETS OF SCORES

Pearson product moment correlation coefficient

As was noted earlier, the Pearson is the parametric equivalent of the Spearman test, in that it is used for correlational designs which compare two sets of data for their degree of association. It may be used when the prerequisite conditions for a parametric test can be fulfilled, in particular interval/ratio data (see p. 81).

As long as the data is of an interval/ratio level, it does not matter whether one variable is measured in yards, feet etc. and the other kilos, percentages, minutes. The Pearson formula can accommodate different sorts of measurement as long as they are of an interval/ratio level.

Example

Let us suppose you were interested in finding out whether there is a correlation between maternal body weight and general physical condition. Your hypothesis is:

H_1 There is a negative correlation between maternal body weight at term and general physical condition (i.e. high body weights

at term are associated with poor general condition). This is a one-tailed hypothesis as it is predicting the *type* of correlation expected i.e. negative.

In order to test your hypothesis, you select ten pregnant women at term who represent a range of body weights. You measure their general physical condition, as indicated by a number of key criteria as a score out of 50. The results are shown in Table 17.7.

Calculating the Pearson test

The Pearson formula involves some rather large numbers, as you will see. These may look very off-putting initially, but you should be all right as long as you have a calculator.

1. Add up all the scores on variable A to give ΣA, i.e.

$$\Sigma A = 1471$$

2. Add up all the scores on variable B to give ΣB, i.e.

$$\Sigma B = 365$$

3. Multiply each subject's variable A score by their variable B score, i.e.

$$\text{Subject 1} = 140 \times 40$$
$$= 5600$$
$$\text{Subject 2} = 128 \times 45$$
$$= 5760$$

Enter each result in Column '$A \times B$'

4. Add up all the scores in Column $A \times B$ to give $\Sigma(A \times B)$, i.e.

$$\Sigma(A \times B) = 52\,910$$

5. Square each subject's variable A score and enter the result in column 'A^2', e.g.

$$\text{Subject 1} = 140^2$$
$$= 19\,600$$

6. Square each subject's variable B score and enter the result in column 'B^2', e.g.

$$\text{Subject 1} = 40^2$$
$$= 1600$$

Table 17.7

Subject	Results from the experiment		Calculations from the statistical test		
	Variable A Maternal weight in lb at term	Variable B General physical condition	$A \times B$	A^2	B^2
1	140	40	5600	19 600	1600
2	128	45	5760	16 384	2025
3	170	25	4250	28 900	625
4	132	40	5280	17 424	1600
5	154	30	4620	23 716	900
6	135	35	4725	18 225	1225
7	143	45	6435	20 449	2025
8	149	50	7450	22 201	2500
9	158	30	4740	24 964	900
10	162	25	4050	26 244	625
Σ	$\Sigma A = 1471$	$\Sigma B = 365$	$\Sigma(A \times B) =$ 52 910	$\Sigma A^2 =$ 218 107	$\Sigma B^2 =$ 14 025

7. Add up all the scores in column A^2 to give ΣA^2, i.e.

$$\Sigma A^2 = 218\ 107$$

8. Add up all the scores in column B^2 to give ΣB^2, i.e.

$$\Sigma B^2 = 14\ 025$$

9. Find the value of r from the following formula:

$$r = \frac{N\Sigma(A \times B) - \Sigma A \times \Sigma B}{\sqrt{[N\Sigma A^2 - (\Sigma A)^2][N\Sigma B^2 - (\Sigma B)^2]}}$$

Where N = number of subjects, i.e. 10
$\Sigma(A \times B)$ = the total of the scores in the column $A \times B$
= 52 910
ΣA = the total of the scores in the variable A column = 1471
ΣB = the total of the scores in the variable B column 365
ΣA^2 = the total of the scores in the A^2 column
= 218 107
ΣB^2 = the total of the scores in the B^2 column
= 14 025
$(\Sigma A)^2$ = the total of the scores in the variable A column, squared

= 1471^2
= 2 163 841
$(\Sigma B)^2$ = the total of the scores in the variable B column, squared
= 365^2
= 133 225

Therefore, if we substitute these values in the formula:

$$r = \frac{(10 \times 52\ 910) - (1471 \times 365)}{\sqrt{[(10 \times 218\ 107) - 2\ 163\ 841][(10 \times 14\ 025) - 133\ 225]}}$$

$$= \frac{529\ 100 - 536\ 915}{\sqrt{[2\ 181\ 070 - 2\ 163\ 841][140\ 250 - 133\ 225]}}$$

$$= \frac{-7815}{\sqrt{11\ 001.533}}$$

$$r = -0.710$$

Looking up the value of r

To find out whether r is significant, you also need a d.f. value, which here is the number of subjects minus 2, i.e. $N - 2$

$$= 10 - 2$$
$$= 8$$

Turn to Table A2.11. Down the left-hand

column you will see a number of d.f. values. Find our d.f. = 8. You will see five numbers, called critical values of r to the right of d.f. = 8:

   0.5494   0.6319   0.7155   0.7646   0.8721

Each of these is associated with the level of significance indicated at the top of its column, e.g. 0.5494 is associated with a level of significance for a one-tailed test of 0.05 and for a two-tailed test of 0.10.

To be significant at one of these levels, our r value has to be equal to or larger than the corresponding critical value. Ignoring the minus sign in front of our r value for the time being, we can see that our r of 0.71 is larger than 0.6319 but smaller than 0.7155. Since we have a one-tailed test, our r value has an associated probability which is less than 0.025 (or 2½%) but greater than 0.01 (1%). According to convention we must say that our r has a p value of *less than* 0.025, (rather than saying it is greater than 0.01). This is expressed as:

$$p < 0.025$$

This means that there is less than a 2.5% chance that our results are due to random error. Had our r value been the same as the critical value of 0.6319 the associated probability value would have been exactly 0.025. This is expressed as:

$$p = 0.025$$

Interpreting the results

Our r value has an associated probability value of < 0.025, which means that the chance of random error being responsible for the results is less than 2.5 in 100.

Because the standard cut-off point for claiming results to be significant is 5% we can conclude that the results here are significant. But before we can definitely state that they support the experimental hypothesis, we must check that the direction of the results was the one predicted. In other words did we obtain the negative correlation between the two variables that we anticipated? Our r value was *minus* 0.71 which means that the results do, in fact, confirm the hypothesis and

that there is a negative correlation between maternal body weight at term and general physical condition. We can therefore reject the null hypothesis and accept the experimental hypothesis. This can be expressed in the following way:

Using a Pearson product moment correlation test on the data ($r = -0.71$, d.f. = 8), the results were significant ($p < 0.025$ for a one-tailed test). This means that there is a negative correlation in women at term between maternal weight and general physical condition (the higher the weight, the worse the general physical condition). The null hypothesis can therefore be rejected.

Activity 17.3   (Answers on page 241)

1. To practise looking up r values, look up the following and state whether or not they are significant and at what level.

(i)	$r = 0.632$	d.f. = 6	one-tailed	p
(ii)	$r = 0.567$	d.f. = 10	two-tailed	p
(iii)	$r = 0.779$	d.f. = 8	one-tailed	p
(iv)	$r = 0.612$	d.f. = 12	two-tailed	p
(v)	$r = 0.784$	d.f. = 13	two-tailed	p

2. Calculate a Pearson on the following data:
   H_1 There is a positive correlation between direct entry midwifery students' marks on their 1st year examination and their averaged continuous assessment mark throughout the year.
   Method: Randomly select eight first year direct entry midwifery students to represent a range of examination marks. Average their continuous assessment marks for the year's assignments.
   The results are shown in Table 17.8.

Table 17.8

Subject	Variable A Examination	Variable B Continuous assessment
1	70	66
2	60	64
3	49	54
4	54	50
5	66	70
6	72	68
7	40	49
8	62	65

State your r and p values in the suggested format.

NON-PARAMETRIC STATISTICAL TEST WHICH COMPARES THREE OR MORE SETS OF SCORES

Both the Spearman and the Pearson test are used for correlational designs which look for the degree of association between two sets of scores only, for instance, comparing the theory and practice exam marks for a group of students to see if they correlate.

However, there will be many occasions when you may want to see if three or more sets of scores are associated in some way.

For example, you may be involved in chairing an interview panel of four people which is concerned with appointing a new midwifery sister for the Special Care Baby Unit. There are six candidates for the post. You decide to ask each member of the panel to rank order these candidates in terms of their suitability for the job. Obviously, if there were consensus in terms of choice the decision would be easy, but you know that is unlikely to be the case. So, you will have to analyse the rankings in order to see whether there is overall agreement. In other words, you have one group of six candidates, each of whom is ranked by four people. You need to assess the four sets of rankings given to each candidate to see how far the opinions of the panel agree.

Therefore, in this case, rather than having two sets of scores to analyse for correlations, you have four sets. Such a design requires a test called the *Kendall coefficient of concordance*.

Kendall coefficient of concordance

This is a non-parametric test which can only be used when the data is ordinal, i.e. when you have three or more sets of rank orderings. This does not, of course, mean that you cannot use this test when you have interval/ratio data; all you would do here is to rank order your data and use the rank orderings in the test.

A further point to remember is that this particular formula of the Kendall coefficient of concordance can only be used if the number of people or objects being ranked is seven or less. So, for instance, you might ask four midwives to rank order six neonates in terms of how alert they are following delivery by mothers who have had Pethidine during labour. Thus there are four judges (or sets of rankings) and six objects or people being ranked. If you want to design an

experiment where more than seven objects or people are being ranked, you will need another formula and you are referred to Siegel (1956). However, you should find the formula provided here sufficient for most purposes. One other point to note about this test: both the Spearman and Pearson tests produce a correlation coefficient which may be somewhere between −1 (negative correlation) through 0 (no correlation) to +1 (positive correlation) whereas the Kendall coefficient of concordance only gives us a value from 0 to +1, i.e. an indication of whether there is no correlation at all between the sets of scores (0) or a positive correlation (+1). It does not give a negative correlation. If we think about this a bit more, the reason for this becomes clear. Where three or more sets of rankings are being compared, they cannot all disagree completely. So in the previous example, Interviewer A may produce a set of rankings which are absolutely the reverse of Interviewer B's. If we only had two interviewers, we could analyse this with a Spearman and we would end up with a negative correlation between the scores. But here, if Interviewers A and B disagree so completely, with each other, what about Interviewers C and D? If C also disagrees with A, it means by definition she must agree with B and hence there is some measure of agreement among the rankings. If D disagrees with C, it means these rankings must agree with those of A, because C disagrees with A. Therefore, all we may conclude from the Kendall coefficient of concordance is whether there is a positive correlation between the scores or whether there is no relationship. Because the Kendall coefficient of concordance only tells us whether or not there is a positive correlation between our results, our hypothesis must be one-tailed.

When calculating the Kendall coefficient of concordance, the value of s is found. This is then looked up in the probability table associated with the Kendall coefficient of concordance, to see whether the value of s represents a significant agreement among the rankings. Remember that because the Kendall only deals with positive correlations, any hypothesis associated with it must be one-tailed.

Example

Let us imagine you are wanting to study the effects on the neonate of different forms of analgesia administered during labour. You select six neonates within the first 5 minutes of delivery, each of whom has been born to a woman using a different form of analgesia (Epidural, Entonox, Trilene, Pethidine, Amytal and TENS). You ask three midwives to rank order these babies in terms of alertness. By doing this, you can assess whether there is any agreement among the midwives as to the impact on the neonates of different forms of analgesia. Therefore, you have three judges and six people being ranked.

Your H_1, therefore, is

H_1 There is significant agreement between the three midwives' judgements of the alertness of neonates born to women using different types of analgesia.

You ask the midwives to rank all the neonates, giving a rank of 1 to the baby most alert and of 6 to the least alert baby. The results you obtain are shown in Table 17.9.

Calculating the Kendall coefficient of concordance

1. For each baby add up the total of the ranks assigned, i.e.

$$
\begin{aligned}
1 &= 18 \\
2 &= 11 \\
3 &= 8 \\
4 &= 6 \\
5 &= 6 \\
6 &= 14
\end{aligned}
$$

Table 17.9

| | | Neonate | | | | |
	1	2	3	4	5	6
Midwife						
1	6	4	2	1	3	5
2	6	2	3	4	1	5
3	6	5	3	1	2	4
Total of ranks for each baby	18	11	8	6	6	14

(When calculating the Kendall coefficient of concordance, always set the results out such that the rank orderings from each judge go across the page.)

Obviously, if all three midwives had been in perfect agreement, the baby most alert would have been assigned three ranks of 1 (total 3), the baby next most alert, three ranks of 2 (total 6), etc. right up to the baby least alert who would have had three ranks of 6 (18). On the other hand, had there been no agreement whatever, every baby would theoretically have ended up with an identical rank total. Therefore, we would have six tied ranks:

$$\text{Ranks} \quad \frac{1 + 2 + 3 + 4 + 5 + 6}{6} = 3.5$$

Thus each baby would have got three ratings of 3.5 = 10.5. What the formula aims to do is to assess how far the actual rankings accord with the rankings for total agreement between judges.

2. Add up all the rank totals to give ΣR, i.e.

$$
\begin{aligned}
\Sigma R &= 18 + 11 + 8 + 6 + 6 + 14 \\
\Sigma R &= 63
\end{aligned}
$$

3. Divide ΣR by the number of babies being ranked to obtain the average rank, ($\bar{x}_R$)

$$
\begin{aligned}
&\text{i.e. } 63 \div 6 \\
&\bar{x}_R = 10.5
\end{aligned}
$$

4. Take each rank total away from the average rank and square the result, i.e.

$$
\begin{aligned}
1. \ (10.5 - 18)^2 &= 56.25 \\
2. \ (10.5 - 11)^2 &= 0.25 \\
3. \ (10.5 - \ 8)^2 &= 6.25 \\
4. \ (10.5 - \ 6)^2 &= 20.25 \\
5. \ (10.5 - \ 6)^2 &= 20.25 \\
6. \ (10.5 - 14)^2 &= 12.25
\end{aligned}
$$

5. Add up all these squared differences to give s, i.e. 115.5

6. Find W from the formula:

$$W = \frac{s}{\frac{1}{12}n^2(N^3 - N)}$$

Where s = the total of all the squared differences between each individual rank total and the average rank, i.e.

$$= \ 115.5$$

n = the number of judges or *sets* of rankings, i.e.

$$= 3$$

N = the number of people or objects *being* ranked, i.e.

$$= 6$$

Substituting these values

$$W = \frac{115.5}{\frac{1}{12}3^2(6^3 - 6)}$$

$$= \frac{115.5}{\frac{1}{12}9 \times 210}$$

$$= \frac{115.5}{157.5}$$

$$W = 0.733$$

Looking up the value of s for significance

To find out whether these results are significant you need the s value (the total of squared differences between each individual rank total and the average rank), the n value (the number of judges or sets of rankings) and N (the number of objects or people ranked).

$$s = 115.5$$
$$n = 3$$
$$N = 6$$

Turn to Table A2.12. This gives critical values of s associated with particular values of p. You will see that two tables are presented, one for p values of 0.05, and one for p values of 0.01. (Note again that because this test only tells you whether or not there is a positive correlation between the scores, these values are associated with one-tailed hypotheses only.) Down the left-hand column you will see values of n, while across the top there are values of N. Taking the $p = 0.05$ table first, locate your n and N values and identify the number at the intersection point, i.e. 103.9. To be significant at the 0.05 level, our s value must be equal to or larger than 103.9. Our s value is larger

(115.5) which means that our results are associated with a probability value of 0.05. But are they significant at the 0.01 level? Repeat the process. You will find the figure at the intersection point is 122.8. Our s value is smaller than this, so the results are not significant at the 0.01 level. So, we must go back to the first table. Now, because our s value is larger than the value at the intersection point, it means that the associated probability comes between the 0.05 probability of the first table and the 0.01 probability of the second. In other words, for our s of 115.5, the associated probability is less than 5% (or 0.05) but greater than 1% (or 0.01). To comply with convention we have to say that our probability is less than 0.05 or 5%. This is expressed as $p < 0.05$.

This means that the probability of random error being responsible for the results is less than 5%. Had our s value been exactly the same as the number at the intersection point, our results would have been associated with a probability value which equalled 0.05. This is stated as $p = 0.05$.

Interpreting the results

Our results have an associated probability value of < 0.05, which means that there is less than a 5% chance that random error could account for the outcome of the experiment. If we use the usual cut-off point of 5% to claim significance, we can state that the results here are, in fact, significant, and that we can reject the null hypothesis and accept the experimental hypothesis. This can be stated thus:

> Using a Kendall's coefficient of concordance on the data ($s = 115.5$, $W = 0.733$, $n = 3$, $N = 6$) the results were found to be significant ($p < 0.05$ for a one-tailed test). This means that there is significant agreement among the midwives as to which neonates were most alert following delivery using different types of analgesia. The null hypothesis can therefore be rejected.

Should you ever have a situation where there are a number of tied ranks, i.e. where, for instance, a judge has ranked three objects or people equally, this will have the effect of reducing the significance of your results. Try, then, to ensure that your data does not contain too many tied ranks.

One final point. Many students ask why W is calculated, since it is not used to look up the significance of the results. The answer is that W is the correlation coefficient, and the researcher often finds it useful to know this value in order to assess, in absolute terms, the extent of the correlation between results. In other words, the correlation coefficient is often as meaningful as the actual probability to the experimenter.

Activity 17.4   (Answers on page 241)

1. To practise looking up s values, look up the following s values and state whether or not they are significant and at what level.

    (i) $s = 96.1$ $n = 4$ $N = 5$ p
    (ii) $s = 117.5$ $n = 5$ $N = 6$ p
    (iii) $s = 124.5$ $n = 3$ $N = 6$ p
    (iv) $s = 103.7$ $n = 6$ $N = 4$ p
    (v) $s = 619.2$ $n = 10$ $N = 7$ p

2. Calculate a Kendall coefficient of concordance on the following data. You are concerned about the variability in marking of student midwives' exam papers. You decide to put this to the test.

    H_1 There is a significant agreement between midwife tutors' marking of students' examination scripts.

    Brief method: Five midwife tutors each blind mark the exam scripts of four students. The marks given to each student are recorded.

The results are shown in Table 17.10. *(Remember the data must be rank ordered!)*

Table 17.10

Midwife tutor	Student 1	Student 2	Student 3	Student 4
1	45	30	50	65
2	45	40	55	70
3	25	30	65	55
4	50	55	30	60
5	60	50	65	80

State your s, W and p values in the format outlined earlier.

LINEAR REGRESSION (PREDICTING THE SCORES ON ONE VARIABLE FROM KNOWLEDGE OF SCORES ON THE OTHER)

We have already seen that correlational designs are used when we want to find out whether two variables are associated with each other, that is, whether high scores on one variable are related to high scores on the other, or alternatively, whether high scores on one variable are related to low scores on the other. This is a particularly valuable sort of approach in medical research because ethical issues are rarely involved. Correlational designs can tell us whether, for example, maternal blood pressure and fetal heart rate are related, or whether the number of units of alcohol consumed and fetal size are associated, although they cannot say which of the two variables causes an effect on the other; all they tell us is whether or not two variables co-vary together in a related way.

Now, there will be occasions when you might be quite happy to leave your research at this point, having found out whether or not the variables are correlated. For example, in the earlier illustration, you may be content with the knowledge that maternal blood pressure and fetal heart rate are negatively correlated, i.e. that the higher the maternal blood pressure, the lower the fetal heart rate.

However, let us suppose that having completed this research, you are faced with a woman whose blood pressure reading is 170/90. Now, from the results of your correlational design, you will know that the fetal reaction is likely to be adverse. Clearly this is useful information since appropriate interventions can be made to safeguard the baby should heart rate fall to a critical level. It would be extremely useful to you to be able to predict this fetus's reaction more precisely from your knowledge of maternal blood pressure. In other words, what you want to be able to do is to predict with some degree of accuracy the scores on one variable from your knowledge of the scores on the other. What you need, therefore, is a formula whereby you can calculate the unknown score. This formula is known as a regression formula or equation and is of enormous use in medical research. For example, as long as you know that the two variables are correlated, it can tell you:

- The birth weight of a baby born to a woman who smokes 55 cigarettes a day.

- The heart rate of a woman who gains excess weight during pregnancy.
- The theory exam performance of a student who achieved 32% in the clinical exam.

So, providing you know that two variables are related, you can make predictions about one variable from your knowledge of scores on the other, using a regression formula. The Linear Regression technique can be used in conjunction with either the Pearson or the Spearman test, but the data should be of a type which assumes equal intervals. In other words it should be interval ratio or a point-scale which implies comparable distances between the points (see p. 27).

The convention when using regression formulae is to call the variable whose score you are trying to predict, Y, and the variable whose scores you already know, X. Therefore, in the above example, we are trying to predict the fetal heart rate (Y) from our knowledge of his maternal blood pressure (X).

Now, it is important to reiterate that you can only use a regression equation if the two variables you are interested in have been shown to be correlated. If you look back to pages 56–60 you will see that there are two types of correlation, a positive correlation whereby high scores on one variable are associated with high scores on the other; and a negative correlation whereby high scores on one variable are associated with low scores on the other. If scattergrams are plotted for both of these, we find that a positive correlation is represented by an uphill slope, while a negative correlation is represented by a downhill one. Furthermore, it was pointed out that a perfect one-to-one correlation would produce an absolutely smooth, straight line although there are very few things in this world which produce a perfect correlation. However, supposing we found that the amount of time spent waiting in an ante-natal clinic produced a one-to-one correlation with the woman's reported dissatisfaction with her care (on a 9-point scale) such that the longer the time spent, the greater the dissatisfaction. If we plotted the data from this, we might end up with the scattergram shown in Figure 17.1.

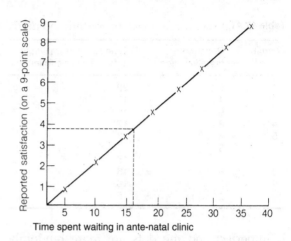

Figure 17.1 Scattergram showing relationship between patient satisfaction and time spent in the ante-natal clinic supposing the correlation were perfect.

For the sake of the example, we shall treat this 9-point scale as though it was interval data and assume that the distances between each point are equal (see p. 27).

We can draw a perfectly straight line through all the dots and it is this line which is used in your future predictions. For example, you would know from this scattergram that if a woman waited for 17 minutes, the degree of reported dissatisfaction would be 3.8, because all you would have to do would be to locate the appropriate time along the bottom axis, and trace it vertically up to the sloping line and then move horizontally across to the satisfaction scores (see dotted line above).

You could also predict that if a woman waited for 3 minutes, her dissatisfaction would be 0.6; again you simply take the 3 minute time along the bottom axis, trace this up to the slope and then move left from the slope to the dissatisfaction scores. In other words, from your existing knowledge that these two variables are related, you can predict on the basis of waiting time how dissatisfied women will be.

You can see that this sloping line is obviously extremely important if you need to make this sort of prediction and therefore it has to be drawn in. However, while it is easy to draw it in when the correlation is perfect because all the dots are lined up, it is not as easy when the correlation

Table 17.11

Woman	Reported dissatisfaction	Time spent in waiting in ante-natal clinic (minutes)
1	7	29
2	4	10
3	6	18
4	8	17
5	2	8
6	3	5
7	5	15
8	6	16
9	5	16
10	1	5

is imperfect and the dots are more randomly scattered.

However, as has already been pointed out, very little in life conforms to a perfect correlation. It would be far more likely in the previous example that the data were as shown in Table 17.11.

Statistical analysis using the Pearson test (see previous section) shows that the data are correlated ($r = 0.836$ $p < 0.005$).

If these data were plotted on a scattergram, we would find the pattern shown in Figure 17.2.

There is still a general upward slope but it is far from smooth. In this case, if you had to draw a straight line through the dots so that you could perform the same sort of prediction as before, where would you draw it? You obviously cannot connect all the dots as you would with the perfect

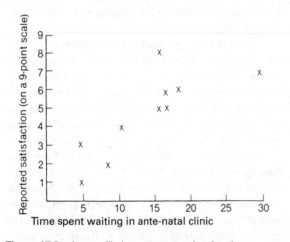

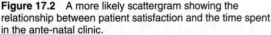

Figure 17.2   A more likely scattergram showing the relationship between patient satisfaction and the time spent in the ante-natal clinic.

correlation and still obtain a straight line, so you need to make a decision about where to put the line so that it achieves the *'best fit'*. The line of best fit is the straight sloping line which when drawn in, means that every dot is as close as possible to the line, and consequently produces fewest errors when predicting the value of variable Y from knowledge of variable X.

Now, if you look at the last scattergram, you can see that it is almost impossible to draw in the line of best fit by eye, and if you cannot draw in this line, then how can you make predictions? For instance, if a woman waited for 12 minutes, what would her level of dissatisfaction be? If you only have the scattergram and no line of best fit, you can't answer this question.

What you need, then, is a regression formula such that this line of best fit can be calculated and the prediction made. This equation is

$$Y = bX + a$$

where Y is the variable to be predicted
X is the known score
a and b are constants which have to be calculated.

(Note that the regression we are dealing with is called linear regression, because it is concerned with simple linear relationships; see the scattergram.)

Calculating the linear regression equation

In order to calculate these constants, take the following steps:

1. Calculate the Spearman or Pearson test (whichever is appropriate) on your data to establish whether or not there is a significant correlation. If there is not a significant correlation, do not proceed any further, since you cannot make any predictions from variables which do not correlate.

2. Having established that the data are correlated, make a note of whether the correlation is positive or negative. If you wish, you can plot a scattergram of the data, but it is not essential.

3. Set out your data in the format shown in Table 17.12, remembering that Y is the variable

to be predicted and X is the variable from which the prediction will be made. Here, we will take the sample data already provided for the last scattergram. So, the $X \times Y$ column is: variable score X multiplied by variable score Y, i.e.

$$\text{for subject 1: } 7 \times 29$$
$$= 203$$

The X^2 column is simply the squared variable X score. Therefore, for subject 1, $29 \times 29 = 841$.

4. Add each column up to give the totals (Σ)

$$\Sigma Y = 47; \quad \Sigma X = 139;$$
$$\Sigma(X \times Y) = 774; \quad \Sigma X^2 = 2405$$

5. To calculate the constants a and b, first find b from the formula:

$$b = \frac{N\Sigma(X \times Y) - (\Sigma X)(\Sigma Y)}{N\Sigma X^2 - (\Sigma X)^2}$$

Where N = the total number of Ss
   = 10
$\Sigma(X \times Y)$ = the total of the $X \times Y$ column
   = 774
ΣX = the total of the variable X column
   = 139
ΣY = the total of the variable Y column
   = 47
ΣX^2 = the total of the X^2 column
   = 2405
$(\Sigma X)^2$ = the total of the variable X column squared
   = 139^2
   = 19 321

Table 17.12

Subject	Variable Y Dis-satisfaction	Variable X Waiting time	X × Y	X²
1	7	29	203	841
2	4	10	40	100
3	6	18	108	324
4	8	17	136	289
5	2	8	16	64
6	3	5	15	25
7	5	15	75	225
8	6	16	96	256
9	5	16	50	256
10	1	5	5	25
Totals	$\Sigma Y = 47$	$\Sigma X = 139$	$\Sigma X \times Y = 774$	$\Sigma X^2 = 2405$

If we substitute our values:

$$b = \frac{(10 \times 774) - (139 \times 47)}{(10 \times 2405) - 19321}$$

$$= \frac{7740 - 6533}{24\,050 - 19\,321}$$

$$= \frac{1207}{4729}$$

$$= 0.255$$

6. Find a from the formula:

$$a = \frac{\Sigma Y}{N} - b\frac{\Sigma X}{N}$$

where N = the total number of Ss
   = 10
ΣY = the total of the variable Y column
   = 47
ΣX = the total of the variable X column
   = 139
b = the result of the earlier calculation
   = 0.255

$$\therefore a = \frac{47}{10} - 0.255 \times \frac{139}{10}$$

$$= 4.7 - (0.255 \times 13.9)$$

$$= 4.7 - 3.545$$

$$= 1.155$$

7. We can now substitute the values of a and b in the regression formula

$$Y = bX + a$$

to find any value of Y we require from the known value of X.

Interpreting the results

Suppose, then, a woman waited for 22 minutes (variable X) we can predict her level of dissatisfaction (variable Y) using the calculated values for the regression equation.

$$Y = (0.255 \times 22) + 1.155$$
$$Y = 5.61 + 1.155$$
$$= 6.765$$

Therefore, this woman's predicted level of dissatisfaction would be 6.765. So it is possible to calculate from any waiting time the associated degree of dissatisfaction.

Activity 17.5   (Answers on page 241)

Imagine that the data in Table 17.13 were obtained from a correlational study which looked at the relationship between the amount of weight gained during pregnancy and length of labour.

Table 17.13

Subject	Weight gain (in lb)	Length of labour (in hours)
1	17	8.3
2	35	16.2
3	28	12.8
4	21	9.9
5	20	10.0
6	30	15.8
7	24	14.0
8	32	17.5
9	20	11.6
10	26	12.2

(The two variables correlate significantly, $p < 0.005$).

Three women come in for the last ante-natal visit. Their weight gains are: (a) 23 lb (b) 16 lb (c) 29 lb.

What is the estimated length of labour for each woman?

18

Estimation

INTRODUCTION

Estimation is a particularly useful statistical technique for any midwife who is involved in resource management or planning. It can be thought of as a sort of statistical 'best guessing' system which, like other methods of inferential statistics, allows us to make predictions about certain characteristics of a population based on our knowledge of a small sample of that population.

However, unlike the statistical tests which we have looked at so far in this book, estimation does not involve testing a hypothesis. Instead, we collect data on the characteristics we are interested in from a sample of people, equipment or whatever, and then, using a statistical formula, we can make predictions or *estimates* about how far the population also possesses these characteristics. (If you are unclear about the terms it might be worth refreshing your memory by re-reading page 20.) The characteristics we are interested in estimating are called *parameters*.

These concepts may be best illustrated by using an example. Let us imagine you are the Principal of a College of Midwifery and each year you have places for 40 new students to start their training. However, over the last 3 years you have had at least five to eight students drop out before the start of the course, which leaves you under the establishment figure. Clearly, if you could make an accurate estimate of potential drop-out for the forthcoming year, you could offer that number of extra places over and above the 40 students you normally take in. This means that when the new course starts, you will have the correct number of students and no resources will be wasted. However, the success of this strategy depends heavily on the accuracy of your estimates. From this example, it can be seen that formal, statistical techniques of estimation are particularly important to any planning activities, whether it be for training places, financial predictions, service delivery or whatever.

However, in order to make good and accurate estimates, the following conditions must be fulfilled:

1. You must define your area of interest clearly, avoiding vague concepts such as 'service delivery', 'patients' etc. If you mean by service delivery the treatment of the umbilicus, then you must say so. In the same way, you must also be precise about the parameters you wish to estimate. For example, if you are managing a budget for the coming year and need to consider how much must be allocated for staff development and top-up training courses, you must specify what type of course you are budgeting for. Are they local one-day events? Are they residential? Over one-week/one-month/one term duration? The characteristics must be properly defined if estimates made about them are to have any value and precision. Therefore, the first rule of estimation is:

Define your terms and focus of interest precisely.

2. The next stage involves the selection of a *random sample,* so that the estimates are based on a reasonably representative sub-group of the population in which you are interested. Random sampling was covered in Chapter 2 but essentially involved ensuring that every member of the relevant population has an equal chance of being selected. This can be achieved using random number tables, pulling names out of hats etc. (see pages 20–22).

The sample should also be of an adequate number in relation to the population size. The concept of adequacy is difficult to define because it depends on the population being studied and the topic under investigation (see page 22).

However a good rule-of-thumb is to select as many subjects as time and your budget will afford. Thus the second rule of estimation is:

Select your subjects randomly and try to ensure that the sample is of an adequate size.

3. The third stage in the estimation process is the data collection phase. Like all other forms of research, it is essential that the data collected is a valid measure of the characteristic you are interested in. Let us imagine you are interested in estimating stress levels among Staff midwives. If you simply monitored blood pressure it would not be an adequate measure since there may be (a) many reasons for elevated blood pressure readings and (b) other additional symptoms such as subjective reports of stress, all of which may be a valuable contribution to your stress indices.

Therefore, the third rule of estimation is:

Ensure the data collected is a suitable and valid measure of the characteristics being studied.

4. The last stage in the estimation process is the application of the appropriate estimation formula. There are different formulae available, and their use is determined by what it is the researcher wishes to find out. These formulae and their functions are described below. The last rule of estimation is therefore:

Apply the appropriate statistical formula for what it is you wish to estimate.

TECHNIQUES OF ESTIMATION

The two main types of estimation procedures are point estimations and interval estimations.

Point estimations

These are simply a single figure (usually a percentage or an average) which is derived from your sample and which is used as an estimate for the relevant population. For example, you might be interested in the take-up of fertility treatment in an out-patient family planning department over the coming year. In order to do this, you select a sample of infertile couples from those who have attended for treatment over the previous year, and calculate the average number of treatments required before discharge. Let us imagine that the average comes out at seven 30-minute treatments per couple (210 minutes in total). On this basis you could estimate the amount of treatment time required for new patients as being 210 minutes. This figure is therefore a *point-estimate* of the average treatment time for patients attending your out-patient fertility clinic.

What you have done here is to select a sample of infertile couples (i.e. a selection from those who attended during the previous year) and you have calculated the average figure for the parameter in which you are interested (i.e. treatment time). From this you have made an estimate for that parameter for the population of couples who are likely to require treatment during the coming year.

However, this may not provide you with all the essential information you might need for accurate planning of resources. What you might also need to know is the proportion or percentage of the total out-patient numbers at the family planning clinic that these couples constitute. By knowing this, you could fine-tune your provision a bit more. Consequently, then, you need to obtain a percentage point-estimate of infertile couples relative to the whole population of out-patients in your clinic. You might find that these patients constituted 12% of the total out-patients for the previous 12 months and therefore you could estimate a similar percentage for the forthcoming year. This percentage point-estimate of 12% coupled with the average point-estimate for treatment (210 minutes per patient) would give you useful information when planning resources and finances in your unit.

I feel sure you are not too impressed by estimation thus far, since it is something that many of us do all the time at a routine and informal level, whether it be estimating our time on domestic tasks so that we know how much can be fitted into a 2-hour slot, or calculating next month's financial outgoings in order to work out whether we can afford new curtains or whatever. However, the accuracy, and thus the *value*, of estima-

tion depends very largely on the quality of the random sample selected for study; in other words, how representative was the particular sample bank-balance you used when predicting next month's expenditure? A truly representative sample is almost impossible to achieve, but even if we managed it, it is still quite possible for any estimates based on the sample to be wrong, if only minutely. Where patient well-being or limited budgets are at stake, even minor inaccuracies in estimates could prove to be disastrous and consequently, it might be useful, in these circumstances, to know what degree of confidence you can place on your estimate.

Interval estimation

The last point leads us into another variant of estimation — *interval estimation* — which involves the calculation of two figures (rather than a single one), between which we can be confident our estimate falls. So, in the example above concerning our infertile couples at the family planning clinic, instead of saying that the estimate for average treatment time is 210 minutes, we would calculate a lower and upper limit of treatment time, for example 150 minutes to 240 minutes, and we could then estimate with a reasonable degree of confidence that the treatments for other infertile couples would fall within this interval.

This procedure clearly allows a bit more leeway in our predictions but it also gives the researcher some confidence about the estimates. This concept of confidence is a crucial one in interval estimation and distinguishes interval estimates from point estimates. The amount of confidence a researcher has in her estimate is expressed as a percentage, and the higher the percentage, the more confident she can be. Therefore an estimate made with 99% confidence should be more reliable than one made with 95%. To illustrate this distinction between the point and interval estimates, it can be seen that the researcher in both cases is asking the same question:

'How much treatment on average are future infertile couples going to need?'

However, a point estimate would answer:

'I do not know precisely, but my guess is an average of 210 minutes of sessions'.

whereas the interval estimate would reply:

'I do not know precisely but I am 95% confident that average treatment needs will be between 150 minutes and 240 minutes of sessions'.

The higher figure in this last answer (i.e. 240 minutes) is called the *upper confidence limit*, while the lower figure i.e. (150 minutes) is called the *lower confidence limit*. The difference between these two numbers is known as the *confidence interval*. How much confidence can be expressed in any given interval estimate depends on the formula used to calculate the estimate. These formulae are given later in the chapter.

The theory behind interval estimates

In order to understand the theoretical basis underpinning interval estimates, it is important that you have read the sections on the normal distribution (pages 42–44) and on the standard deviation (pages 41–42). Just to refresh your memory on the key points, a normal distribution is a frequency distribution graph, which is bell-shaped as in Figure 18.1.

This curve has a number of important properties which are essential to statistics.

The standard deviation is a number which represents how much a set of data varies, on average, from the mean of those data.

It is the relationship between the normal distribution and the standard deviation which is important to estimation. In any set of normally

distributed data, a fixed percentage of that data lies within given areas on either side of the average score.

These 'given areas' are related to the standard deviations of that set of data and are as follows:

- 68% of the scores fall within *one* standard deviation either side of the mean.
- 95% of the scores fall within *two* standard deviations either side of the mean.
- 99.73% of the scores fall within *three* standard deviations either side of the mean.

These figures may be more clearly illustrated by looking back to the diagram on page 43.

If you re-read the example regarding heart rate given beneath the illustration on page 43, then the implications all this has for estimation can be explored further.

On the hypothetical basis that the average heart rate is 72 beats per minute, and the standard deviation is 5, you would know that 68% of the population have heart rates of between 67 and 77 beats per minute, 95% have heart rates between 62 and 82 beats per minute, and 99.73% have heart rates between 57 and 87 beats per minute.

These (fictitious) figures would have been calculated on a *sample* of people. If, for example, you wanted to make an interval estimate on heart rate for the whole population with 95% confidence in that estimate, then you need to use the mean score and add two standard deviations to it to get the upper confidence limit (i.e. 82 beats). You then take two standard deviations away from the mean to get the lower confidence limit (i.e. 62 beats). This would give us the confidence interval of 62–82 beats per minute. Because 95% of any normally distributed data lie within two standard deviations either side of the mean, you could say with 95% confidence that the heart rates of the whole population lie within that interval. This 95% figure is called the *level of confidence* and is a statement of belief that the population's heart rate will fall within the upper and lower confidence limits stated.

In the same way, you could make estimates with 68% confidence by using one standard deviation either side of the mean, or with 99.73% confidence by using three standard deviations

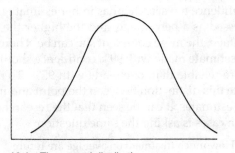

Figure 18.1 The normal distribution curve.

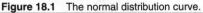

either side of the mean. However, it is more common to use confidence levels of 90% and 99% in addition to 95% and these clearly have no direct correspondence with the standard deviations. Therefore, we need to use the appropriate estimation formulae. These are provided in the next section. These formulae also allow the researcher to make estimates from large samples (over 30) about characteristics which are not normally distributed throughout the population.

Calculating interval estimates

There are several different formulae for calculating interval estimates and which one you use will depend on the following points:

1. Whether your sample size is greater or less than 30.
2. Do you want to estimate the population *average* for the parameter in question (such as the average number of visits the community midwife makes to new mothers) or do you require *proportions* or *percentages* (for example, the proportion of miscarriages classified as incomplete abortions)?
3. The confidence level you need in your estimate. The usual level is 95%, but you may need to have more confidence (i.e. 99%) or less (90%) depending on what it is you are estimating. The more disastrous the effects of an inaccurate estimate, the more confidence you will need.

SAMPLES LARGER THAN THIRTY

Estimating confidence limits for the population average

If you wish to estimate population *averages* from data derived from samples larger than 30, the formulae contained in this section are appropriate. The first formula provided is for the most commonly used 95% confidence level. The other formulae are for the 99% and 90% levels respectively.

Supposing you were interested in the average absenteeism rate of Staff Midwives across your region. To calculate your estimate for this population, you might select a random sample of 75 Staff midwives and work out their average absence rate over the previous 12 months. Let us say this works out at 19.0 units p.a. with a standard deviation of 4.5.

What you have here is:

- a sample larger than 30
- an average or mean score for the parameter in which you are interested (i.e. absenteeism).

The 95% confidence level

If you need the usual 95% confidence level in your estimate, the formula is:

$$1.96 \times \frac{SD}{\sqrt{n}}$$

where 1.96 is a constant for the 95% confidence level

SD is the standard deviation of the population

n is the sample size

$\sqrt{}$ is the square root of the sample size

It is important to note that very often the standard deviation of the population is not known. In such cases you can use the standard deviation of the sample instead.

If we now transfer these figures from the example about Staff Midwives' absenteeism rates, into the formula, we get:

$$1.96 \times \frac{4.5}{\sqrt{75}}$$

$$= 1.96 \times \frac{4.5}{8.66}$$

$$= 1.96 \times 0.52$$

$$= 1.02$$

This figure of 1.02 is then added to the average absenteeism rate of 19.0 units to give the upper confidence limit, i.e.

$$19.0 + 1.02 = 20.02$$

It is then subtracted from the average to give the lower confidence limit, i.e.

$$19.0 - 1.02 = 17.98$$

This gives us the confidence interval of 17.98–20.02. We can therefore say with 95% confidence that average absenteeism rates among the Staff Midwives in the region will fall within these figures.

The 99% confidence level

Should you want to make your estimates with more confidence, the formula becomes

$$2.58 \times \frac{SD}{\sqrt{n}}$$

So, using the above example, and substituting the relevant figures we get

$$2.58 \times \frac{4.5}{\sqrt{75}}$$

$$= 2.58 \times 0.52$$

$$= 1.34$$

The upper confidence limit is then 19.0 + 1.34 = 20.34

and the lower confidence limit is 19.0 – 1.34 = 17.66

So we can now say with 99% confidence that the average absenteeism will fall between 17.66 and 20.34 units.

The 90% confidence level

If we do not need such a high level of confidence in our estimate, we can use the less stringent 90% formula:

$$1.64 \times \frac{SD}{\sqrt{n}}$$

Therefore, using the same data we get

$$1.64 \times \frac{4.5}{\sqrt{75}}$$

$$= 1.64 \times 0.52$$

$$= 0.85$$

The confidence interval is therefore

$$18.15 - 19.85$$

We can estimate with 90% confidence that the average absenteeism rates for the population of Staff Midwives will be between 18.15 and 19.85 units p.a.

Estimating confidence limits for proportions of the population

If, rather than estimating confidence limits for population averages, you wish to calculate population proportions or percentages, you will need the following formulae instead. Three formulae are provided, the first for the 95% confidence limits, the second for the 99% limits and the third for the 90% limits.

Let us imagine you are interested in the topic of carpal tunnel syndrome in pregnancy. You wish to estimate what proportion of the pregnant women population is likely to suffer this problem. You select a sample of 90 pregnant women of 35+ weeks' gestation and find that 27 of them have carpal tunnel syndrome. You therefore have a sample larger than 30 and are concerned with proportion and percentage estimates of the population.

The following formulae are therefore appropriate for this purpose.

The 95% confidence limit

The formula for this calculation is

$$1.96 \times \sqrt{\frac{pq}{n}}$$

Where 1.96 is a constant to be used for the 95% confidence limits
p is the proportion of the sample which possesses the characteristic
q is the proportion of the sample which does *not* possess the characteristic
n is the sample size
$\sqrt{}$ is the square root of the calculations under this sign

The proportion of a sample is calculated by

dividing the actual *number* of people possessing the characteristic by the total number of people in the sample. For example, here the proportion of women *with* carpal tunnel syndrome would be:

$$\frac{27}{90} = 0.3$$

While the proportion of women *without* the syndrome is

$$\frac{63}{90} = 0.7$$

Therefore substituting these figures in the formula we get:

$$1.96 \times \sqrt{\frac{0.3 \times 0.7}{90}}$$

$$= 1.96 \times \sqrt{\frac{0.21}{90}}$$

$$= 1.96 \times \sqrt{0.0023}$$

$$= 1.96 \times 0.05$$

$$= 0.1$$

This figure of 0.1 is now

- *added* to the proportion of the sample who have carpal tunnel syndrome to get the *upper confidence limit*, i.e.

$$0.1 + 0.3 = 0.4$$

- *subtracted* from the proportion of the sample who have carpal tunnel syndrome to get the *lower confidence limit*, i.e.

$$0.3 - 0.1 = 0.2$$

This gives us the confidence interval of 0.2–0.4, which means that we can now estimate with 95% confidence that the proportion of the population of pregnant women who suffer carpal tunnel syndrome will lie between 0.2 and 0.4.

The 99% confidence limit

Should you need to have greater confidence in your estimate then the following formula should be used:

$$2.58 \times \sqrt{\frac{pq}{n}}$$

If we use the example and figures above then we get:

$$2.58 \times \sqrt{\frac{0.3 \times 0.7}{90}}$$

$$= 2.58 \times \sqrt{\frac{0.21}{90}}$$

$$= 2.58 \times \sqrt{0.0023}$$

$$= 2.58 \times 0.05$$

$$= 0.13$$

This number is then:

- *added* to the proportion of the sample who have carpal tunnel syndrome to get the upper confidence limit, i.e.

$$0.3 + 0.13 = 0.43$$

- *subtracted* from the proportion of the sample with carpal tunnel syndrome to get the lower confidence limit, i.e.

$$0.3 - 0.13 = 0.17$$

Therefore, the 99% confidence interval for the proportion of the population of pregnant women with carpal tunnel syndrome is 0.17 to 0.43.

The 90% confidence limit

If you do not need such a high level of confidence in your estimate, you can use the 90% confidence limit formula instead:

$$1.64 \times \sqrt{\frac{pq}{n}}$$

$$1.64 \times \sqrt{\frac{0.3 \times 0.7}{90}}$$

$$= 1.64 \times \sqrt{\frac{0.21}{90}}$$

$$= 1.64 \times \sqrt{0.0023}$$

$$= 1.64 \times 0.05$$

$$= 0.08$$

This number is now

- *added* to the proportion of the sample with carpal tunnel syndrome to give the upper confidence limit i.e. 0.3 + 0.08 = 0.38
- *subtracted* from the proportion of the sample with carpal tunnel syndrome to give the lower confidence limit, i.e.

$$0.3 - 0.08 = 0.22$$

Therefore, it can be predicted with 90% confidence that the proportion of the pregnant women population who have carpal tunnel syndrome falls somewhere between 0.22 and 0.38.

SAMPLE OF FEWER THAN THIRTY SUBJECTS

Before proceeding with estimates for samples of less than 30, it is important to emphasize two points. Firstly, these particular calculations should only be performed if the parent population is known to be normally distributed on the characteristic in question. The second important point to note is that proportions of a population are not usually calculated from samples of less than 30, because the estimates are likely to be unreliable. Consequently, only the formulae associated with estimating means will be provided.

Let us suppose you are interested in the promotion prospects of newly qualified Diplomate midwives. You select a random sample of 15 and follow them up over a 10 year period. You find that the average length of time taken to achieve a Sister's post is 4.7 years. From this sample mean you wish to calculate the population mean. Therefore, your interest is in averages and you have a sample of less than 30. The following formulae are therefore appropriate.

The formula for the 99%, 95% and 90% confidence limits requires that you first calculate the standard deviation from the sample data, thus

$$SD = \sqrt{\frac{\Sigma(x - \bar{x})^2}{N - 1}}$$

where Σ is the total

x is the individual score
$\bar{x}$ is the average score
N is the total number of scores in the sample
$\sqrt{}$ is the square root of all the calculations under this sign

To refresh your memory on how to do this calculation, turn back to page 41. Imagine for the purpose of this example that the standard deviation is 2.1 years.

The estimate calculations for the confidence limits of 99%, 95% and 90% all start off in the same way:

1. Calculate N-1 where N is the number in your sample, i.e.

$$15 - 1 = 14$$

2. Turn to the probability tables associated with the *t*-test (Table A2.5), where you can see that down the left hand column are d.f. values from 1–120. Look down this column until you find our N-1 value of 14. To the right of this are the numbers

    1.345   1.761   2.145   2.624   2.977   4.140

The procedure for calculating the different levels of confidence limits now changes slightly, and each will be dealt with separately.

Calculating the 95% confidence limits

We are only interested in the figure under the heading '0.05 level of significance for a two-tailed test'; see top of the table. This terminology is explained in Chapter 9 but is of no relevance to us here. The figure at the intersection point of this column with N-1 = 14, is 2.145 and is used to provide us with the 95% confidence limit, thus:

$$t \times \frac{SD}{\sqrt{N}}$$

where t is the figure derived from the probability table for t, i.e.

2.145

SD is the standard deviation of the sample's score, i.e.

$$2.1 \text{ years}$$

N is the number of subjects in the sample, i.e.

$$15$$

$\sqrt{}$ is the square root

Therefore, substituting these figures we get:

$$= 2.145 \times \frac{2.1}{\sqrt{15}}$$

$$= 2.145 \times \frac{2.1}{3.87}$$

$$= 2.145 \times 0.54$$

$$= 1.16$$

This figure is:

- *added* to the average sample score to give the *upper confidence limit*, i.e.

$$4.7 + 1.16 = 5.86$$

- *subtracted* from the average sample score to give the *lower confidence limit*, i.e.

$$4.7 - 1.16 = 3.54$$

Therefore we can estimate with 95% confidence that the population of newly qualified Diplomate midwives will achieve a Sister's post between 3.54 and 5.86 years after qualifying.

The 99% confidence limits

To calculate this value we need to look under the '0.01 level of significance for a two-tailed test' heading in Table A2.5 for *N*-1. Our *N*-1 value is 14 and the relevant figure at the intersection point is 2.977.

Using the formula:

$$t \times \frac{SD}{\sqrt{N}}$$

and substituting our values we get

$$= 2.977 \times \frac{2.1}{\sqrt{15}}$$

$$= 2.977 \times \frac{2.1}{3.87}$$

$$= 2.977 \times 0.54$$

$$= 1.61$$

We now:

- *add* 1.61 to the sample mean of 4.7 to get the *upper confidence limit*, i.e.

$$4.7 + 1.61 = 6.31$$

- *subtract* 1.61 from the sample mean of 4.7 to get the *lower confidence limit*, i.e.

$$4.7 - 1.61 = 3.09$$

Therefore the 99% confidence limits are 3.09–6.31 years.

The 90% confidence limits

To obtain the 90% confidence limits we need to select the number under the heading '0.10 level of significance for a two-tailed test' (in Table A2.5), to the right of *N*-1.

Here for our N-1 value of 14, the relevant figure is 1.761

Using the formula:

$$t \times \frac{SD}{\sqrt{N}}$$

and substituting our values we get:

$$1.761 \times \frac{2.1}{\sqrt{15}}$$

$$= 1.761 \times \frac{2.1}{3.87}$$

$$= 1.761 \times 0.54$$

$$= 0.95$$

This figure is now:

- *added* to the sample mean of 4.7 to give the *upper confidence limit*, i.e.

$$4.7 + 0.95 = 5.65$$

- *subtracted* from the sample mean of 4.7 to give the *lower confidence limit,* i.e.

$$4.7 - 0.95 = 3.75$$

The 90% confidence limits for this example are therefore 3.75–5.65 years.

KEY CONCEPTS

1. Estimation is a technique of making scientific 'best guesses' about events.
2. It is particularly useful to anyone who is involved in planning (e.g. budgets, service delivery etc).
3. The technique of estimation involves making predictions about a particular population characteristic known as a *parameter* from knowledge about a small sample of that population.
4. There are two types of estimation: *point estimates* and *interval estimates.*
5. Point estimates make a prediction of a *single* figure about the population parameter, whereas interval estimates make a prediction that the population parameter will fall between *two* figures.
6. These two figures are called *confidence limits* and the gap between them is called the confidence interval.
7. When using interval estimates, the predictions about the population can be made with different levels of confidence.
8. The degree of confidence is dictated by the nature of the research and the formula used to calculate the estimates.

Activity 18.1 (Answers on page 241)

1. You are the midwifery Sister in charge of an ante-natal clinic. The non-attendance levels are becoming increasingly worrying because of resource wastage. If you could make an accurate estimate of non-attendance over the next 6 months, you could adjust staffing levels accordingly.

   You find that the number of non-attenders of a sample of 150 women was 57.

   Estimate the confidence limits for the percentage of non-attenders in the ante-natal clinic population using the 95% confidence level.
2. You are trying to plan care activities in a new Special Care Baby Unit. As many of these babies have multiple problems and are very premature, you will need to estimate how much of the midwife's time on average, will be required per child, per day.

   You select a sample of 25 babies and find that the average amount of midwifery time needed is 3.2 hours, with a SD of 1.7 hours. Estimate the average amount of time that will be required by the babies in this new unit, using the 99% confidence level.
3. You are responsible for the equipment budget in your District Health Authority. One activity involves you in estimating the mean life-expectancy of your ultrasound scanners over the next financial year.

   You look at the life-span of a sample of 40 of these machines and find that the mean length of service is 4.3 years, with a standard deviation of 0.9 years. Using the 90% confidence level, estimate the average life-expectancy of the ultrasound scanning machines in your area, so that you can get some idea of how many replacements will be needed.

References

Cartwright A 1983 Health surveys in practice and potential. King Edward's Hospital Fund for London

Chalmers A F 1983 What is this thing called science? Open University Press, Milton Keynes

Darbyshire P 1986 When the face doesn't fit! Nursing Times 82 (39): 28–30

Ferguson G A 1976 Statistical analysis in psychology and education. McGraw-Hill Kogakusha, Tokyo

Gardener G 1978 Social surveys for social planners. Open University Press, Milton Keynes

Green J & D'Oliveira M 1982 Learning to use statistical tests in psychology. Open University Press, Milton Keynes

Hicks C M 1993 Effects of psychological prejudices on communication and social interaction. British Journal of Midwifery 1 (1): 10–16

Hicks C M 1996 Ethics in midwifery research. In: Firth L (ed) Midwifery and ethics. Butterworth Heinemann, Oxford

McNemar Q 1962 Psychological statistics. Wiley, New York

Peters D P & Ceci S 1982 Peer-review practices of psychological journals – the fate of accepted, published articles submitted again. Behavioural and Brain Sciences 5 (2): 187–195

Polgar S & Thomas S A 1992 Introduction to research in the health sciences. Churchill-Livingstone, Edinburgh

Robson C 1974 Experiment, design and statistics in psychology. Penguin, Harmondsworth

Sanders D H, Eng R J & Murph A F 1985 Statistics: a fresh approach. McGraw-Hill, New York

Siegal S 1956 Nonparametric statistics for the behavioural sciences. McGraw-Hill Kogakusha, Tokyo

Appendices and Glossary

Appendix 1

Basic mathematical principles

BRACKETS

You will not always meet with straightforward calculations in statistical tests. Many of them have quite complex formulae and it is essential to know which part of the formula should be computed first. One way of indicating which part should be dealt with first is by using brackets. Any figures or formulae contained in brackets should be calculated before anything else, or else you will get quite incorrect results. This can be illustrated by the following examples:

$$114 - (15 + 23)$$
$$= 114 - 38$$
$$= 76$$

as opposed to:

$$(114 - 15) + 23$$
$$= 99 + 23$$
$$= 122$$

Brackets can change your answer quite dramatically. Therefore, the first principle you must remember when calculating any statistical tests is:

all calculations contained in brackets must be carried out first.

However, not all formulae are as convenient as this. Some have brackets within brackets, e.g.:

$$14 + [(15 \times 3) - 12]$$

In these cases, you must calculate the formula in the innermost brackets first, then go on to the formula in the next set of brackets and so on. Therefore, the above formula becomes:

$$14 + [45 - 12] = 14 + 33 = 47$$

So:

always calculate the formula in the innermost set of brackets first and then work outwards.

ADDITION, SUBTRACTION, MULTIPLICATION AND DIVISION

Although any formula in brackets must always be calculated first, not all formulae have brackets.

Sometimes you will come across something like this:

$$12 + 19 - 7 - 4 + 8$$

In such cases, where you have a mixure of just additions and subtraction and no brackets, you simply start calculating from the left-hand side and work systematically across to the right. The importance of this principle can be illustrated by the following example:

$$[72 - 34 + 9]$$

If you work systematically from left to right to right, the answer 47. If, however, you do the addition first, the answer is 29 – quite different and quite incorrect. So the next principle to remember is:

When you have a row of additions and substractions only and no brackets, start the calculations at the left-hand side and work systematically across to the right.

Similarly, there will be occasions when you have a row of additions only, e.g.:

$$19 + 17 + 9$$

subtractions only, e.g.:

$$28 - 4 - 16$$

divisions only, e.g.:

$$45 \div 3 \div 5$$

multiplications only, e.g.:

$$7 \times 8 \times 14$$

or a mixture of multiplications and divisions, e.g.:

$$12 \times 8 \div 4$$

While it doesn't matter too much in which order these are carried out, it is easier and less confusing if you stick to the left-to-right rule.

However, quite often you will come across mixtures of addition and/or subtraction with multiplication and/or division, e.g.:

$$\text{a. } 71 + 9 \div 18$$

or

$$\text{b. } 117 - 6 \times 10$$

In these cases you must do the multiplication or division first, followed by the additions or subtractions. The reason for doing this can be ilustrated by the above examples. If they are calculated correctly, the answer to (a) is 71.5 and to (b) 57. If, however, you apply the left to right rule here, you end up with 4.44 and 1110 respectively. So the next rule of basic maths is that:

multiplying and dividing are carried out before adding and subtracting.

To recap on what has been outlined so far:
- First, carry out the calculations in brackets. If there are brackets within brackets, do the calculations in the inside brackets first.
- Second, if there are no brackets, do the multiplications and divisions first.
- Third, if there are no multiplications and divisions, just work from left to right.

Just one final point – sometimes you will see something like 9(12 – 2). This means 9 × (12 – 2), except that the multiplication sign between the 9 and the bracket is *assumed*.

POSITIVE AND NEGATIVE NUMBERS

It's easy to get confused over positive and negative numbers. While 40 – 20 is simple to work out, 20 – 40 starts to cause confusion. Perhaps the easiest way to overcome the problems of plus and minus numbers is to think of the left-hand figure as your 'bank' of money in a Monopoly® game. Obviously, you can add to your bank or you can take away from your bank, but both transactions will alter the resulting amount of money you have to play with. Suppose you started with £200 but then landed on your competitor's Mayfair property, which meant you owed them £300. You have, then £200 – £300. This means that you are £100 in the red, in other words you have –£100. Suppose now that another player landed on your Park Lane property which meant you could receive £200. Because you're already in debt to the tune of £100, half the money you're owed must go towards putting your debt right, which means that you're £100 in credit. In other words you have:

$$- £100 + £200 = £100$$

However, it's often more expensive than this in Monopoly®. Suppose that while you are £100 in debt, you land on the Strand and owe a further £50. This means you have one debt of £100 (–£100) plus another debt of £50 (–£50). This can be expressed as:

$$(-£100) + (-£50) = -£150$$

There are, of course, many occasions when you will be either multiplying or dividing plus and minus numbers, e.g.

$$(+5) \times (-10) \text{ or } (-80) \div (+8)$$

Multiplying or dividing a mixture of plus and minus numbers always gives a minus answer. So in the examples above, the answers are –50 and –10 respectively. Multiplying or dividing positive numbers *only* always results in positive answers, but multiplying or dividing minus numbers only also produces a positive number. If you think about this in terms of double negatives in speech, 'I didn't do nothing' actually means 'I did something'. Similarly, double negatives in maths also mean a positive.

We can state some further mathematical principles now:

1. Adding two negative numbers results in a negative answer, e.g.:

$$(-20) + (-10) = -30$$

2. Adding one plus number to a minus number is the same as taking the minus number from the plus number, e.g.:

$$-24 + 6 = -18$$
$$+6 - 24 = -18$$

3. Multiplying two positive numbers always results in a positive answer.
4. Multiplying one positive number by one negative number always results in a negative answer.
5. Multiplying two negative numbers always results in a positive answer.
6. Dividing two positive numbers always results in a positive answer.
7. Dividing one positive number by one negative number always results in a negative answer.
8. Dividing two negative numbers always results in a positive answer.

SQUARES AND SQUARE ROOTS

Two common calculations you will have to carry out in the statistical tests are squares and square roots.

The **square** of a number is quite simply that number multiplied by itself and is expressed by a small 2 thus:

$$8^2$$

This means that you multiply 8 by 8. So whenever you see the small ^{2} to the top right of a number, you simply multiply that number by itself. The answer you will obtain will always be a positive number, since if you square $+8$ you multiply $+8 \times +8$ which will give you $+64$, while if you square -8, you multiply -8×-8 which will still give you $+64$, since multiplying two negative numbers always gives a positive number.

The **square root** of a number is actually the opposite of the square, in that the square root of any given number is a number which multiplied by itself gives the number you already have. It is expressed by the symbol $\sqrt{\ }$. Therefore $\sqrt{25} = 5$, since $5 \times 5 = 25$.

While your calculator will almost certainly have a square root function (which you should not hesitate to use), this is a good example of an occasion when you should be 'eyeballing' the result. For example, while you cannot easily work out in your head what the square root of 14 is, you do know that it must be somewhere between 3 and 4, since 3 is the square root of 9 and 4 is the square root of 16; if you come out with something larger or smaller, something has gone wrong somewhere!

In many of the formulae in this book, you will find that the square root sign extends over more than one number, e.g.:

$$\sqrt{45 + 19} = \sqrt{64} = 8$$

Do make sure that you complete all the calculations under the square root symbol before computing the square root.

ROUNDING UP DECIMAL PLACES

When using decimals in fairly complicated calculations, you can often end up with a whole row of figures to the right of the decimal point. To continue your calculations with all these numbers is both cumbersome and unnecessarily accurate. Therefore, it is easier to limit the number of figures to the right of the decimal point to 2 or 3. In order to do this correctly, we do not simply chop off the excess figures, but **round them up**.

This is done by starting with the figure on the extreme right of the decimal point. If this figure is equal to 5 or larger, then the number to its immediate left is increased by 1. If the end figure is less than 5, then number to its left remains the same, e.g.:

9.14868125 becomes
9.1486813

If you wish to drop the 3, the same rule applies, so that the above decimal becomes:

9.149681

If you wish to cut down the number of decimal places to 2, the process is:

9.148681 becomes
9.14868 which becomes
9.1487 which becomes
9.149 which becomes
9.15

While this process is relatively straightforward in the above example, look at the following decimal number, which we wish to round up to two places:

7.19498

Here, dropping the last number changes the 9 to a 10, and this automatically changes the 4 to 5 which in turn changes the next 9 into a 10, such that the end result is 7.2, even though we were rounding up to 2 decimal places, thus:

7.19498 becomes
7.195   which becomes
7.2

Throughout this book, the figures have been rounded to three decimal places. If you have chosen to round up to two decimal places throughout the calculations, you will find that the end result is slightly different. Don't worry about this unless there is a massive discrepancy which will probably mean that something has gone wrong somewhere in your calculations.

Statistical probability tables

Table A2.1 Critical values of χ^2 at various levels of probability. For your χ^2 value to be significant at a particular probability level, it should be *equal to* or *larger than* the critical values associated with the df in your study. (Reproduced From Lindley DV, Scott WF (1984) New Cambridge Elementary Statistical Tables, 10th edn. Cambridge University Press, with permission.)

Level of significance for a two-tailed test				
df	.10	.05	.02	.01	.001
1	2.71	3.84	5.41	6.64	10.83
2	4.60	5.99	7.82	9.21	13.82
3	6.25	7.82	9.84	11.34	16.27
4	7.78	9.49	11.67	13.28	18.46
5	9.24	11.07	13.39	15.09	20.52
6	10.64	12.59	15.03	16.81	22.46
7	12.02	14.07	16.62	18.48	24.32
8	13.36	15.51	18.17	20.09	26.12
9	14.68	16.92	19.68	21.67	27.88
10	15.99	18.31	21.16	23.21	29.59
11	17.28	19.68	22.62	24.72	31.26
12	18.55	21.03	24.05	26.22	32.91
13	19.81	22.36	25.47	27.69	34.53
14	21.06	23.68	26.87	29.14	36.12
15	22.31	25.00	28.26	30.58	37.70
16	23.54	26.30	29.63	32.00	39.29
17	24.77	27.59	31.00	33.41	40.75
18	25.99	28.87	32.35	34.80	42.31
19	27.20	30.14	33.69	36.19	43.82
20	28.41	31.41	35.02	37.57	45.32
21	29.62	32.67	36.34	38.93	46.80
22	30.81	33.92	37.66	40.29	48.27
23	32.01	35.17	38.97	41.64	49.73
24	33.20	36.42	40.27	42.98	51.18
25	34.38	37.65	41.57	44.31	52.62
26	35.56	38.88	42.86	45.64	54.05
27	36.74	40.11	44.14	46.97	55.48
28	37.92	41.34	45.42	48.28	56.89
29	39.09	42.56	46.69	49.59	58.30
30	40.26	43.77	47.96	50.89	59.70

NB If you have a one-tailed hypothesis, look up your value as usual and simply *halve* the associated *p* value shown for a two-tailed hypothesis.

Table A2.2 **Critical values of** *T* (Wilcoxon test) at various levels of probability. (For your *T* value to be significant at a particular probability level, it should be *equal to* or *less than* critical values associated with the *N* in your study)

	Level of significance for one-tailed test					Level of significance for one-tailed test			
	.05	.025	.01	.005		.05	.025	.01	.005
	Level of significance for two-tailed test					Level of significance for two-tailed test			
N	.10	.05	.02	.01	*N*	.10	.05	.02	.01
5	1	-	-	-	28	130	117	102	92
6	2	1	-	-	29	141	127	111	100
7	4	2	0	-	30	152	137	120	109
8	6	4	2	0	31	163	148	130	118
9	8	6	3	2	32	175	159	141	128
10	11	8	5	3	33	188	171	151	138
11	14	11	7	5	34	201	183	162	149
12	17	14	10	7	35	214	195	174	160
13	21	17	13	10	36	228	208	186	171
14	26	21	16	13	37	242	222	198	183
15	30	25	20	16	38	256	235	211	195
16	36	30	24	19	39	271	250	224	208
17	41	35	28	23	40	287	264	238	221
18	47	40	33	28	41	303	279	252	234
19	54	46	38	32	42	319	295	267	248
20	60	52	43	37	43	336	311	281	262
21	68	59	49	43	44	353	327	297	277
22	75	66	56	49	45	371	344	313	292
23	83	73	62	55	46	389	361	329	307
24	92	81	69	61	47	408	379	345	323
25	101	90	77	68	48	427	397	362	339
26	110	98	85	76	49	446	415	380	356
27	120	107	93	84	50	466	434	398	373

Dashes in the table indicate that no decision is possible at the stated level of significance.

Table A2.3   Critical values of χ_r^2 (Friedman test) at various levels of probability. (For your χ_r^2 value to be significant at a particular probability level, it should be *equal to* or *larger than* the critical values associated with the C and N in your study)
a.Critical values for three conditions ($C = 3$)

N = 2		N = 3		N = 4		N = 5		N = 6		N = 7		N = 8		N = 9	
χr^2	p	χr^2	p	χr^2	p	χr^2	p	χr^2	p	χr^2	p	χr^2	p	χr^2	p
0	1.000	.000	1.000	.0	1.000	.0	1.000	.00	1.000	.000	1.000	.00	1.000	.000	1.000
1	.833	.667	.944	.5	.931	.4	.954	.33	.956	.286	.964	.25	.967	.222	.971
3	.500	2.000	.528	1.5	.653	1.2	.691	1.00	.740	.857	.768	.75	.794	.667	.814
4	.167	2.667	.361	2.0	.431	1.6	.522	1.33	.570	1.143	.620	1.00	.654	.889	.865
		4.667	.194	3.5	.273	2.8	.367	2.33	.430	2.000	.486	1.75	.531	1.556	.569
		6.000	.028	4.5	.125	3.6	.182	3.00	.252	2.571	.305	2.25	.355	2.000	.398
				6.0	.069	4.8	.124	4.00	.184	3.429	.237	3.00	.285	2.667	.328
				6.5	.042	5.2	.093	4.33	.142	3.714	.192	3.25	.236	2.889	.278
				8.0	.0046	6.4	.039	5.33	.072	4.571	.112	4.00	.149	3.556	.187
						7.6	.024	6.33	.052	5.429	.085	4.75	.120	4.222	.154
						8.4	.0085	7.00	.029	6.000	.052	5.25	.079	4.667	.107
						10.0	.00077	8.33	.012	7.143	.027	6.25	.047	5.556	.069
								9.00	.0081	7.714	.021	6.75	.038	6.000	.057
								9.33	.0055	8.000	.016	7.00	.030	6.222	.048
								10.33	.0017	8.857	.0084	7.75	.018	6.889	.031
								12.00	.00013	10.286	.0036	9.00	.0099	8.000	.019
										10.571	.0027	9.25	.0080	8.222	.016
										11.143	.0012	9.75	.0048	8.667	.010
										12.286	.00032	10.75	.0024	9.556	.0060
										14.000	.000021	12.00	.0011	10.667	.0035
												12.25	.00086	10.889	.0029
												13.00	.00026	11.556	.0013
												14.25	.000061	12.667	.00066
												16.00	.0000036	13.556	.00035
														14.000	.00020
														14.222	.000097
														14.889	.000054
														16.222	.000011
														18.000	.0000006

NB These values are all for a two-tailed test only.

Table A2.3 (contd) Critical values of χ_r^2 (Friedman test). (For your χ_r^2 value to be significant at a particular probability level, it should be *equal to* or *larger than* the critical values associated with the C and N in your study.)
b. **Critical values for four conditions ($C = 4$)**

χ_r^2	p	χ_r^2	p	χ_r^2	p	χ_r^2	p
				$N = 2$			
.0	1.000	.0	1.000	.0	1.000	5.7	.141
.6	.958	.6	.958	.3	.992	6.0	.105
1.2	.834	1.0	.910	.6	.928	6.3	.094
1.8	.792	1.8	.727	.9	.900	6.6	.077
2.4	.625	2.2	.608	1.2	.800	6.9	.068
3.0	.542	2.6	.524	1.5	.754	7.2	.054
3.6	.458	3.4	.446	1.8	.677	7.5	.052
4.2	.375	3.8	.342	2.1	.649	7.8	.036
4.8	.208	4.2	.300	2.4	.524	8.1	.033
5.4	.167	5.0	.207	2.7	.508	8.4	.019
6.0	.042	5.4	.175	3.0	.432	8.7	.014
		5.8	.148	3.3	.389	9.3	.012
		6.6	.075	3.6	.355	9.6	.0069
		7.0	.054	3.9	.324	9.9	.0062
		7.4	.033	4.5	.242	10.2	.0027
		8.2	.017	4.8	.200	10.8	.0016
		9.0	.0017	5.1	.190	11.1	.00094
				5.4	.158	12.0	.000072

Column group headers: $N = 2$ (cols 1–2), $N = 3$ (cols 3–4), $N = 4$ (cols 5–8)

NB These values are all for a two-tailed test only.

Table A2.4 Critical values of L (Page's L trend test) at various levels of probability. (For your L value to be significant at a particular probability level, it should be *equal to* or *larger* than the critical values associated with the C and N in your study.)

N	C (no. of conditions)				p<
	3	4	5	6	
2	-	-	109	178	.001
	-	60	106	173	.01
	28	58	103	166	.05
3	-	89	160	260	.001
	42	87	155	252	.01
	41	84	150	244	.05
4	56	117	210	341	.001
	55	114	204	331	.01
	54	111	197	321	.05
5	70	145	259	420	.001
	68	141	251	409	.01
	66	137	244	397	.05
6	83	172	307	499	.001
	81	167	299	486	.01
	79	163	291	474	.05
7	96	198	355	577	.001
	93	193	346	563	.01
	91	189	338	550	.05
8	109	225	403	655	.001
	106	220	393	640	.01
	104	214	384	625	.05
9	121	252	451	733	.001
	119	246	441	717	.01
	116	240	431	701	.05
10	134	278	499	811	.001
	131	272	487	793	.01
	128	266	477	777	.05
11	147	305	546	888	.001
	144	298	534	869	.01
	141	292	523	852	.05
12	160	331	593	965	.001
	156	324	581	946	.01
	153	317	570	928	.05

NB These values are for a one-tailed test only.

Table A2.5 Critical values of t (related and unrelated t tests) at various levels of probability. For your t value to be significant at a particular probability level, it should be *equal to* or *larger than* critical values associated with the df in your study. (Reproduced from Lindley DV, Scott WF (1984) New Cambridge Elementary Statistical Tables, 10th edn. Cambridge University Press, with permission.)

df	Level of significance for one-tailed test					
	.10	.05	.025	.01	.005	.0005
	Level of significance for two-tailed test					
	.20	.10	.05	.02	.01	.001
1	3.078	6.314	12.706	31.821	63.657	636.619
2	1.886	2.920	4.303	6.965	9.925	31.598
3	1.638	2.353	3.182	4.541	5.841	12.941
4	1.533	2.132	2.776	3.747	4.604	8.610
5	1.476	2.015	2.571	3.365	4.032	6.859
6	1.440	1.943	2.447	3.143	3.707	5.959
7	1.415	1.895	2.365	2.998	3.499	5.405
8	1.397	1.860	2.306	2.896	3.355	5.041
9	1.383	1.833	2.262	2.821	3.250	4.781
10	1.372	1.812	2.228	2.764	3.169	4.587
11	1.363	1.796	2.201	2.718	3.106	4.437
12	1.356	1.782	2.179	2.681	3.055	4.318
13	1.350	1.771	2.160	2.650	3.012	4.221
14	1.345	1.761	2.145	2.624	2.977	4.140
15	1.341	1.753	2.131	2.602	2.947	4.073
16	1.337	1.746	2.120	2.583	2.921	4.015
17	1.333	1.740	2.110	2.567	2.898	3.965
18	1.330	1.734	2.101	2.552	2.878	3.922
19	1.328	1.729	2.093	2.539	2.861	3.883
20	1.325	1.725	2.086	2.528	2.845	3.850
21	1.323	1.721	2.080	2.518	2.831	3.819
22	1.321	1.717	2.074	2.508	2.819	3.792
23	1.319	1.714	2.069	2.500	2.807	3.767
24	1.318	1.711	2.064	2.492	2.797	3.745
25	1.316	1.708	2.060	2.485	2.787	3.725
26	1.315	1.706	2.056	2.479	2.779	3.707
27	1.314	1.703	2.052	2.473	2.771	3.690
28	1.313	1.701	2.048	2.467	2.763	3.674
29	1.311	1.699	2.045	2.462	2.756	3.659
30	1.310	1.697	2.042	2.457	2.750	3.646
40	1.303	1.684	2.021	2.423	2.704	3.551
60	1.296	1.671	2.000	2.390	2.660	3.460
120	1.289	1.658	1.980	2.358	2.617	3.373
∞	1.282	1.645	1.960	2.326	2.576	3.291

NB When there is no exact df use the next lowest number, except for very large dfs (well over 120), when you should use the infinity row. This is marked ∞.

Table A2.6 Critical values of F (anovas) at various levels of probability. For your F value to be significant at a particular probability level, it should be *equal to* or *larger than* the critical values associated with v_1 and v_2 in your study. (Reproduced from Lindley DV, Scott WF (1984) New Cambridge Elementary Statistical Tables, 10th edn. Cambridge University Press, with permission.)
a. Critical value of F at $p < .05$

v_2	1	2	3	4	5	6	7	8	10	12	24	∞
1	161.4	199.5	215.7	224.6	230.2	234.0	236.8	238.9	241.9	243.9	249.0	254.3
2	18.5	19.0	19.2	19.2	19.3	19.3	19.4	19.4	19.4	19.4	19.5	19.5
3	10.13	9.55	9.28	9.12	9.01	8.94	8.89	8.85	8.79	8.74	8.64	8.53
4	7.71	6.94	6.59	6.39	6.26	6.16	6.09	6.04	5.96	5.91	5.77	5.63
5	6.61	5.79	5.41	5.19	5.05	4.95	4.88	4.82	4.74	4.68	4.53	4.36
6	5.99	5.14	4.76	4.53	4.39	4.28	4.21	4.15	4.06	4.00	3.84	3.67
7	5.59	4.74	4.35	4.12	3.97	3.87	3.79	3.73	3.64	3.57	3.41	3.23
8	5.32	4.46	4.07	3.84	3.69	3.58	3.50	3.44	3.35	3.28	3.12	2.93
9	5.12	4.26	3.86	3.63	3.48	3.37	3.29	3.23	3.14	3.07	2.90	2.71
10	4.96	4.10	3.71	3.48	3.33	3.22	3.14	3.07	2.98	2.91	2.74	2.54
11	4.84	3.98	3.59	3.36	3.20	3.09	3.01	2.95	2.85	2.79	2.61	2.40
12	4.75	3.89	3.49	3.26	3.11	3.00	2.91	2.85	2.75	2.69	2.51	2.30
13	4.67	3.81	3.41	3.18	3.03	2.92	2.83	2.77	2.67	2.60	2.42	2.21
14	4.60	3.74	3.34	3.11	2.96	2.85	2.76	2.70	2.60	2.53	2.35	2.13
15	4.54	3.68	3.29	3.06	2.90	2.79	2.71	2.64	2.54	2.48	2.29	2.07
16	4.49	3.63	3.24	3.01	2.85	2.74	2.66	2.59	2.49	2.42	2.24	2.01
17	4.45	3.59	3.20	2.96	2.81	2.70	2.61	2.55	2.45	2.38	2.19	1.96
18	4.41	3.55	3.16	2.93	2.77	2.66	2.58	2.51	2.41	2.34	2.15	1.92
19	4.38	3.52	3.13	2.90	2.74	2.63	2.54	2.48	2.38	2.31	2.11	1.88
20	4.35	3.49	3.10	2.87	2.71	2.60	2.51	2.45	2.35	2.28	2.08	1.84
21	4.32	3.47	3.07	2.84	2.68	2.57	2.49	2.42	2.32	2.25	2.05	1.81
22	4.30	3.44	3.05	2.82	2.66	2.55	2.46	2.40	2.30	2.23	2.03	1.78
23	4.28	3.42	3.03	2.80	2.64	2.53	2.44	2.37	2.27	2.20	2.00	1.76
24	4.26	3.40	3.01	2.78	2.62	2.51	2.42	2.36	2.25	2.18	1.98	1.73
25	4.24	3.39	2.99	2.76	2.60	2.49	2.40	2.34	2.24	2.16	1.96	1.71
26	4.23	3.37	2.98	2.74	2.59	2.47	2.39	2.32	2.22	2.15	1.95	1.69
27	4.21	3.35	2.96	2.73	2.57	2.46	2.37	2.31	2.20	2.13	1.93	1.67
28	4.20	3.34	2.95	2.71	2.56	2.45	2.36	2.29	2.19	2.12	1.91	1.65
29	4.18	3.33	2.93	2.70	2.55	2.43	2.35	2.28	2.18	2.10	1.90	1.64
30	4.17	3.32	2.92	2.69	2.53	2.42	2.33	2.27	2.16	2.09	1.89	1.62
32	4.15	3.29	2.90	2.67	2.51	2.40	2.31	2.24	2.14	2.07	1.86	1.59
34	4.13	3.28	2.88	2.65	2.49	2.38	2.29	2.23	2.12	2.05	1.84	1.57
36	4.11	3.26	2.87	2.63	2.48	2.36	2.28	2.21	2.11	2.03	1.82	1.55
38	4.10	3.24	2.85	2.62	2.46	2.35	2.26	2.19	2.09	2.02	1.81	1.53
40	4.08	3.23	2.84	2.61	2.45	2.34	2.25	2.18	2.08	2.00	1.79	1.51
60	4.00	3.15	2.76	2.53	2.37	2.25	2.17	2.10	1.99	1.92	1.70	1.39
120	3.92	3.07	2.68	2.45	2.29	2.18	2.09	2.02	1.91	1.83	1.61	1.25
∞	3.84	3.00	2.60	2.37	2.21	2.10	2.01	1.94	1.83	1.75	1.52	1.00

NB When there is no exact number for the df, use the next lowest number. For very large dfs (well over 120) you should use the row for infinity. This is indicated ∞.

These values are all for a two-tailed test only.

Table A2.6 (contd) Critical values of F (anovas) at various levels of probability. (For your F value to be significant at a particular probability level, it should be *equal to* or *larger than* the critical values associated with v_1 and v_2 in your study.)
b. Critical values of F at $p < .025$

v_2	v_1 1	2	3	4	5	6	7	8	10	12	24	∞
1	648	800	864	900	922	937	948	957	969	977	997	1018
2	38.5	39.0	39.2	39.2	39.3	39.3	39.4	39.4	39.4	39.4	39.5	39.5
3	17.4	16.0	15.4	15.1	14.9	14.7	14.6	14.5	14.4	14.3	14.1	13.9
4	12.22	10.65	9.98	9.60	9.36	9.20	9.07	8.98	8.84	8.75	8.51	8.26
5	10.01	8.43	7.76	7.39	7.15	6.98	6.85	6.76	6.62	6.52	6.28	6.02
6	8.81	7.26	6.60	6.23	5.99	5.82	5.70	5.60	5.46	5.37	5.12	4.85
7	8.07	6.54	5.89	5.52	5.29	5.12	4.99	4.90	4.76	4.67	4.42	4.14
8	7.57	6.06	5.42	5.05	4.82	4.65	4.53	4.43	4.30	4.20	3.95	3.67
9	7.21	5.71	5.08	4.72	4.48	4.32	4.20	4.10	3.96	3.87	3.61	3.33
10	6.94	5.46	4.83	4.47	4.24	4.07	3.95	3.85	3.72	3.62	3.37	3.08
11	6.72	5.26	4.63	4.28	4.04	3.88	3.76	3.66	3.53	3.43	3.17	2.88
12	6.55	5.10	4.47	4.12	3.89	3.73	3.61	3.51	3.37	3.28	3.02	2.72
13	6.41	4.97	4.35	4.00	3.77	3.60	3.48	3.39	3.25	3.15	2.89	2.60
14	6.30	4.86	4.24	3.89	3.66	3.50	3.38	3.29	3.15	3.05	2.79	2.49
15	6.20	4.76	4.15	3.80	3.58	3.41	3.29	3.20	3.06	2.96	2.70	2.40
16	6.12	4.69	4.08	3.73	3.50	3.34	3.22	3.12	2.99	2.89	2.63	2.32
17	6.04	4.62	4.01	3.66	3.44	3.28	3.16	3.06	2.92	2.82	2.56	2.25
18	5.98	4.56	3.95	3.61	3.38	3.22	3.10	3.01	2.87	2.77	2.50	2.19
19	5.92	4.51	3.90	3.56	3.33	3.17	3.05	2.96	2.82	2.72	2.45	2.13
20	5.87	4.46	3.86	3.51	3.29	3.13	3.01	2.91	2.77	2.68	2.41	2.09
21	5.83	4.42	3.82	3.48	3.25	3.09	2.97	2.87	2.73	2.64	2.37	2.04
22	5.79	4.38	3.78	3.44	3.22	3.05	2.93	2.84	2.70	2.60	2.33	2.00
23	5.75	4.35	3.75	3.41	3.18	3.02	2.90	2.81	2.67	2.57	2.30	1.97
24	5.72	4.32	3.72	3.38	3.15	2.99	2.87	2.78	2.64	2.54	2.27	1.94
25	5.69	4.29	3.69	3.35	3.13	2.97	2.85	2.75	2.61	2.51	2.24	1.91
26	5.66	4.27	3.67	3.33	3.10	2.94	2.82	2.73	2.59	2.49	2.22	1.88
27	5.63	4.24	3.65	3.31	3.08	2.92	2.80	2.71	2.57	2.47	2.19	1.85
28	5.61	4.22	3.63	3.29	3.06	2.90	2.78	2.69	2.55	2.45	2.17	1.83
29	5.59	4.20	3.61	3.27	3.04	2.88	2.76	2.67	2.53	2.43	2.15	1.81
30	5.57	4.18	3.59	3.25	3.03	2.87	2.75	2.65	2.51	2.41	2.14	1.79
32	5.53	4.15	3.56	3.22	3.00	2.84	2.72	2.62	2.48	2.38	2.10	1.75
34	5.50	4.12	3.53	3.19	2.97	2.81	2.69	2.59	2.45	2.35	2.08	1.72
36	5.47	4.09	3.51	3.17	2.94	2.79	2.66	2.57	2.43	2.33	2.05	1.69
38	5.45	4.07	3.48	3.15	2.92	2.76	2.64	2.55	2.41	2.31	2.03	1.66
40	5.42	4.05	3.46	3.13	2.90	2.74	2.62	2.53	2.39	2.29	2.01	1.64
60	5.29	3.93	3.34	3.01	2.79	2.63	2.51	2.41	2.27	2.17	1.88	1.48
120	5.15	3.80	3.23	2.89	2.67	2.52	2.39	2.30	2.16	2.05	1.76	1.31
∞	5.02	3.69	3.12	2.79	2.57	2.41	2.29	2.19	2.05	1.94	1.64	1.00

NB When there is no exact number for the df, use the next lowest number. For very large dfs (i.e. well over 120) you should use the row for infinity, marked ∞.

These values are all for a two-tailed test only.

Table A2.6 (contd) Critical values of F (anovas) at various levels of probability. (For your F value to be significant at a particular probability level, it should be *equal to* or *larger* than the critical values associated with v_1 and v_2 in your study.)
c. Critical values of F at $p < .01$

v_2	v_1 1	2	3	4	5	6	7	8	10	12	24	∞
1	4052	5000	5403	5625	5764	5859	5928	5981	6056	6106	6235	6366
2	98.5	99.0	99.2	99.2	99.3	99.3	99.4	99.4	99.4	99.4	99.5	99.5
3	34.1	30.8	29.5	28.7	28.2	27.9	27.7	27.5	27.2	27.1	26.6	26.1
4	21.2	18.0	16.7	16.0	15.5	15.2	15.0	14.8	14.5	14.4	13.9	13.5
5	16.26	13.27	12.06	11.39	10.97	10.67	10.46	10.29	10.05	9.89	9.47	9.02
6	13.74	10.92	9.78	9.15	8.75	8.47	8.26	8.10	7.87	7.72	7.31	6.88
7	12.25	9.55	8.45	7.85	7.46	7.19	6.99	6.84	6.62	6.47	6.07	5.65
8	11.26	8.65	7.59	7.01	6.63	6.37	6.18	6.03	5.81	5.67	5.28	4.86
9	10.56	8.02	6.99	6.42	6.06	5.80	5.61	5.47	5.26	5.11	4.73	4.31
10	10.04	7.56	6.55	5.99	5.64	5.39	5.20	5.06	4.85	4.71	4.33	3.91
11	9.65	7.21	6.22	5.67	5.32	5.07	4.89	4.74	4.54	4.40	4.02	3.60
12	9.33	6.93	5.95	5.41	5.06	4.82	4.64	4.50	4.30	4.16	3.78	3.36
13	9.07	6.70	5.74	5.21	4.86	4.62	4.44	4.30	4.10	3.96	3.59	3.17
14	8.86	6.51	5.56	5.04	4.70	4.46	4.28	4.14	3.94	3.80	3.43	3.00
15	8.68	6.36	5.42	4.89	4.56	4.32	4.14	4.00	3.80	3.67	3.29	2.87
16	8.53	6.23	5.29	4.77	4.44	4.20	4.03	3.89	3.69	3.55	3.18	2.75
17	8.40	6.11	5.18	4.67	4.34	4.10	3.93	3.79	3.59	3.46	3.08	2.65
18	8.29	6.01	5.09	4.58	4.25	4.01	3.84	3.71	3.51	3.37	3.00	2.57
19	8.18	5.93	5.01	4.50	4.17	3.94	3.77	3.63	3.43	3.30	2.92	2.49
20	8.10	5.85	4.94	4.43	4.10	3.87	3.70	3.56	3.37	3.23	2.86	2.42
21	8.02	5.78	4.87	4.37	4.04	3.81	3.64	3.51	3.31	3.17	2.80	2.36
22	7.95	5.72	4.82	4.31	3.99	3.76	3.59	3.45	3.26	3.12	2.75	2.31
23	7.88	5.66	4.76	4.26	3.94	3.71	3.54	3.41	3.21	3.07	2.70	2.26
24	7.82	5.61	4.72	4.22	3.90	3.67	3.50	3.36	3.17	3.03	2.66	2.21
25	7.77	5.57	4.68	4.18	3.86	3.63	3.46	3.32	3.13	2.99	2.62	2.17
26	7.72	5.53	4.64	4.14	3.82	3.59	3.42	3.29	3.09	2.96	2.58	2.13
27	7.68	5.49	4.60	4.11	3.78	3.56	3.39	3.26	3.06	2.93	2.55	2.10
28	7.64	5.45	4.57	4.07	3.75	3.53	3.36	3.23	3.03	2.90	2.52	2.06
29	7.60	5.42	4.54	4.04	3.73	3.50	3.33	3.20	3.00	2.87	2.49	2.03
30	7.56	5.39	4.51	4.02	3.70	3.47	3.30	3.17	2.98	2.84	2.47	2.01
32	7.50	5.34	4.46	3.97	3.65	3.43	3.26	3.13	2.93	2.80	2.42	1.96
34	7.45	5.29	4.42	3.93	3.61	3.39	3.22	3.09	2.90	2.76	2.38	1.91
36	7.40	5.25	4.38	3.89	3.58	3.35	3.18	3.05	2.86	2.72	2.35	1.87
38	7.35	5.21	4.34	3.86	3.54	3.32	3.15	3.02	2.83	2.69	2.32	1.84
40	7.31	5.18	4.31	3.83	3.51	3.29	3.12	2.99	2.80	2.66	2.29	1.80
60	7.08	4.98	4.13	3.65	3.34	3.12	2.95	2.82	2.63	2.50	2.12	1.60
120	6.85	4.79	3.95	3.48	3.17	2.96	2.79	2.66	2.47	2.34	1.95	1.38
∞	6.63	4.61	3.78	3.32	3.02	2.80	2.64	2.51	2.32	2.18	1.79	1.00

NB When there is no exact number for the df, use the next lowest number. For very large dfs (i.e. well over 120) you should use the row for infinity, marked ∞.

These values are all for a two-tailed test only.

Table A2.6 (contd) Critical values of F (anovas) at various level of probability. (For your F value to be significant at a particular probability level, it should be *equal to* or *larger than* the critical values associated with v_1 and v_2 in your study.)
d. Critical values of F at $p < .001$

v_2	v_1 1	2	3	4	5	6	7	8	10	12	24	∞
1	*4053	5000	5404	5625	5764	5859	5929	5981	6056	6107	6235	6366*
2	998.5	999.0	999.2	999.2	999.3	999.3	999.4	999.4	999.4	999.4	999.5	999.5
3	167.0	148.5	141.1	137.1	134.6	132.8	131.5	130.6	129.2	128.3	125.9	123.5
4	74.14	61.25	56.18	53.44	51.71	50.53	49.66	49.00	48.05	47.41	45.77	44.05
5	47.18	37.12	33.20	31.09	29.75	28.83	28.16	27.65	26.92	26.42	25.14	23.79
6	35.51	27.00	23.70	21.92	20.80	20.03	19.46	19.03	18.41	17.99	16.90	15.75
7	29.25	21.69	18.77	17.20	16.21	15.52	15.02	14.63	14.08	13.71	12.73	11.70
8	25.42	18.49	15.83	14.39	13.48	12.86	12.40	12.05	11.54	11.19	10.30	9.34
9	22.86	16.39	13.90	12.56	11.71	11.13	10.69	10.37	9.87	9.57	8.72	7.81
10	21.04	14.91	12.55	11.28	10.48	9.93	9.52	9.20	8.74	8.44	7.64	6.76
11	19.69	13.81	11.56	10.35	9.58	9.05	8.66	8.35	7.92	7.63	6.85	6.00
12	18.64	12.97	10.80	9.63	8.89	8.38	8.00	7.71	7.29	7.00	6.25	5.42
13	17.82	12.31	10.21	9.07	8.35	7.86	7.49	7.21	6.80	6.52	5.78	4.97
14	17.14	11.78	9.73	8.62	7.92	7.44	7.08	6.80	6.40	6.13	5.41	4.60
15	16.59	11.34	9.34	8.25	7.57	7.09	6.74	6.47	6.08	5.81	5.10	4.31
16	16.12	10.97	9.01	7.94	7.27	6.80	6.46	6.19	5.81	5.55	4.85	4.06
17	15.72	10.66	8.73	7.68	7.02	6.56	6.22	5.96	5.58	5.32	4.63	3.85
18	15.38	10.39	8.49	7.46	6.81	6.35	6.02	5.76	5.39	5.13	4.45	3.67
19	15.08	10.16	8.28	7.27	6.62	6.18	5.85	5.59	5.22	4.97	4.29	3.51
20	14.82	9.95	8.10	7.10	6.46	6.02	5.69	5.44	5.08	4.82	4.15	3.38
21	14.59	9.77	7.94	6.95	6.32	5.88	5.56	5.31	4.95	4.70	4.03	3.26
22	14.38	9.61	7.80	6.81	6.19	5.76	5.44	5.19	4.83	4.58	3.92	3.15
23	14.19	9.47	7.67	6.70	6.08	5.65	5.33	5.09	4.73	4.48	3.82	3.05
24	14.03	9.34	7.55	6.59	5.98	5.55	5.23	4.99	4.64	4.39	3.74	2.97
25	13.88	9.22	7.45	6.49	5.89	5.46	5.15	4.91	4.56	4.31	3.66	2.89
26	13.74	9.12	7.36	6.41	5.80	5.38	5.07	4.83	4.48	4.24	3.59	2.82
27	13.61	9.02	7.27	6.33	5.73	5.31	5.00	4.76	4.41	4.17	3.52	2.75
28	13.50	8.93	7.19	6.25	5.66	5.24	4.93	4.69	4.35	4.11	3.46	2.69
29	13.39	8.85	7.12	6.19	5.59	5.18	4.87	4.64	4.29	4.05	3.41	2.64
30	13.29	8.77	7.05	6.12	5.53	5.12	4.82	4.58	4.24	4.00	3.36	2.59
32	13.12	8.64	6.94	6.01	5.43	5.02	4.72	4.48	4.14	3.91	3.27	2.50
34	12.97	8.52	6.83	5.92	5.34	4.93	4.63	4.40	4.06	3.83	3.19	2.42
36	12.83	8.42	6.74	5.84	5.26	4.86	4.56	4.33	3.99	3.76	3.12	2.35
38	12.71	8.33	6.66	5.76	5.19	4.79	4.49	4.26	3.93	3.70	3.06	2.29
40	12.61	8.25	6.59	5.70	5.13	4.73	4.44	4.21	3.87	3.64	3.01	2.23
60	11.97	7.77	6.17	5.31	4.76	4.37	4.09	3.86	3.54	3.32	2.69	1.89
120	11.38	7.32	5.78	4.95	4.42	4.04	3.77	3.55	3.24	3.02	2.40	1.54
∞	10.83	6.91	5.42	4.62	4.10	3.74	3.47	3.27	2.96	2.74	2.13	1.00

*Critical values to the right of V_2 = 1 should all be multiplied by 100, i.e. 4053 should be 40 5300.

NB When there is no exact number for the df, use the next lowest number. For very large dfs (i.e. well over 120) you should use the row for infinity, marked ∞.

These values are all for a two-tailed test only.

Table A2.7 Critical values of U (Mann–Whitney U test) at various levels of probability. For your U value to be significant at a particular probability level, it should be *equal to* or *less than* the critical value associated with n_1 and n_2 in your study. (Reproduced from Runyon R, Haber A (1991) Fundamentals of Behavioral Statistics 7th edn. with permission of McGraw-Hill Inc.)

a. Critical values of U for a one-tailed test at .005; two-tailed test at .01*

n_2	n_1 1	2	3	4	5	6	7	8	9	10	11	12	13	14	15	16	17	18	19	20
1	-	-	-	-	-	-	-	-	-	-	-	-	-	-	-	-	-	-	-	-
2	-	-	-	-	-	-	-	-	-	-	-	-	-	-	-	-	-	-	0	0
3	-	-	-	-	-	-	-	-	0	0	0	1	1	1	2	2	2	2	3	3
4	-	-	-	-	-	0	0	1	1	2	2	3	3	4	5	5	6	6	7	8
5	-	-	-	-	0	1	1	2	3	4	5	6	7	7	8	9	10	11	12	13
6	-	-	-	0	1	2	3	4	5	6	7	9	10	11	12	13	15	16	17	18
7	-	-	-	0	1	3	4	6	7	9	10	12	13	15	16	18	19	21	22	24
8	-	-	-	1	2	4	6	7	9	11	13	15	17	18	20	22	24	26	28	30
9	-	-	0	1	3	5	7	9	11	13	16	18	20	22	24	27	29	31	33	36
10	-	-	0	2	4	6	9	11	13	16	18	21	24	26	29	31	34	37	39	42
11	-	-	0	2	5	7	10	13	16	18	21	24	27	30	33	36	39	42	45	48
12	-	-	1	3	6	9	12	15	18	21	24	27	31	34	37	41	44	47	51	54
13	-	-	1	3	7	10	13	17	20	24	27	31	34	38	42	45	49	53	56	60
14	-	-	1	4	7	11	15	18	22	26	30	34	38	42	46	50	54	58	63	67
15	-	-	2	5	8	12	16	20	24	29	33	37	42	46	51	55	60	64	69	73
16	-	-	2	5	9	13	18	22	27	31	36	41	45	50	55	60	65	70	74	79
17	-	-	2	6	10	15	19	24	29	34	39	44	49	54	60	65	70	75	81	86
18	-	-	2	6	11	16	21	26	31	37	42	47	53	58	64	70	75	81	87	92
19	-	0	3	7	12	17	22	28	33	39	45	51	56	63	69	74	81	87	93	99
20	-	0	3	8	13	18	24	30	36	42	48	54	60	67	73	79	86	92	99	105

*Dashes in the table mean that no decision is possible for those n values at the given level of significance.

b. Critical values of U for a one-tailed test at .01; two-tailed test at .02*

n_2	n_1 1	2	3	4	5	6	7	8	9	10	11	12	13	14	15	16	17	18	19	20
1	-	-	-	-	-	-	-	-	-	-	-	-	-	-	-	-	-	-	-	-
2	-	-	-	-	-	-	-	-	-	-	-	-	0	0	0	0	0	0	1	1
3	-	-	-	-	-	-	0	0	1	1	1	2	2	2	3	3	4	4	4	5
4	-	-	-	-	0	1	1	2	3	3	4	5	5	6	7	7	8	9	9	10
5	-	-	-	0	1	2	3	4	5	6	7	8	9	10	11	12	13	14	15	16
6	-	-	-	1	2	3	4	6	7	8	9	11	12	13	15	16	18	19	20	22
7	-	-	0	1	3	4	6	7	9	11	12	14	16	17	19	21	23	24	26	28
8	-	-	0	2	4	6	7	9	11	13	15	17	20	22	24	26	28	30	32	34
9	-	-	1	3	5	7	9	11	14	16	18	21	23	26	28	31	33	36	38	40
10	-	-	1	3	6	8	11	13	16	19	22	24	27	30	33	36	38	41	44	47
11	-	-	1	4	7	9	12	15	18	22	25	28	31	34	37	41	44	47	50	53
12	-	-	2	5	8	11	14	17	21	24	28	31	35	38	42	46	49	53	56	60
13	-	0	2	5	9	12	16	20	23	27	31	35	39	43	47	51	55	59	63	67
14	-	0	2	6	10	13	17	22	26	30	34	38	43	47	51	56	60	65	69	73
15	-	0	3	7	11	15	19	24	28	33	37	42	47	51	56	61	66	70	75	80
16	-	0	3	7	12	16	21	26	31	36	41	46	51	56	61	66	71	76	82	87
17	-	0	4	8	13	18	23	28	33	38	44	49	55	60	66	71	77	82	88	93
18	-	0	4	9	14	19	24	30	36	41	47	53	59	65	70	76	82	88	94	100
19	-	1	4	9	15	20	26	32	38	44	50	56	63	69	75	82	88	94	101	107
20	-	1	5	10	16	22	28	34	40	47	53	60	67	73	80	87	93	100	107	114

*Dashes in the table mean that no decision is possible for those n values at the given level of significance.

Table A2.7 Critical values of U (Mann-Whitney U test) at various levels of probability. (For your U value to be significant at a particular probability level, it should be *equal to* or *less than* the critical value associated with n_1 and n_2 in your study.)

c. Critical values of U for a one-tailed test at .025; two-tailed test at .05*

n_2																				
	1	2	3	4	5	6	7	8	9	10	11	12	13	14	15	16	17	18	19	20
1	-	-	-	-	-	-	-	-	-	-	-	-	-	-	-	-	-	-	-	-
2	-	-	-	-	-	-	-	0	0	0	0	1	1	1	1	1	2	2	2	2
3	-	-	-	-	0	1	1	2	2	3	3	4	4	5	5	6	6	7	7	8
4	-	-	-	0	1	2	3	4	4	5	6	7	8	9	10	11	11	12	13	13
5	-	-	0	1	2	3	5	6	7	8	9	11	12	13	14	15	17	18	19	20
6	-	-	1	2	3	5	6	8	10	11	13	14	16	17	19	21	22	24	25	27
7	-	-	1	3	5	6	8	10	12	14	16	18	20	22	24	26	28	30	32	34
8	-	0	2	4	6	8	10	13	15	17	19	22	24	26	29	31	34	36	38	41
9	-	0	2	4	7	10	12	15	17	20	23	26	28	31	34	37	39	42	45	48
10	-	0	3	5	8	11	14	17	20	23	26	29	33	36	39	42	45	48	52	55
11	-	0	3	6	9	13	16	19	23	26	30	33	37	40	44	47	51	55	58	62
12	-	1	4	7	11	14	18	22	26	29	33	37	41	45	49	53	57	61	65	69
13	-	1	4	8	12	16	20	24	28	33	37	41	45	50	54	59	63	67	72	76
14	-	1	5	9	13	17	22	26	31	36	40	45	50	55	59	64	67	74	78	83
15	-	1	5	10	14	19	24	29	34	39	44	49	54	59	64	70	75	80	85	90
16	-	1	6	11	15	21	26	31	37	42	47	53	59	64	70	75	81	86	92	98
17	-	2	6	11	17	22	28	34	39	45	51	57	63	67	75	81	87	93	99	105
18	-	2	7	12	18	24	30	36	42	48	55	61	67	74	80	86	93	99	106	112
19	-	2	7	13	19	25	32	38	45	52	58	65	72	78	85	92	99	106	113	119
20	-	2	8	13	20	27	34	41	48	55	62	69	76	83	90	98	105	112	119	127

*Dashes in the table mean that no decision is possible for those n values at the given level of significance.

d. Critical values of U for a one-tailed test at .05; two-tailed test at .10*

n_2	1	2	3	4	5	6	7	8	9	10	11	12	13	14	15	16	17	18	19	20
1	-	-	-	-	-	-	-	-	-	-	-	-	-	-	-	-	-	-	0	0
2	-	-	-	-	0	0	0	1	1	1	1	2	2	2	3	3	3	4	4	4
3	-	-	0	0	1	2	2	3	3	4	5	5	6	7	7	8	9	9	10	11
4	-	-	0	1	2	3	4	5	6	7	8	9	10	11	12	14	15	16	17	18
5	-	0	1	2	4	5	6	8	9	11	12	13	15	16	18	19	20	22	23	25
6	-	0	2	3	5	7	8	10	12	14	16	17	19	21	23	25	26	28	30	32
7	-	0	2	4	6	8	11	13	15	17	19	21	24	26	28	30	33	35	37	39
8	-	1	3	5	8	10	13	15	18	20	23	26	28	31	33	36	39	41	44	47
9	-	1	3	6	9	12	15	18	21	24	27	30	33	36	39	42	45	48	51	54
10	-	1	4	7	11	14	17	20	24	27	31	34	37	41	44	48	51	55	58	62
11	-	1	5	8	12	16	19	23	27	31	34	38	42	46	50	54	57	61	65	69
12	-	2	5	9	13	17	21	26	30	34	38	42	47	51	55	60	64	68	72	77
13	-	2	6	10	15	19	24	28	33	37	42	47	51	56	61	65	70	75	80	84
14	-	2	7	11	16	21	26	31	36	41	46	51	56	61	66	71	77	82	87	92
15	-	3	7	12	18	23	28	33	39	44	50	55	61	66	72	77	83	88	94	100
16	-	3	8	14	19	25	30	36	42	48	54	60	65	71	77	83	89	95	101	107
17	-	3	9	15	20	26	33	39	45	51	57	64	70	77	83	89	96	102	109	115
18	-	4	9	16	22	28	35	41	48	55	61	68	75	82	88	95	102	109	116	123
19	0	4	10	17	23	30	37	44	51	58	65	72	80	87	94	101	109	116	123	130
20	0	4	11	18	25	32	39	47	54	62	69	77	84	92	100	107	115	123	130	138

*Dashes in the table mean that no desicison is possible for those n values at the given level of significance.

Table A2.8 Critical values of *H* (Kruskal-Wallis test) at various levels of probability. (For your *H* value to be significant at a particular probability level, it should be *equal to* or *larger than* the critical values associated with the *ns* in your study.)

Size of groups					Size of groups				
n_1	n_2	n_3	*H*	*p*	n_1	n_2	n_3	*H*	*p*
2	1	1	2.7000	.500	4	3	1	5.8333	.021
2	2	1	3.6000	.200				5.2083	.050
2	2	2	4.5714	.067				5.0000	.057
			3.7143	.200				4.0556	.093
3	1	1	3.2000	.300				3.8889	.129
3	2	1	4.2857	.100	4	3	2	6.4444	.008
			3.8571	.133				6.3000	.011
3	2	2	5.3572	.029				5.4444	.046
			4.7143	.048				5.4000	.051
			4.5000	.067				4.5111	.098
			4.4643	.105				4.4444	.102
3	3	1	5.1429	.043	4	3	3	6.7455	.010
			4.5714	.100				6.7091	.013
			4.0000	.129				5.7909	.046
3	3	2	6.2500	.011				5.7273	.050
			5.3611	.032				4.7091	.092
			5.1389	.061				4.7000	.101
			4.5556	.100	4	4	1	6.6667	.010
			4.2500	.121				6.1667	.022
3	3	3	7.2000	.004				4.9667	.048
			6.4889	.011				4.8667	.054
			5.6889	.029				4.1667	.082
			5.6000	.050				4.0667	.102
			5.0667	.086	4	4	2	7.0364	.006
			4.6222	.100				6.8727	.011
4	1	1	3.5714	.200				5.4545	.046
4	2	1	4.8214	.057				5.2364	.052
			4.5000	.076				4.5545	.098
			4.0179	.114				4.4455	.103
4	2	2	6.0000	.014	4	4	3	7.1439	.010
			5.3333	.033				7.1364	.011
			5.1250	.052				5.5985	.049
			4.4583	.100				5.5758	.051
			4.1667	.105				4.5455	.099
								4.4773	.102
					4	4	4	7.6538	.008
								7.5385	.011
								5.6923	.049
								5.6538	.054
								4.6539	.097
								4.5001	.104

NB These values are all for a two-tailed test only.

Table A2.8 (contd) Critical values of H (Kruskal-Wallis test) at various levels of probability. (For your H values to be significant at a particular probability level, it should be *equal to* or *larger than* the critical values associated with the ns in your study.)

Size of groups					Size of groups				
n_1	n_2	n_3	H	p	n_1	n_2	n_3	H	p
5	1	1	3.8571	.143	5	4	3	7.4449	.010
5	2	1	5.2500	.036				7.3949	.011
			5.0000	.048				5.6564	.049
			4.4500	.071				5.6308	.050
			4.2000	.095				4.5487	.099
			4.0500	.119				4.5231	.103
5	2	2	6.5333	.008	5	4	4	7.7604	.009
			6.1333	.013				7.7440	.011
			5.1600	.034				5.6571	.049
			5.0400	.056				5.6176	.050
			4.3733	.090				4.6187	.100
			4.2933	.122				4.5527	.102
5	3	1	6.4000	.012	5	5	1	7.3091	.009
			4.9600	.048				6.8364	.011
			4.8711	.052				5.1273	.046
			4.0178	.095				4.9091	.053
			3.8400	.123				4.1091	.086
5	3	2	6.9091	.009				4.0364	.105
			6.8218	.010	5	5	2	7.3385	.010
			5.2509	.049				7.2692	.010
			5.1055	.052				5.3385	.047
			4.6509	.091				5.2462	.051
			4.4945	.101				4.6231	.097
5	3	3	7.0788	.009				4.5077	.100
			6.9818	.011	5	5	3	7.5780	.010
			5.6485	.049				7.5429	.010
			5.5152	.051				5.7055	.046
			4.5333	.097				5.6264	.051
			4.4121	.109				4.5451	.100
5	4	1	6.9545	.008				4.5363	.102
			6.8400	.011	5	5	4	7.8229	.010
			4.9855	.044				7.7914	.010
			4.8600	.056				5.6657	.049
			3.9873	.098				5.6429	.050
			3.9600	.102				4.5229	.099
5	4	2	7.2045	.009				4.5200	.101
			7.1182	.010	5	5	5	8.0000	.009
			5.2727	.049				7.9800	.010
			5.2682	.050				7.7800	.049
			4.5409	.098				5.6600	.051
			4.5182	.101				4.5600	.100
								4.5000	.102

NB These values are all for a two-tailed test only.

Table A2.9 Critical values of S (Jonckheere trend test) at various levels of probability.
(For your S value to be significant at a particular probability level, it should be *equal to* or *larger than* the critical values associated with C and n in your study.)

a. Significance level $p < .05$

					n				
C	2	3	4	5	6	7	8	9	10
3	10	17	24	33	42	53	64	76	88
4	14	26	38	51	66	82	100	118	138
5	20	34	51	71	92	115	140	166	194
6	26	44	67	93	121	151	184	219	256

b. Significance level $p < .01$

3	-	23	32	45	59	74	90	106	124
4	20	34	50	71	92	115	140	167	195
5	26	48	72	99	129	162	197	234	274
6	34	62	94	130	170	213	260	309	361

NB These values are all for a one-tailed test only.

Table A2.10 Critical values of r_s (Spearman test) at various levels of probability.
(For your r_s value to be significant at a particular probability level, it should be *equal to* or *larger* than the critical values associated with N in your study.)

N (number of subjects)	Level of significance for one-tailed test			
	.05	.025	.01	.005
	Level of significance for two-tailed test			
	.10	.05	.02	.01
5	.900	1.000	1.000	-
6	.829	.886	.943	1.000
7	.714	.786	.893	.929
8	.643	.738	.833	.881
9	.600	.683	.783	.833
10	.564	.648	.746	.794
12	.506	.591	.712	.777
14	.456	.544	.645	.715
16	.425	.506	.601	.665
18	.399	.475	.564	.625
20	.377	.450	.534	.591
22	.359	.428	.508	.562
24	.343	.409	.485	.537
26	.329	.392	.465	.515
28	.317	.377	.448	.496
30	.306	.364	.432	.478

NB When there is no exact number of subjects use the next lowest number.

Table A2.11 Critical values of r (Pearson test) at various levels of probability. (For your r value to be significant at a particular probability level, it should be *equal to* or *larger* than the critical values associated with the *df* in your study. (Reproduced with kind permission of Longman Group Limited.)

df = N – 2	Level of significance for one-tailed test				
	.05	.025	.01	.005	.0005
	Level of significance for two-tailed test				
	.01	.05	.02	.01	.001
1	.9877	.9969	.9995	.9999	1.0000
2	.9000	.9500	.9800	.9900	.9990
3	.8054	.8783	.9343	.9587	.9912
4	.7293	.8114	.8822	.9172	.9741
5	.6694	.7545	.8329	.8745	.9507
6	.6215	.7067	.7887	.8343	.9249
7	.5822	.6664	.7498	.7977	.8982
8	.5494	.6319	.7155	.7646	.8721
9	.5214	.6021	.6851	.7348	.8471
10	.4973	.5760	.6581	.7079	.8233
11	.4762	.5529	.6339	.6835	.8010
12	.4575	.5324	.6120	.6614	.7800
13	.4409	.5139	.5923	.6411	.7603
14	.4259	.4973	.5742	.6226	.7420
15	.4124	.4821	.5577	.6055	.7246
16	.4000	.4683	.5425	.5897	.7084
17	.3887	.4555	.5285	.5751	.6932
18	.3783	.4438	.5155	.5614	.6787
19	.3687	.4329	.5034	.5487	.6652
20	.3598	.4227	.4921	.5368	.6524
25	.3233	.3809	.4451	.4869	.5974
30	.2960	.3494	.4093	.4487	.5541
35	.2746	.3246	.3810	.4182	.5189
40	.2573	.3044	.3578	.3932	.4896
45	.2428	.2875	.3384	.3721	.4648
50	.2306	.2732	.3218	.3541	.4433
60	.2108	.2500	.2948	.3248	.4078
70	.1954	.2319	.2737	.3017	.3799
80	.1829	.2172	.2565	.2830	.3568
90	.1726	.2050	.2422	.2673	.3375
100	.1638	.1946	.2301	.2540	.3211

NB When there is no exact df use the next lowest number.

Table A2.12 Critical values of s (Kendall's coefficient of concordance) at various levels of probability. (For your s value to be significant at a particular probability level, it should be *equal to* or *larger than* the critical values associated with C and N in your study.)

a. Critical values of s at p = 0.05

C	$N = 3$	$N = 4$	$N = 5$	$N = 6$	$N = 7$
3	-	-	64.4	103.9	157.3
4	-	49.5	88.4	143.3	217.0
5	-	62.6	112.3	182.4	276.2
6	-	75.7	136.1	221.4	335.2
8	48.1	101.7	183.7	299.0	453.1
10	60.0	127.8	231.2	376.7	571.0
15	89.8	192.9	349.8	570.5	864.9
20	119.7	258.0	468.5	764.4	1158.7

b. Critical values of s at p = 0.01

C	$N = 3$	$N = 4$	$N = 5$	$N = 6$	$N = 7$
3	-	-	75.6	122.8	185.6
4	-	61.4	109.3	176.2	265.0
5	-	80.5	142.8	229.4	343.8
6	-	99.5	176.1	282.4	422.6
8	66.8	137.4	242.7	388.3	579.9
10	85.1	175.3	309.1	494.0	737.0
15	131.0	269.8	475.2	758.2	1129.5
20	177.0	364.2	641.2	1022.2	1521.9

NB The values are all for a one-tailed test only.

A dash in the table means that no decision can be made at this level.

Appendix 3

Answers to Activities

Chapter 1

Activity 1.1

1. 46
2. –2
3. 43
4. 253
5. 65
6. 49
7. 54
8. 11
9. 104
10. 47
11. –6
12. –8
13. –48
14. –44
15. 42
16. –48
17. 45
18. –13
19. +7
20. –240

Chapter 4

Activity 4.1

The following are examples of nominal levels of measurement. Any variation on these which still involved allocating patients to a category is acceptable.

1. You might measure improvement in incontinence by asking the woman 'Did you experience any improvement following therapy?'
   Yes/No
2. This might be measured by categorizing the reported pain levels for a breech delivery as (a) no reduction in pain or (b) reduction in pain.
3. You assess whether or not a woman experienced a reduction in perineal pain following a warm bath by allocating her to either (a) reduction in pain category or (b) no reduction in pain category.

4. Women could be classified as those who kept appointments and those who did not.
5. This might be assessed by asking women to answer the following question. Did you find the ante-natal care

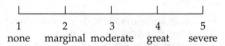

acceptable [   ]   not acceptable [   ]

Activity 4.2

Again, any variation on the answers suggested below is acceptable as long as you are rank ordering your data according to the dimension you are interested in.

1. Improvement in incontinence might be measured by asking the women to answer the following question:
   To what extent did your incontinence improve following therapy?

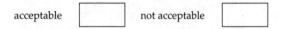

1	2	3	4	5
very much	better	about the	worse	very much
better		same		worse

   Alternatively, you could rank order your subjects according to how much they improved.

2. This might be measured by assessing the reported pain along a scale thus: the level of pain during a breech delivery was:

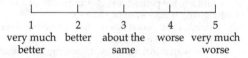

| 1 | 2 | 3 | 4 | 5 |
| none | marginal | moderate | great | severe |

   Similarly you could rank order the patients according to their reported pain.

3. Reduction in pain could be assessed by either rank ordering the subjects from the greatest reduction in pain to the smallest reduction, or alternatively you could use a point scale thus:

The reduction in pain following a warm bath was:

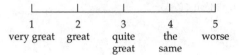

1	2	3	4	5
very great	great	quite great	the same	worse

4. Likelihood of keeping appointments could be assessed by a point scale thus: how likely is this woman to keep an appointment at the outpatients' clinic?

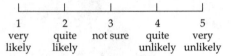

1	2	3	4	5
very likely	quite likely	not sure	quite unlikely	very unlikely

5. Assessing the quality of ante-natal care could be conducted along similar lines: How would you rate the quality of the ante-natal care you received?

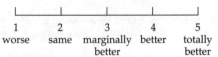

1	2	3	4	5	6	7
excellent	very good	good	average	poor	very poor	appalling

Activity 4.3

1. You could measure incontinence on an interval/ratio scale simply by monitoring the number of times a woman was incontinent or the number of ccs of urine voided accidentally.
2. Reported pain during a breech delivery could be assessed by noting the amount of analgesia used.
3. Perineal pain could be measured as above or on a visual analogue scale.
4. The number of appointments kept and missed could be monitored for each woman.
5. You could ask the patients to rate the quality of ante-natal care by giving it marks out of 20 or 100.
6. (i) Efficiency of breast shells for correcting inverted nipples could be measured
   — on a nominal scale by allocating the results to either (a) improved or (b) not improved
   — on an ordinal scale by assessing the level of improvement on, say, a 5-point scale:

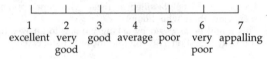

1	2	3	4	5
worse	same	marginally better	better	totally better

   — on an interval/ratio scale by measuring the extent of nipple protrusion in mm.
   (ii) Improvement in carpal tunnel syndrome 3 months post-delivery could be measured:
   — on a nominal scale by classifying the women according to whether they:
   a. experienced an improvement or
   b. experienced no improvement
   — on an ordinal scale using a point scale thus:
   What degree of improvement did this woman experience?

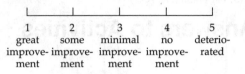

1	2	3	4	5
great improvement	some improvement	minimal improvement	no improvement	deteriorated

   — on an interval/ratio scale by measuring the strength of grasp on a pressure scale.
   (iii) Experience of pain during stitching of an episiotomy could be measured
   — on a nominal scale by classifying women according to whether they experienced pain, or did not experience pain
   — on an ordinal scale by using a point scale thus:
   How much pain did you experience during stitching?

1	2	3	4
very great pain	great pain	some pain	no pain

   — on an interval/ratio scale by finding out the amount of analgesia required.

7. (i) Nominal
   (ii) Ordinal (or interval if equal distances between points are assumed)
   (iii) Interval/ratio
   (iv) Interval/ratio
   (v) Interval/ratio

Chapter 5

Activity 5.1

1. (a) Histogram (Fig. A3.1)

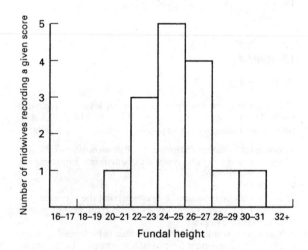

Figure A3.1

(b) Bar graph (Fig. A3.2)

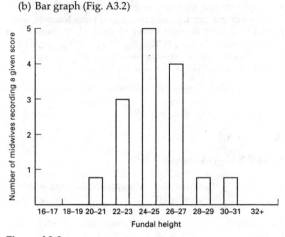

Figure A3.2

(c) Frequency polygon (Fig. A3.3)

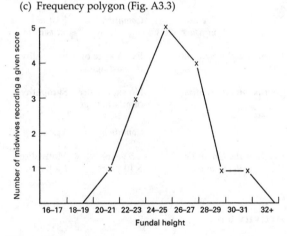

Figure A3.3

2. Frequency polygon with reduced number of units along horizontal axis (Fig. A3.4)

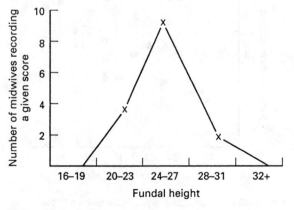

Figure A3.4

Activity 5.2

1. (i) Mean: 70.333
        Median: 76
        Mode: 76
    (ii) Mean: 28.667
         Median: 27
         Mode: 17
    (iii) Mean: 50.1
          Median: 47.5
          Mode: 43
2. Set of data (i) has the largest range of scores while (ii) has the smallest.

Activity 5.3

1. (i) Range: 24
         Deviation: 14 – 19.444 = – 5.444
                      9 – 19.444 = –10.444
                     21 – 19.444 = +1.556
                     23 – 19.444 = +3.556
                     18 – 19.444 = –1.444
                     17 – 19.444 = –2.444
                     33 – 19.444 = +13.556
                     28 – 19.444 = +8.556
                     12 – 19.444 = –7.444
         Variance: 52.691
         Standard deviation: 7.259

    (ii) Range: 33
          Deviation: 71 – 67.571 = +3.429
                      50 – 67.571 = –17.571
                      48 – 67.571 = –19.571
                      64 – 67.571 = –3.571
                      80 – 67.571 = +12.429
                      81 – 67.571 = +13.429
                      79 – 67.571 = +11.429
          Variance: 168.816
          Standard deviation: 12.993

2. You might assess the reliability of the scales by taking five neonates and asking ten different midwives to weigh them. For each set of ten readings you might calculate the mean and the median to assess the homogeneity or similarity of the scores. You might also wish to calculate the range and the standard deviation to find out how disparate the readings are.

Activity 5.4

1. 95% of women will have heart rates of between 66 and 98 during weeks 10–20 of pregnancy.
2. 2.36% of women will have heart rates of between 99 and 106.
3. This woman comes in 0.135% of the population in terms of heart rate.

Chapter 6

Activity 6.1

The two variables in each hypothesis are:

1. Incidence of placenta praevia and parity.
2. Use of alkaline preparations and the chance of developing anaemia.
3. Social class and likelihood of breast feeding.
4. Incidence of costal margin pain and maternal height.
5. Intake of calcium-rich foods and incidence of cramp.

Activity 6.2

The null hypotheses are:
1. There is no relationship between the incidence of placenta praevia and parity.
2. There is no relationship between the use of alkaline preparations and the chance of developing anaemia.
3. There is no relationship between social class and likelihood of breast feeding.
4. There is no relationship between the incidence of costal margin pain and maternal height.
5. There is no relationship between the intake of calcium-rich foods and the incidence of cramp.

Activity 6.3

1. IV = type of birth.
   DV = incidence of UTI.
   IV manipulated by selecting one group of women having water births and one group of women having 'land' deliveries.
2. IV = treatment.
   DV = reduction of round ligament pain.
   IV manipulated by selecting a number of women having round ligament pain and randomly allocating half to the heat treatment group and the remainder to the no-treatment group.
3. IV = length of wait.
   DV = blood pressure.
   IV manipulated by selecting one group of women who have waited less than 2 hours at the ante-natal clinic and another group who have waited more than 2 hours.
4. IV = type of induction.
   DV = neonatal outcome.
   IV manipulated by selecting one group of women who have had artificial rupture of the membranes and a second group who have had prostaglandin pessaries.
5. IV = use of electronic fetal monitoring.
   DV = caesarean section.
   IV manipulated by selecting a number of women who have had electronic fetal monitoring and a further group who have not.

Activity 6.4

Other possible explanations for a more tolerant attitude amongst these midwives might be:

1. Simply the fact that they were a bit older and therefore a bit wiser and perhaps as a result a bit more tolerant.
2. Having a baby themselves which made them more aware of the woman's perspective.
3. Reading a book on attitude change.
4. Attending another sort of course.

Plus, of course, many other possible reasons.

Activity 6.5

Designs for hypotheses on page 53.

1.

	Pre-test measure of DV	Condition	Post-test measure of DV
Experimental Group	Compliance	Information	Compliance
Control Group	Compliance	No Information	Compliance

2.

	Pre-test measure of DV	Condition	Post-test measure of DV
Experimental	Sympathy	Experience of miscarriage	Sympathy
Control Group	Sympathy	No experience of miscarriage	Sympathy

3.

	Condition	Measure of DV
Experimental Group 1	< 5 years	Motivation
Experimental Group 2	> 10 years	Motivation

Activity 6.6

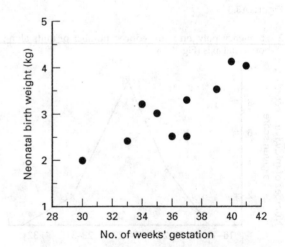

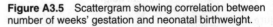

Figure A3.5 Scattergram showing correlation between number of weeks' gestation and neonatal birthweight.

Activity 6.7

1. (i) A positive correlation is predicted, with high scores on age being associated with high scores on labour time. This would be represented by a general upward slope on a scattergram and a correlation coefficient of around +1.0.
   (ii) A negative correlation is predicted with high scores on distance being associated with low scores on attendance. This would be represented by a general downward slope on a scattergram and a correlation coefficient of around −1.0.
   (iii) A positive correlation is predicted with low scores on GCSEs being associated with low final exam scores. An upward slope and a correlation coefficient of around +1.0 would be anticipated.
   (iv) A negative correlation is predicted with high scores on fibre intake being associated with low scores on incidence of constipation during the third trimester. A general downward slope and a correlation coefficient of around −1.0 would be predicted.

2. From strongest to weakest, the coefficients are:

   $-0.73 \quad +0.61 \quad -0.42 \quad +0.21 \quad -0.17 \quad +0.09$

Chapter 8

Activity 8.1

Some of the constant and random errors involved in these experiments are outlined in Tables A3.1 and A3.2. You may have thought of many more.

Table A3.1 Hypothesis: Premature babies nursed on sheepskins gain weight more quickly than those nursed on cotton sheeting

Constant error	Solution	Random error	Solution
1. Weeks gestational	Ensure both groups are of comparable gestation	1. Individual personality differences	Random Selection of babies in each group
2. Condition	Ensure both groups in comparable condition	2. Subtle differences in staff treatment/ attitudes	
3. Birth weight	Both groups of similar birth weight	3. Biochemical make-up	
4. Gender	Ensure both groups have had similar number of male: females	4. Inherent and undetected lung defects	
5. Mother a smoker/ non-smoker	Ensure that no mother of either group smokes		

Table A3.2 Hypothesis: Mothers who drink more than 14 units of alcohol per week during pregnancy are more likely to deliver pre-term

Constant error	Solution	Random error	Solution
1. Age of mother	Ensure both groups of women are of comparable age	1. Unidentified physiological/ anatomical causes	
2. Raised blood pressure	Ensure there is no raised blood pressure in either group	2. Personality of woman	
3. Health of woman	Ensure comparability of health in both groups	3. Attitude of woman	Randomly select patients from each situation to take part in the experiment
4. Previous premature deliveries	Ensure both groups have had no previous premature deliveries	4. Biochemical make-up	
5. Placental insufficiency	Ensure that there is no evidence of placental insufficiency in either group	5. Shock/Stress	

Activity 8.2

From greatest support to least:

$p = 0.01\% \quad p = 3\% \quad p = 5\% \quad p = 7\% \quad p = 15\% \quad p = 19\%$

Converted to a decimal:
$p = 0.0001 \quad p = 0.03 \quad p = 0.05 \quad p = 0.07 \quad p = 0.15 \quad p = 0.19$

Activity 8.3

See Table A3.3

Table A3.3

	% probability that the results are due to chance
$p = 0.01$	1%
$p = 0.07$	7%
$p = 0.03$	3%
$p = 0.05$	5%
$p = 0.50$	50%

Chapter 9

Activity 9.1

1. Chi-squared test (data are nominal).
2. Related *t*-test or Wilcoxon.
3. Pearson or Spearman.
4. Mann-Whitney U test (data are ordinal).
5. Friedman or one-way anova for related samples.
6. Kruskal-Wallis.

Activity 9.2

1. one-tailed (*more* effective)
2. two-tailed (*different* effects)
3. one-tailed (*more* likely to have an operative delivery)
4. two-tailed (*difference* in length)
5. one-tailed (*greater* take-up)

Converting the one-tailed hypotheses to two-tailed.
1. There is a difference in the effectiveness of parent craft classes according to whether one or both partners attend.
2. There is a difference in the number of operative deliveries according to maternal weight at conception.
3. There is a relationship between pre-conceptual counselling and the take-up of ante-natal services.

Converting the two-tailed hypotheses to one-tailed.
1. Forceps deliveries have a better effect on maternal well-being than ventouse extractions.
2. White Caucasian women have longer second-stage labours than African-Caribbean women.

Chapter 13

Activity 13.1

1. (i) $p < 0.025$ significant
   (ii) $p < 0.005$ significant
   (iii) $p = 0.02$ significant
   (iv) p is *greater than* 0.05, and is therefore not significant
   (v) $p < 0.001$ significant
   (vi) $p < 0.05$ significant

2. $\chi^2 = 9.6$; $p < 0.01$
   Using the McNemar test ($\chi^2 = 9.6$) the results were significant $p < 0.01$ (two-tailed). These results suggest that providing information about the reasons for changing the shift system significantly modifies midwives' opinions.

Activity 13.2

1. See Table A3.4

Table A3.4

Subject	Condition A	Condition B	d	Rank
1	10	9	+ 1	3.5
2	8	9	− 1	3.5
3	9	7	+ 2	7
4	6	7	− 1	3.5

Table A3.4   *(cont'd)*

Subject	Condition A	Condition B	d	Rank
5	5	4	+ 1	3.5
6	8	3	+ 5	11
7	7	6	+ 1	3.5
8	9	9	0	omit
9	9	6	+ 3	8
10	5	6	− 1	3.5
11	7	3	+ 4	9.5
12	8	4	+ 4	9.5

2. (i) $p < 0.05$ significant
   (ii) $p < 0.01$ significant
   (iii) $p < 0.025$ significant
   (iv) $p < 0.01$ significant
   (v) $p < 0.1$ not significant
   (vi) $p < 0.05$ significant
   (vii) $p = 0.01$ significant
   (viii) $p < 0.01$ significant

3. $T = 0$
   $N = 9$
   $p < 0.005$, one-tailed
   Using a Wilcoxon on the data ($T = 0$, $N = 9$) the results were found to be significant at $p < 0.005$ (one-tailed). These results support the hypothesis that reported satisfaction with care is significantly greater when the mother has taken an active role in managing her labour, than when she has been passive or peripheral.

Activity 13.3

1. (i) $p = 0.033$ significant
   (ii) $p < 0.02$ significant
   (iii) $p < 0.072$ not significant
   (iv) $p < 0.001$ significant
   (v) $p < 0.008$ significant
   (If you got any of these wrong, or are confused about the answers, do check that you were using the correct table, see p. 133).
2. $\chi r^2 = 2.658$, $p < 0.305$; not significant
   Using a Friedman test to analyse the data, the results were not significant ($\chi r^2 = 2.658$, $p < 0.305$). This suggests that there is no significant difference in the reported pain during labour according to whether the mother was mobile, in a bathing chair or supine. The null hypothesis can therefore be accepted.

Activity 13.4

1. (i) $p < 0.01$ significant
   (ii) $p = 0.05$ significant
   (iii) $p < 0.05$ significant
   (iv) $p < 0.001$ significant
   (v) p is greater than 0.05 and is therefore not significant.

2. $L = 105$ $p < 0.05$
   Using the Page's L trend test to analyse the data, the results were significant ($L = 105$, $p < 0.05$). These results support the experimental hypothesis that sheepskins are

more effective than terry-towelling, which in turn is more effective than cotton sheeting in reducing crying amongst premature babies.

Chapter 14

Activity 14.1

1. (i) $p < 0.025$ significant
   (ii) $p < 0.1$ not significant
   (iii) $p < 0.01$ significant
   (iv) $p < 0.001$ significant
   (v) $p < 0.02$ significant

2. $t = 2.362$; d.f. = 11; $p < 0.025$
   Using a related t-test to analyse the data, the results were found to be significant at $p < 0.025$ ($t = 2.362$, d.f. = 11). This suggests that direct entry student midwives with 'A'- level biology do better in their 1st year theory exam marks, than students without 'A'-level biology. The null hypothesis can therefore be rejected in favour of the experimental hypothesis.

Activity 14.2

1. (i) $p < 0.05$ significant
   (ii) $p < 0.01$ significant
   (iii) p is greater than 0.05 and is therefore not significant
   (iv) $p < 0.025$ significant
   (v) $p < 0.05$ significant
   (vi) $p < 0.025$ significant

2. See Table A3.5

Table A3.5

Source of variation in scores	SS	d.f.	MS	F ratios
Variation in scores (*between conditions*)	31.445	2	15.723	3.529
Variation in scores (*between subjects*)	76.278	5	15.256	3.424
Variation in scores due to *random error*	44.555	10	4.456	
Total	152.278	17		

F ratio = 3.529; d.f.$_{bet}$ = 2; d.f.$_{error}$ = 10;
p is not significant.
F ratio$_{subj}$ = 3.424; d.f.$_{subj}$ = 5; d.f.$_{error}$ = 10
$p < 0.05$; significant

These results suggest that there is no significant effect from the different types of analgesia used, but that the sets of matched subjects *were* significantly different from one another, and were therefore an atypical sample. These results can be expressed in the following way:

Using a one-way anova for related samples, no significant differences were found between the three treatment condi-tions ($F = 3.529$, d.f.$_{bet}$ = 2, d.f.$_{error}$ = 10). This suggests that the type of analgesia used during labour has no significant effect on length of the second stage. However, significant differences were found between the sets of matched subjects, ($F = 3.424$, d.f.$_{subj}$ = 5, d.f.$_{error}$ = 10, $p < 0.05$). This indicates that the subject sample was an atypical group and may represent a flaw in the sampling procedure. The null hypothesis must therefore be accepted.

Activity 14.3

Comparisons:
   a. *Condition 1* (role play) × *Condition 2* (film)
      ($F^1 = (C - 1)\,3.29 = 9.87$)
      $F = 2.8\ p < 0.05$ not significant
   This suggests that the role play method is not significantly more effective than films as teaching medium in parentcraft classes.
   b. *Condition 1* (role play) × *Condition 3* (lecture)
      ($F^1 = (C - 1)\,3.29 = 9.87$)
      $F = 0.194$; not significant
   This suggests that there is no difference in the effective-ness of role play or lecture methods as a teaching medium in parentcraft classes.
   c. *Condition 1* (role play) × *Condition 4* (reading)
      ($F^1 = (C - 1)\,3.29 = 9.87$
      $F = 6.078$; not significant
   This suggests that role play is not more effective than reading as a teaching medium in parentcraft classes.
   d. *Condition 2* (film) × *Condition 3* (lecture)
      ($F^1 = (C - 1)\,3.29 = 9.87$
      $F = 4.465$; not significant
   These results indicate that films are no more effective than lectures as a teaching medium in parentcraft classes.
   e. *Condition 2* (film) × *Condition 4* (reading)
      ($F^1 = (C - 1)\,5.42 = 16.26$
      $F = 17.124\ p < 0.01$, significant
   These results suggest that films are significantly more effective than reading as a teaching medium in parentcraft classes.
   f. *Condition 3* (lecture) × *Condition 4* (reading)
      ($F^1 = (C - 1)\,3.29 = 9.87$
      $F = 4.101$ not significant
   These results suggest that lectures are no more effective than reading as a teaching medium in parentcraft classes.

Chapter 15

Activity 15.1

1. (i) $p < 0.025$ significant
   (ii) $p < 0.02$ significant
   (iii) $p < 0.05$ significant
   (iv) p is greater than 0.10 and is therefore not significant
   (v) $p < 0.005$ significant
2. χ^2 8.377 d.f. = 1, $p < 0.005$
   Using a χ^2 to analyse the data ($\chi^2 = 8.377$, d.f. = 1) the results were significant ($p < 0.005$, one-tailed). This means that the null hypothesis can be rejected and that midwife tutors are more likely to undertake research than are clini-cal midwives.

Activity 15.2

1. (i) $p < 0.05$ significant
   (ii) $p = 0.05$ significant
   (iii) $p < 0.01$ significant
   (iv) $p < 0.005$ significant
   (v) $p < 0.05$ significant
   (vi) p is larger than 0.10 and is therefore not significant.
2. $U = 45$, $p < 0.01$, one-tailed test.
   Using a Mann-Whitney U test on the data ($U = 45$, $N_1 = 14$, $N_2 = 14$) the results were found to be significant at $p < 0.01$ for a one-tailed hypothesis. This suggests that the experimental hypothesis has been supported and that women who eat a high fat diet are more likely to experience severe carpal tunnel syndrome during the third trimester than are women who eat a vegetarian diet.

Activity 15.3

1. (i) $p < 0.046$ significant
   (ii) $p = 0.049$ significant
   (iii) $p < 0.05$ significant
   (iv) $p < 0.011$ significant
   (v) $p < 0.01$ significant
   (vi) p is larger than 0.05 and is therefore not significant.
2. $H = 6.26$, $N_1 = 5$, $N_2 = 5$, $N_3 = 5$ $p < 0.049$
   Using a Kruskal-Wallis test on the data ($H = 6.26$, $N_1 = 5$, $N_2 = 5$, $N_3 = 5$), the results were found to be significant at $p < 0.049$ for a one-tailed test). This suggests that the three methods of giving postnatal exercise instructions are differentially effective. This means the null hypothesis can be rejected and the experimental hypothesis supported.

Activity 15.4

1. (i) $p < 0.01$ significant
   (ii) p is greater than 0.05 and so the results are not significant.
   (iii) $p < 0.05$ significant
   (iv) $p < 0.01$ significant
   (v) $p < 0.05$ significant
   (vi) p is greater than 0.05 and therefore the results are not significant.
2. $A = 128$, $B = 192$, $S = 64$, $C = 3$, $n = 8$, $p < 0.05$
   Using a Jonckheere trend test to analyse the results ($S = 64$, $C = 3$, $n = 8$) the results were found to be significant ($p < 0.05$, one-tailed). This suggests that there is a significant trend in the probability of keeping ante-natal appointments, according to social class, with social class 3 being the most likely to keep them, followed by social class 2, and finally class 4. The null hypothesis can be rejected.

Activity 15.5

1. (i) p is greater than 10% and so the results are not significant.
   (ii) $p < 0.05$ significant
   (iii) $p < 0.05$ significant
   (iv) p is greater than 0.05, and is therefore not significant.
   (v) $p < 0.02$ significant

2. $\chi^2 = 5.095$, d.f. = 2, p is greater than 5% and so is not significant.
   Using an extended χ^2 on the data, ($\chi^2 = 5.096$, d.f. = 2) the results were found to be not significant (p is greater than 5%). Therefore the null hypothesis is accepted; there is no significant relationship between keeping an ante-natal appointment and ease of journey, using public transport.

Chapter 16

Activity 16.1

1. (i) $p < 0.05$ significant
   (ii) $p < 0.02$ significant
   (iii) $p < 0.01$ significant.
   (iv) p is larger than 5% and so the results are not significant.
   (v) $p < 0.01$ significant
2. $t = 2.43$; d.f. = 25; $p < 0.025$
   Using an unrelated t-test on the data ($t = 2.43$, d.f. = 25), the results were significant ($p < 0.025$ for a one-tailed test). The null hypothesis can be rejected. This suggests that absenteeism is significantly greater amongst midwives working under the traditional random allocation system than amongst those operating as 'named midwives'.

Activity 16.2

1. (i) $p < 0.01$ significant
   (ii) $p < 0.001$ significant
   (iii) $p = 0.05$ significant
   (iv) $p < 0.01$ significant
2. $F = 2.171$, p is greater than 5% and is therefore not significant.

Table A3.6

Source of variation	SS	d.f.	MS	F ratio
Variation due to treatment, i.e. *between conditions*	180.952	2	90.476	2.171
Variation due to *random error*	750	18	41.667	
Total	930.952	20		

Using a one-way anova (see Table A3.6) for unrelated subject designs on the data ($F = 2.171$, d.f.$_{bet}$ = 2, d.f.$_{error}$ = 18) the results were found to be not significant (p is greater than 5%). This means that the null hypothesis must be accepted and that there is no relationship between parity and weight gain during months 3–5.

Activity 16.3

1. a. Comparison of strong vs. moderate contractions
      $F = 4.982$
      p is not significant
      i.e. There is no difference in length of labour depending on whether contractions are strong or moderate.

b. Comparison of strong vs. light contractions
$F = 35.124$
$p < 0.01$
i.e. Length of labour was significantly greater for women who had light contractions as opposed to strong ones.
c. Comparison of moderate vs. light contractions
$F = 13.649$
$p < 0.01$
i.e. Length of labour was significantly greater for women who had light contractions as opposed to moderate ones.

Chapter 17

Activity 17.1

1. H_1 There is a relationship between the age of the woman and time taken to conceive.
   a. *Correlational design*
   You would select one group of women who represented a whole range of ages (e.g. 18–45). You would then assess how long it took them to conceive, to see if there was a correlation between these variables.
   b. *Experimental design*
   You have two possible options here.
   Firstly, you might select two groups of women one being at the young/ish end of the age range and the other being at the older end.

Group 1	18–30 years (for example)
Group 2	31–45 years (for example)

   You would measure the length of time taken to conceive to see if there was any difference between the groups. Alternatively, you might select a third group who represented a mid-age range thus:

Group 1	18–25 years (for example)
Group 2	26–35 years (for example)
Group 3	36–45 years (for example)

   Again you would compare the times taken to conceive for differences between the groups.

Activity 17.2

1. $p < 0.01$
   p = not significant
   $p = 0.02$
   p = not significant
   $p < 0.005$
2. Results of the calculation of the Spearman rho:
   $r_s = -0.827$
   $p < 0.01$ (two-tailed)
   Using a Spearman test on the data, $(r_s = -0.827, N = 10)$ the results were found to be significant ($p < 0.01$ for a two-tailed test). This suggests that there is a significant negative correlation between the length of waiting time in an antenatal clinic and degree of satisfaction with care. The null hypothesis can therefore be rejected.

Activity 17.3

1. (i) $p < 0.05$
   (ii) p = not significant
   (iii) $p < 0.005$
   (iv) $p = 0.02$
   (v) $p < 0.001$
2. Results of the calculation of the Pearson product moment correlation:
   $r = +0.899$
   $p < 0.005$ (one-tailed)
   Using a Pearson product moment correlation test on the data ($r = +0.899$, d.f. = 6), the results were found to be significant ($p < 0.005$, for a one-tailed test). This means that there is a significant positive correlation between students' marks on their 1st year exam and their averaged continuous assessment mark through the year. The null hypothesis can therefore be rejected.

Activity 17.4

1. (i) $p < 0.05$
   (ii) p is greater than 5% and is therefore not significant.
   (iii) $p < 0.01$
   (iv) $p < 0.01$
   (v) p is greater than 5% and is therefore not significant.
2. Results of the calculation of the Kendall coefficient of concordance.
   $s = 77, W = 0.616$
   $p < 0.05$
   Using the Kendall coefficient of concordance on the data ($s = 77, W = 6.61, n = 5, N = 4$) the results were found to be significant ($p < 0.05$ for a one-tailed test).
   This suggests that there is significant agreement between midwife tutors' marks on examination scripts. The null hypothesis can be rejected.

Activity 17.5

1. a = 0.939, b = 0.47
   a. This patient would be in labour for 11.1749 hours.
   b. This patient would be in labour for 8.459 hours.
   c. This patient would be in labour for 14.569 hours.

Chapter 18

Activity 18.1

1. The proportion of non-attenders in the outpatient clinic will be somewhere between 0.3–0.46 (for 95% confidence level).
2. The average amount of midwifery time the premature babies will require will be between 2.25–4.15 hours, per baby, per week (99% confidence level).
3. The average life expectancy of your ultrasound scanners is estimated with 90% confidence to fall within the confidence interval of 4.07–4.53 years.

Glossary

abstract (Also called a summary) a résumé usually found at the beginning of journal articles, which summarises the key features of the study.

analysis of variance (anova) a statistical technique which allows the simultaneous comparison of three or more sets of data derived from experimental designs. There are a number of variants on this technique which allow the researcher to analyse data from different-, same- and matched-subject designs, or a mixture of both. While there are non-parametric analyses of variance tests, the term anova is commonly taken to mean the parametric variety, while the non-parametric tests are referred to by specific names (e.g. Kruskal–Wallis test).

apparatus any equipment used in a research project.

bar graph a graph used to show the frequency of a given event by the height of vertically arranged bars or columns. These bars have spaces between them.

baseline a stage in a research project when the subjects receive no treatment or intervention.

bias any distortion in results due to flaws in the design of the study. (See also *experimenter bias*.)

central tendency a description of a set of results which typically makes use of the average score, the most commonly occurring score and the mid-score of that set of data.

characteristic this is some feature of a population for which the researcher wishes to make an estimate from a sample of that population.

chi-squared test (χ^2) a non-parametric statistical test used to analyse two sets of nominal data from different subject designs which employ two groups of subjects only. (See also *extended χ^2 test*.)

clinical significance the degree to which a set of results have some clinical meaning or relevance.

Sometimes results can be statistically significant but clinically meaningless.

closed-response question any question which is framed in such a way that only a limited number of answers are possible.

confidence interval a range in a set of scores derived from a sample in which the population characteristic is confidently expected to fall.

confidence level the degree of confidence which can be placed in an estimate of a population characteristic. It is expressed as a percentage and the most commonly used levels are 90%, 95% and 99%.

confidence limits the upper and lower figures of the confidence interval

constant errors any sources of bias and error in a research project which will influence the results in a constant and predictable way. They must be controlled or eliminated: if they are not then the conclusions may be wrong, misleading and possibly dangerous.

control group a group of subjects in an experimental design which does not receive any treatment or intervention. This group can then be compared with the experimental group which does receive some intervention, in order to establish the effects of the independent variable.

correlation coefficient a numerical value somewhere between -1.0 and $+1.0$ which indicates the degree and nature of the association between sets of data derived from a correlational design.

correlational designs designs which test an experimental hypothesis by collecting data on both the variables in the hypothesis to see if the data is related in some way. The two relationships which are of interest are *positive correlations* and *negative correlations* (see entries under these headings).

counterbalancing a technique used in research design to overcome the bias caused by order effects. It involves ensuring that the order of testing a group of subjects is alternated so that any results will not be influenced by the sequence of testing.

data the facts and figures collected during a research project.

degrees of freedom a complex concept involved in some statistical tests which refers to the extent to which data have the capacity to vary once certain limits have been imposed. It is abbreviated to df and is very easy to calculate.

dependent variable the variable in an experimental hypothesis which changes as a result of manipulating the independent variable. The changes in the dependent variable constitute the data in a study and can be thought of as the effects of the manipulation of the independent variable.

descriptive statistics methods of describing a set of results in terms of their most interesting characteristics.

different-subject design experimental designs which use two or more separate or different groups of subjects each of which is tested once. The groups are then compared for any differences between them. Sometimes known as a between- or unrelated-subjects design.

discussion a section of a research report which discusses the findings of that research.

double-blind technique an aspect of research design whose aim is to minimise the biasing effect that subjects and experimenters may have on the results by knowing what the aims of the study are. The double-blind procedure involves keeping the subjects ignorant of the project's aims until after the data has been collected, as well as using someone other than the main researcher to collect the data. This person will also be unaware of the purpose of the research project.

estimation a form of scientific 'best guessing' where estimates of a population characteristic are made on the basis of knowledge of the sample characteristic. It is a useful tool in planning.

ethics a set of guidelines imposed on a study to ensure that the project will not compromise or upset the subjects in any way.

experimental condition a group of subjects in an experimental design which receives some form of intervention or level of the independent variable. This group may be compared with other experimental groups who receive a different form of intervention or with a control group who receive no intervention at all.

experimental design a method of testing hypotheses which involves manipulating the independent variable(s) in the experimental hypothesis and monitoring what impact this has on the dependent variable. By doing this cause and effect can be established.

experimental hypothesis a prediction of a consistent and reliable relationship between two or more variables. The experimental hypothesis is the starting point of any piece of experimental research and is often referred to in the literature as H_1.

experimenter bias effects a source of bias to the results which results from the experimenter (usually unwittingly) influencing subjects' responses so that they fulfil the experimenter's aims. It can be counteracted to some extent by using a naive data collector (see single-blind procedures).

extended chi-squared (χ^2) test a non-parametric statistical test for use with nominal data and different subject designs. It is used with more than two nominal categories and/or more than two groups of subjects.

fatigue effects an aspect of order problems where subjects do worse on the second or subsequent testing because of fatigue. This can mask the real effects of the independent variable.

frequency distribution graph a graph which presents the frequency with which any given event occurs. These graphs can be bar graphs, histograms and frequency polygons (see separate entries).

frequency polygon a frequency distribution graph which is characterised by the single continuous line drawn between the points on the graph.

Friedman test a non-parametric analysis of variance for use with same- or matched-subject design, using more than two testing conditions. The data can be ordinal or interval/ratio, but this test is most likely to be used with ordinal data.

histogram a frequency distribution graph characterised by the use of adjacent vertical columns.

incidental sample a method of selecting subjects for study which involves using the most easily available people.

independent variable that variable in the experimental hypothesis which is manipulated so that the impact of this on the dependent variable can be observed. It can be thought of as the cause of something happening.

inferential statistics a statistical technique whereby results derived from a sample of subjects are also inferred to apply to the population from which they come.

interobserver reliability the degree to which two or more people agree in their observations of an event.

interval level of measurement usually linked with the ratio level of measurement, this is a level of data which: (a) allows parametric statistical tests to be performed; (b) assumes equal intervals in measurement between the data; (c) has no absolute zero (i.e. a score of 0 does not mean the absence of that characteristic).

interview a conversation between the researcher and the subject which aims to elicit information relevant to the research topic. This interview may follow prescribed topics (structured interview) or may be entirely open (unstructured interview).

introduction (to a research report) the section of a research report which reviews the relevant literature, and provides a rationale and the aims of the study in question.

Jonckheere trend test a non-parametric statistical analysis which is used with three or more separate groups of subjects (a different-subject design), ordinal or interval/ratio data, and where the results are expected to be in a specified trend.

Kendall's coefficient of concordance a non-parametric statistical test used with correlational designs and ordinal data which assesses the extent of agreement between three or more sets of data.

Kruskal–Wallis test a non-parametric analysis of variance test used with three or more separate groups of subjects (a different-subject design) and ordinal or interval/ratio data.

levels of measurement the data collected from a piece of research fall into one of four levels of measurement, which differ in their sophistication and the type of calculation that can be performed on them. These levels are (in order of sophistication from least to most):
Nominal (least)
Ordinal
Interval
Ratio (most)

linear regression a statistical technique used with sets of data known to be correlated, such that values on one variable can be calculated from knowledge of the values on the other.

literature review a survey of all the research relevant to the topic in question, which allows the researcher to establish what has already been carried out.

Mann–Whitney *U*-test a non-parametric statistical test used with two separate groups of subjects (a different-subject design) and ordinal or interval/ratio data.

matched-subject designs types of experimental designs which involve matching subjects on all those factors which may affect the results. While these designs have the advantage of not being affected by individual differences and order effects, they are very difficult to carry out properly.

materials any non-mechanical items used in a piece of research, e.g. questionnaires, blood pressure sheets etc.

McNemar test a non-parametric statistical test used with same- or matched-subject designs, two testing conditions and nominal data. It assesses the significance of any changes noted over the two testings.

mean the average score in a set of data, calculated by adding all the scores up and dividing this total by the number of scores in the set of data.

median the middle score in a set of data, such that there are as many scores above it as below.

method the section of a research report which describes in detail what was done, how and with whom, in a piece of research. It should be sufficiently detailed that anyone who reads this section should be able to replicate the study exactly.

mode the most frequently occurring score in a set of data.

negative correlation the relationship between two sets of data derived from a correlational design, whereby high scores on one set of data are associated with low scores on the other.

negative skew a frequency distribution distorted to one side because too many subjects recorded high scores (see Fig. 5.11).

nominal level of measurement a very basic level of measurement (sometimes referred to as categorical data) which simply allocates subjects or their responses to named categories. It is characterised by the following:
(a) Only non-parametric statistical analyses can be performed on this data.
(b) The categories are mutually exclusive.
(c) There is no commonly understood value attached to the category labels.

non-parametric tests these are techniques of data analysis which are less sensitive and rather cruder than parametric tests. They can be used, in principle, with all levels of measurement, but are most commonly associated with the nominal and ordinal levels.

normal distribution a symmetrical bell-shaped curve which has certain properties which are critical to statistical inference.

null hypothesis the prediction which counters the claim made by the experimental hypothesis in a study. The null hypothesis predicts there is no relationship between the variables in the experimental hypothesis. It is often referred to in the literature as H_0.

observation a technique of conducting research which involves the researcher simply observing what goes on in naturalistic settings.

one-tailed hypotheses or tests these refer to hypotheses where a prediction is made that the results of the study will be in a specific direction.

open-ended questions questions which allow the respondent to reply in a free and unstructured way to any given question.

order effects a source of bias usually found in same-subject designs where the order in which the subjects were tested rather than the independent variable produces the results. This can be overcome by counterbalancing the order of testing.

ordinal level of measurement a type of data which allows the researcher to rank order subjects along the dimension of interest (e.g. least improvement–most improvement). An important feature of this scale is that while it allows the researcher to impose a numerical score on the subject's response, the differences between the points on the scale are not equal.

Page's L trend test a non-parametric test used with same- or matched-subject designs which yields three or more sets of ordinal or interval/ratio data. A particular characteristic is that a trend in the results is specifically predicted.

parametric tests techniques of statistical analysis which are said to be robust and sensitive. They require certain conditions or parameters to be fulfilled before they can be applied, the most important of which is that the data must be interval/ratio.

Pearson test a parametric test for use with correlational designs and interval/ratio data.

pilot study a preliminary run of the main study to highlight any problems which can then be corrected.

placebo effect an interesting phenomenon whereby subjects show a significant degree of improvement even though their treatment is known to have no use.

point estimation a statistical 'best guess' which provides a single figure estimate (usually an average or percentage figure) of a population characteristic based on information about the sample's characteristic.

population a group of people all of whom have a characteristic in common which is of interest to the researcher, e.g. talipes. The sample for study in the research is drawn from this parent population.

population characteristic see *characteristic*.

positive correlation the degree of relationship between the data from two or more variables derived from a correlational design, such that high scores on one variable are associated with high scores from the other(s), and similarly low scores are associated with low scores.

positive skew a frequency distribution where the data are distorted towards the lower scores, for example, where students perform badly on an exam which is too difficult (see Fig. 5.10).

post–test a measurement of the dependent variable which takes place after the intervention has occurred.

practice effects a variety of order effects whereby subjects perform better on second and subsequent testings and this improved performance masks the effects of the independent variable.

pre-test a measurement of the dependent variable which takes place before any intervention has occurred.

probability the likelihood that random error is producing the results in a study. It is expressed as a percentage or decimal and is usually abbreviated to 'p'.

qualitative research techniques of research investigation which collect non-numerical information from subjects.

quantitative research techniques of research which collect numerical information from subjects.

questionnaires a method of collecting information whereby subjects answer a set of questions usually predefined by the researcher.

quota sample a process of selecting a sample to participate in a research study, such that pre-set quotas of subjects will be selected to represent categories deemed to be important.

random errors any sources of bias or error in a piece of research which will affect the results in a random and unpredictable way. They include a variety of individual differences and cannot be eliminated completely.

random number tables tables of randomly generated numbers which can be used to select a random sample of subjects for study.

random selection/sample a method of selecting subjects to take part in a study, such that every member of the parent population has an equal chance of being chosen.

range the difference between the lowest score and the highest score in a set of data.

ratio level of measurement the 'highest' level of data which is characterised by equal intervals between the data points and an absolute zero which represents an absence of the quality in question.

references a section in a research report which lists all the research articles referred to in the body of the report.

related *t* test a parametric statistical test for use with same- or matched-subject designs and two sets of interval/ratio data.

representative sample a sample which is typical or accurately reflects the population from which it comes.

research proposal an outline of an anticipated piece of research covering background literature, aims, objectives, methodology, proposed analysis, and a cost/benefit analysis. A research proposal is often required by ethical committees or when funding is applied for.

same-subject designs a variant of experimental design which involves testing the same group of subjects on two or more occasions. They are typically used in before/after designs.

sample a group of subjects selected from a parent population, who are used in a piece of research.

scattergram a technique of plotting data derived from correlational studies in a graph. A general upward slope to the graph indicates a positive correlation, while a general downward slope indicates a negative correlation.

Scheffé multiple range test a statistical technique used in conjunction with parametric anovas which have yielded significant results. The Scheffe test allows the researcher to make an objective scrutiny of the data in order to establish which parts were responsible for the significant anova results.

significance level A cut-off point, usually of 5% or less, such that if the results from a piece of research have a probability of 5% or less of being due to random error, then they are said to be significant.

The null (no relationship) hypothesis can then be rejected in favour of the experimental hypothesis.

Spearman test a non-parametric test for use with correlational designs and ordinal or interval/ratio data.

standard deviation a measure of the average amount that a set of scores varies or deviates from the mean.

stratified random sample a method of selecting a sample from a population, so that subgroups of that population are represented in the sample.

subjects the individual people who take part in a study.

surveys a method of collecting data which involves the researcher measuring relevant sample variables (often using a questionnaire) without any form of manipulation or systematic intervention.

systematic sample a method of selecting a sample for study by choosing every fourth, fifth or whatever, member of the parent population.

two-tailed hypothesis or test an experimental hypothesis which, simply predicts that the variables in the hypothesis are related, but does not specify the precise nature of that relationship.

Type I error a conclusion that there is a relationship between the variables in the hypothesis, when in fact there is not.

Type II error a conclusion that there is no relationship between the variables in the hypothesis when, in fact, there is.

Unrelated *t* test a parametric statistical test used with two different groups of subjects and interval/ratio data.

variable any event or characteristic which has the capacity to vary (e.g. weight, age etc.).

variance the degree to which a set of scores vary or are dispersed

Wilcoxon test a non-parametric statistical test used with same- or matched-subject designs, and two sets of ordinal or interval/ratio data.

Index